Addiction: A Global Overview

Addiction: A Global Overview

Edited by **Don Boles**

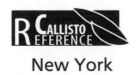

New York

Published by Callisto Reference,
106 Park Avenue, Suite 200,
New York, NY 10016, USA
www.callistoreference.com

Addiction: A Global Overview
Edited by Don Boles

© 2016 Callisto Reference

International Standard Book Number: 978-1-63239-634-1 (Hardback)

Printed in the United States of America.

Contents

Chapter 12   **Therapist's Gender and Gender Roles: Impact on Attitudes toward Clients in Substance Abuse Treatment**   92
Tytti Artkoski and Pekka Saarnio

Chapter 13   **Measuring Problematic Mobile Phone Use: Development and Preliminary Psychometric Properties of the PUMP Scale**   98
Lisa J. Merlo, Amanda M. Stone and Alex Bibbey

Chapter 14   **Controlling Chaos: The Perceptions of Long-Term Crack Cocaine Users in Vancouver, British Columbia, Canada**   105
Steven Persaud, Despina Tzemis, Margot Kuo, Vicky Bungay and Jane A. Buxton

Chapter 15   **The AC-OK Cooccurring Screen: Reliability, Convergent Validity, Sensitivity and Specificity**   114
Andrew L. Cherry and Mary E. Dillon

Chapter 16   **Everyday prospective Memory and Executive function deficits Associated with Exposure to Second-Hand Smoke**   122
Thomas M. Heffernan and Terence S. O'Neill

Chapter 17   **Pattern and Trend of Substance Abuse in Eastern Rural Iran: A Household Survey in a Rural Community**   129
Hasan Ziaaddini, Tayebeh Ziaaddini and Nouzar Nakhaee

Chapter 18   **Exploring Spatial Associations between On-Sale Alcohol Availability, Neighborhood Population Characteristics, and Violent Crime in a Geographically Isolated City**   135
Daikwon Han and Dennis M. Gorman

Chapter 19   **Smoking and Other Drug Characteristics of Aboriginal and Non-Aboriginal Prisoners in Australia**   141
Robyn L. Richmond, Devon Indig, Tony G. Butler, Kay A. Wilhelm, Vicki A. Archer and Alex D. Wodak

Chapter 20   **Early Adolescents and Substance Use**   150
Raimondo Maria Pavarin and Dario Consonni

Chapter 21   **Involvement in Specific HIV Risk Practices among Men Who Use the Internet to Find Male Partners for Unprotected Sex**   156
Hugh Klein

Chapter 22   **Evaluation of a Low-Threshold/High-Tolerance Methadone Maintenance Treatment Clinic in Saint John, New Brunswick, Canada: One Year Retention Rate and Illicit Drug Use**   176
Timothy K. S. Christie, Alli Murugesan, Dana Manzer, Michael V. O'Shaughnessey and Duncan Webster

Chapter 23   **Parental Factors Associated with Mexican American Adolescent Alcohol Use**   181
Cristina Mogro-Wilson

              Permissions

              List of Contributors

Preface

It is often said that books are a boon to mankind. They document every progress and pass on the knowledge from one generation to the other. They play a crucial role in our lives. Thus I was both excited and nervous while editing this book. I was pleased by the thought of being able to make a mark but I was also nervous to do it right because the future of students depends upon it. Hence, I took a few months to research further into the discipline, revise my knowledge and also explore some more aspects. Post this process, I began with the editing of this book.

Some of us knowingly or unknowingly indulge into some habits which eventually lead to addiction over a period of time. Addiction is the stronger form of habit which can be referred to as a compulsive disorder. This book aims to bring fourth some of the unexplored aspects of addiction and recent researches in this field. Different approaches, evaluations, methodologies and advanced studies have been included in it. This book serves as a reference to a wide spectrum of readers. It aims to understand the various factors that stimulate and facilitate addiction. It also sheds light on behavioral addiction along with methods for diagnosis and treatment therapies. It covers some existent theories and innovative concepts revolving around addiction.

I thank my publisher with all my heart for considering me worthy of this unparalleled opportunity and for showing unwavering faith in my skills. I would also like to thank the editorial team who worked closely with me at every step and contributed immensely towards the successful completion of this book. Last but not the least, I wish to thank my friends and colleagues for their support.

Editor

1

The Relationship between Endorsing Gambling as an Escape and the Display of Gambling Problems

Jeffrey N. Weatherly

Department of Psychology, University of North Dakota, Grand Forks, ND 58202-8380, USA

Correspondence should be addressed to Jeffrey N. Weatherly; jeffrey.weatherly@und.edu

Academic Editor: Ingmar Franken

Previous research has reported a strong relationship between endorsing gambling as an escape and problem/pathological gambling as measured by the South Oaks Gambling Screen (SOGS). The present study recruited 249 university students to complete the Gambling Functional Assessment-Revised (GFA-R), which measures the function of the respondent's gambling, as well as the SOGS and the Problem Gambling Severity Index (PGSI), which was designed to identify gambling problems in the general population. Endorsing gambling as an escape on the GFA-R was again predictive of SOGS scores. The function of one's gambling was also predictive of the respondents' PGSI scores, but whether gambling for positive reinforcement or as an escape was the significant predictor differed between male and female respondents. Scores on the GFA-R subscales also accounted for a significant amount of variance in PGSI scores above and beyond that accounted for by SOGS scores. The present results support the idea that both practitioners and researchers should be interested in the function of an individual's gambling as well as the presence or the absence of pathology. They also suggest that differences in the function of gambling might also exist between the sexes.

1. Introduction

Problem and pathological gambling are recognized as being major societal problems, with millions of individuals suffering from them (e.g., see [1]). Because of this fact, a great deal of effort has been exerted trying to identify who might have such problems. Numerous examples of diagnostic screens can be found in the literature, including the South Oaks Gambling Screen (SOGS, [2]), the NORC DSM-IV screen for problem gamblers [3], and the Canadian Problem Gambling Index [4, 5]. The rationale behind these attempts is that if one can determine who might be experiencing problems with gambling, one is in a better position to treat, and potentially prevent, such problems.

Far less effort has been focused on an equally important issue—why people might gamble. In other words, what contingencies might be maintaining a gambler's behavior? Having such information would seem important because it seems reasonable to believe that different individuals might gamble for different reasons. It may also be the case that certain contingencies are more closely associated with gambling problems than are others. Further, it is quite possible

that the reason why someone begins to gamble is different than the reason why the same person continues to gamble. Instruments designed to assess the contingencies reinforcing gambling behavior are, therefore, necessary to obtain this information.

Dixon and Johnson [6] were the first to introduce a screening instrument designed for this purpose when they forwarded the Gambling Functional Assessment (GFA). The GFA was patterned off of a similar measure designed to ascertain the contingencies maintaining self-injurious behavior [7] and was proposed to measure four potential maintaining contingencies: gambling for tangible gain, for the sensory experience, for social attention, or as an escape. Subsequent psychometric research, however, suggested that the GFA was not measuring four distinct maintaining contingencies [8]. Rather, it was only measuring two—gambling for positive reinforcement and/or as an escape—and was not cleanly parsing those two.

Because the GFA did not appear to be operating as designed, Weatherly et al. [9] revised the GFA (GFA-R) with the intention of cleanly measuring gambling maintained by positive reinforcement and escape. The GFA-R contains 16 items, each eight designed to measure gambling maintained by those two contingencies. Weatherly et al. [9] reported that the GFA-R had sound psychometric properties and cleanly parsed those two contingencies. Likewise, Weatherly et al. [10] demonstrated that the GFA-R displayed good temporal reliability and internal consistency. Overall, the research to date suggests that the psychometric properties of the GFA-R are superior to the original GFA.

In terms of the contingencies maintaining gambling behavior, research using the original GFA uncovered a potentially interesting relationship between gambling problems and endorsing gambling as an escape [8, 11]. Specifically, Miller et al. [8, 11] reported that most respondents on the GFA displayed higher scores for gambling for positive reinforcement than for gambling as an escape. However, gambling as an escape, but not gambling for positive reinforcement, was strongly predictive of potential gambling problems as measured by scores on the SOGS. Subsequent research with the GFA-R has replicated both of these findings [10, 12]. It has likewise shown that endorsing gambling as an escape is associated with both executive function and emotional regulation deficits that have been linked to gambling problems [13].

Thus, there appears to be a strong relationship between gambling problems and endorsing gambling as an escape. This relationship may not be completely surprising given that gambling as an escape is an official symptom of pathological gambling [14]. Gambling as an escape has, in fact, been a central tenant in some theories of pathological gambling (e.g., [15]). Still, what might be considered surprising is the strength of the potential relationship. For instance, Weatherly and Derenne [12] reported a correlation of 0.689 between endorsing gambling as an escape on the GFA-R and scores on the SOGS in their sample of 177 participants.

One potential criticism of such research is that it has relied on the association between the scores on the GFA-R (or the GFA) and the SOGS. Although the SOGS is a widely used screening measure within the research literature, it has been criticized on a number of fronts (e.g., see [16, 17]). One criticism is that the SOGS overestimates the prevalence of pathological gambling. A second criticism is that the SOGS was developed based on a prior, not the most recent, version of the diagnostic criteria for pathological gambling (i.e., [14]). The SOGS also focuses on the respondent's gambling history, not necessarily the severity of the issues that face the respondent. In the light of these criticisms, one cannot necessarily conclude that a strong relationship between GFA-R escape scores and SOGS scores is equivalent to predicting the severity of the respondents' gambling problems. It is possible that such a relationship might exist, but research to date has not established it beyond using the SOGS. Attempting to do so was the goal of the present study.

In the present study, respondents were recruited to complete three measures: the GFA-R, SOGS, and Problem Gambling Severity Index (PGSI), which is part of the Canadian Problem Gambling Index [4, 5]. The PGSI measures both gambling behavior and consequences and has been shown to have sound psychometric properties (e.g., [18]).

Furthermore, unlike the SOGS, the PGSI was designed for the use with the general population [19].

Based on previous research, the following hypotheses were made. First, participants would endorse gambling for positive reinforcement on the GFA-R to a greater extent than they would endorse gambling as an escape. Second, endorsing gambling as an escape on the GFA-R would be a stronger predictor of SOGS scores than would be the endorsing gambling for positive reinforcement. Third, endorsing gambling as an escape on the GFA-R would be a stronger predictor of PGSI scores than would be the endorsing gambling for positive reinforcement. Finally, it was predicted that SOGS scores would be significant predictors of PGSI scores, but GFA-R escape scores would explain a significant amount of the variance in PGSI scores above and beyond that account for by SOGS scores.

2. Methods

2.1. Participants. The participants were 249 (180 females and 69 males) students enrolled in psychology courses at the University of North Dakota. The mean age of the participants was 19.8 years (SD = 3.6 years), and their self-reported grade point average was 3.4 out of 4.0 (SD = 0.5). The vast majority of the participants reported as Caucasian (229, 92.0%). All participants received (extra) course credit in their psychology class in return for their participation.

2.2. Materials and Procedure. Participants completed the study online using an experiment management system (SONA Systems, Ltd, Version 2.72; Tallinn, Estonia). This system guaranteed that participants could complete the materials only one time even if they were enrolled in multiple psychology courses.

The first item presented to all participants was an informed consent document that outlined the study and the participant's rights. Continuation beyond this document constituted the granting of informed consent.

After the informed consent document, participants completed four different measures. One of them was a brief demographic survey that asked them about their sex, age, grade point average, and race. They also completed the GFA-R [9], which consists of 16 items that respondents respond to on a scale that ranges from 0 (Never) to 6 (Always). Both eight-item subscales (i.e., positive reinforcement and escape) are summed to provide a score for that particular subscale. No items are reverse coded. Research has shown that the internal consistency of the GFA-R is high [10]. GFA-R scores have also been shown to have good temporal reliability ($r = 0.80$ at four weeks and $r = 0.81$ at 12 weeks [10]).

Participants also completed the SOGS [2], which consists of 20 items pertaining to the respondent's gambling history. A score of 3 or 4 suggests possible problem gambling, and a score of 5 or more suggests the probable presence of pathology. Original research [2] reported that the SOGS had high internal consistency ($\alpha = 0.97$), and subsequent research has reported that it has fair ($\alpha = 0.69$, [17]) to good ($\alpha = 0.81$, [20]) internal consistency. Research has also shown that the

SOGS has good temporal reliability ($r = 0.89$ at four weeks and $r = 0.67$ at 12 weeks [10]).

Finally, the participants completed the PGSI [4, 5]. The PGSI consists of 12 items, only nine of which are included when calculating respondents' scores. Research indicates that these nine items are associated with a single construct [21]. All items are answered on a four-point scale that ranges from 0 (Never) to 3 (Almost always). Scores from the nine counted items are summed, with scores of 0 indicating no gambling problems, 1-2 indicating a low level of gambling problems with few negative consequences, 3–7 indicating a moderate level of gambling problems with some negative consequences as a result, and 8 or more indicating problem gambling that includes negative consequences. Initial research on the PGSI [4] indicated that internal consistency was good ($\alpha = 0.84$), and subsequent research (e.g., [19]) has replicated that finding. Ferris and Wynne [4] also reported that the PGSI had good temporal reliability ($r = 0.78$).

The order of presentation of the demographic form, the GFA-R, the SOGS, and the PGSI varied randomly across participants.

3. Results

Table 1 presents the descriptive statistics for each gambling measure. Because females constituted a majority of the sample and because the prevalence of gambling problems varies as a function of sex (see [1]), scores of the female and male participants are reported. Furthermore, 47 participants (18.9%) scored 0 on the GFA-R, suggesting that these participants either did not gamble or gambled for reasons not measured by the GFA-R (scores on the GFA-R, rather than the SOGS or PGSI, were used to make this distinction because the GFA-R was the focus of the current study. Data from participants scoring 0 on the GFA were included to provide information about the observed relationships when using a sample that may be representative of the general population, some of whom do not gamble). Thus, Table 1 also presents the descriptive statistics for the different groups when the data from these potential nongamblers were excluded.

3.1. Hypothesis 1.
The data in Table 1 appear to support the first hypothesis; that respondents would endorse gambling for positive reinforcement to a greater extent than they would endorse gambling as an escape. When analyzing the data from the entire sample, results from Wilcoxon signed rank tests indicated that scores on the GFA-R positive reinforcement subscale were higher than scores on the escape subscale for both females ($Z = -10.03$, $P < .001$) and males ($Z = -6.95$, $P < .001$). When the nongamblers (i.e., GFA-R = 0) were excluded, scores remained significantly higher on the positive reinforcement subscale than on the escape subscale for both females ($Z = -10.03$, $P < .001$) and males ($Z = -6.95$, $P < .001$) (the Z values are identical for the two sets of analyses because, in the original analysis, nonresponders scored 0 on both subscales resulting in a tie score between the subscales). Thus, participants endorsed gambling for positive reinforcement to a greater extent than they did gambling as an escape. In these analyses, and all that follow, statistical significance that was considered met at $P < .05$.

3.2. Hypothesis 2.
Table 2 presents the bivariate correlations that were observed between scores on the different measures for females and males in both the entire sample and for only those respondents who scored above 0 on the GFA-R. The correlations in Table 2 would seem to support the second hypothesis in that, in all cases, stronger correlations were observed between GFA-R escape subscales scores and SOGS scores than were observed between GFA-R positive reinforcement subscale scores and SOGS scores. These differences, however, were not always statistically significant. Tests of differences between two nonindependent rs [22] indicated that the correlation between the scores on the GFA-R escape subscale and on the SOGS was significantly stronger than the correlation between the GFA-R positive reinforcement subscale and the SOGS for both female samples. However, the correlations were not significantly different for either male sample. Thus, stronger correlations were observed between endorsing gambling as an escape and SOGS scores than between endorsing gambling for positive reinforcement and SOGS scores for the female respondents, but not for the male respondents.

One could argue that these results are influenced by the fact that both GFA-R escape subscale scores and SOGS scores were positively skewed. To assess this possibility, GFA-R escape subscale scores were transformed into a categorical variable, with scores of 0 coded as 0, scores between 1 and 5 coded as 1, and scores of 6 or more coded as 2 (these categories were informed by previous research [11, 13]). SOGS scores were similarly coded into a categorical variable, with scores between 0 and 2 coded as 0, between 3 and 4 coded as 1, and 5 or more coded as 2. Simultaneous linear regressions were then conducted with the transformed SOGS scores serving as the dependent measure and participants' GFA-R positive reinforcement subscale scores, which were not skewed, and the transformed GFA-R escape subscale scores serving as the potential predictor variables. Simultaneous regressions were conducted because these analyses allow for an assessment of the variance of that accounted for by each predictor variable independent of the other.

For the entire sample of female participants, the overall regression model was significant, $F(2, 177) = 34.17, P < .001$, and $R^2 = .279$. In this model, the transformed escape subscale scores were a significant predictor of the transformed SOGS scores, $\beta = .449$, $P < .001$, but the positive reinforcement subscales were not, $\beta = .132$, $P = .076$. When the data from the females who scored 0 on the GFA-R were excluded, the regression model was again significant $F(2, 135) = 24.98, P < .001$, and $R^2 = .270$. Both the escape, $\beta = .434$, $P < .001$, and positive reinforcement subscale scores, $\beta = .168$, $P = .036$, were significant predictors of SOGS scores, although the escape scores were the stronger predictor.

For the entire sample of male participants, the overall regression model was significant, $F(2, 65) = 8.81, P < .001$, and $R^2 = .213$. In this model, the transformed escape subscale scores were a significant predictor of the transformed SOGS

TABLE 1: Means scores on the GFA-R and its two subscales, the SOGS, and the PGSI for females, males, and all participants in either the entire sample and only for those participants who scored above 0 on the GFA-R (with standard deviations in parentheses).

Group (n)	GFA-R	GFA-R pos.	GFA-R esc	SOGS	PGSI
		Total sample			
Females (180)	18.7 (16.4)	16.1 (13.1)	2.6 (5.9)	1.1 (1.8)	1.0 (2.6)
Males (69)	24.9 (12.5)	22.1 (10.1)	2.8 (4.0)	1.5 (1.6)	1.4 (2.4)
Total (249)	20.5 (15.6)	17.8 (12.6)	2.7 (5.4)	1.2 (1.8)	1.1 (2.5)
		Respondents scoring > 0 on the GFA-R only			
Females (138)	24.4 (14.5)	21.0 (11.0)	3.4 (6.5)	1.4 (2.0)	1.3 (2.8)
Males (64)	26.8 (10.7)	23.9 (8.2)	3.0 (4.1)	1.6 (1.6)	1.5 (2.5)
Total (202)	25.2 (13.4)	21.9 (10.3)	3.3 (5.9)	1.4 (1.9)	1.4 (2.7)

TABLE 2: Bivariate correlations on the untransformed scores from each of the scales for the total sample and the subsample of respondents who scored above 0 on the GFA-R.

	GFA-R	GFA-R pos.	GFA-R esc	SOGS	PGSI
		Total sample: females ($n = 180$)			
GFA-R	—	0.94**	0.67**	0.58**	0.55**
GFA-R Pos.		—	0.39**	0.43**	0.34**
GRA-R Esc.			—	0.64**	0.76**
SOGS				—	0.73**
		Total sample: males ($n = 69$)			
GFA-R	—	0.96**	0.71**	0.47**	0.50**
GFA-R Pos.		—	0.47**	0.40**	0.41**
GRA-R Esc.			—	0.46**	0.54**
SOGS				—	0.72**
		Respondents scoring > 0 on the GFA-R only: females ($n = 138$)			
GFA-R	—	0.90**	0.69**	0.55**	0.54**
GFA-R Pos.		—	0.31**	0.35**	0.27*
GRA-R Esc.			—	0.62**	0.75**
SOGS				—	0.73**
		Respondents scoring > 0 on the GFA-R only: males ($n = 64$)			
GFA-R	—	0.94**	0.74**	0.43**	0.50**
GFA-R Pos.		—	0.46**	0.34*	0.40**
GRA-R Esc.			—	0.44**	0.52**
SOGS				—	0.72**

*$P < .01$; **$P < .001$.

scores, $\beta = .429$, $P = .001$, but the positive reinforcement subscales were not, $\beta = .062$, $P = .622$. When the data from the males who scored 0 on the GFA-R were excluded, the regression model was again significant $F(2, 60) = 7.79$, $P = .001$, and $R^2 = .206$, and escape subscale scores, $\beta = .413$, $P = .002$, but not positive reinforcement subscale scores, $\beta = .086$, $P = .496$, were significant predictors of SOGS scores.

Thus, results from these regression analyses would suggest that, for both females and males, escape scores on the GFA-R were stronger predictors of SOGS scores than were the positive reinforcement subscale scores.

3.3. Hypothesis 3. The correlations in Table 2 would also seem to support the third hypothesis in that, in all cases, stronger correlations were observed between GFA-R escape subscales scores and PGSI scores than were observed between GFA-R

positive reinforcement subscale scores and PGSI scores. Like the correlations with the SOGS, however, these differences were not always statistically significant. Tests of differences between two nonindependent rs indicated that the correlation between the scores on the GFA-R escape subscale and the PGSI was significantly stronger than the correlation between the scores on the GFA-R positive reinforcement subscale and the PGSI for both female samples. The correlations were not significantly different for either male sample. Thus, as with the SOGS, whether GFA-R escape subscales scores were significantly more correlated with PGSI scores than were GFA-R positive reinforcement subscale scores varied as a function of sex.

As with the SOGS scores, PGSI scores were positively skewed (see Table 1). Thus, these scores were transformed into a categorical variable, with scores of 0 coded as 0, of between 1 and 2 coded as 1, of between 3 and 7 coded as 2, and of 8 or more coded as 3 (as suggested by [4]). A series of simultaneous linear regressions was then conducted with the transformed PGSI scores serving as the dependent measure and participants' GFA-R positive reinforcement subscale scores and their transformed GFA-R escape subscale scores serving as the predictor variables.

For the entire sample of female participants, the overall regression model was significant, $F(2, 177) = 57.04$, $P < .001$, $R^2 = .392$. In this model, both the transformed escape subscale scores, $\beta = .522$, $P < .001$, and the positive reinforcement subscales, $\beta = .171$, $P = .012$, were significant predictors of the transformed PGSI scores, with the escape scores being the stronger predictor. When the data from females scoring 0 on the GFA-R were excluded, the identical results were observed. The regression model was significant $F(2, 135) = 35.72$, $P < .001$, and $R^2 = .346$, and both the escape, $\beta = .510$, $P < .001$, and positive reinforcement subscale scores, $\beta = .159$, $P = .036$, were significant predictors of the PGSI scores, with the escape scores being the stronger predictor.

For the entire sample of male participants, the overall regression model was significant, $F(2, 65) = 11.64$, $P < .001$, $R^2 = .264$. In this model, both the transformed escape subscale, $\beta = .244$, $P = .048$, and the positive reinforcement subscales scores, $\beta = .350$, $P = .005$, were significant predictors of the transformed PGSI scores. In this instance, the positive reinforcement subscale scores were the stronger predictor. When the data from males scoring 0 on the GFA-R were excluded, the regression model was again significant $F(2, 60) = 8.49$, $P = .001$, and $R^2 = .221$. Escape subscale scores did not significantly predict PGSI scores, $\beta = .240$, $P = .058$, but positive reinforcement subscale scores did, $\beta = .319$, $P = .013$.

Thus, GFA-R subscale scores were significant predictors of PGSI scores. Which subscale was the better predictor, however, varied as a function of sex. For females, GFA-R escape subscale scores were the best predictors of PGSI scores. For males, GFA-R positive reinforcement subscale scores were the best predictors.

3.4. *Hypothesis 4.* The SOGS was designed to identify potential pathological gamblers, whereas the PGSI was designed to test for potential gambling problems in the general population. However, one would suspect that there might be a significant overlap between the two. The high correlations between the two measures displayed in Table 2 support that contention. Hypothesis four pertains to the question of whether the GFA-R subscales are related to gambling problems (as measured by the PGSI) independent of potential pathology (as measured by the SOGS). To answer this question, multiple hierarchical linear regressions were conducted using the transformed PGSI scores as the dependent measure and transformed SOGS scores as the initial predictor. The GFA-R positive reinforcement subscale scores and the transformed GFA-R escape subscales scores were then simultaneously entered in the second block as additional predictor variables.

When the data from all female participants were subjected to this analysis, the initial model was significant, $F(1, 178) = 194.99$, $P < .001$, and $R^2 = .523$, and SOGS scores were a significant predictor of PGSI scores, $\beta = .723$, $P < .001$. When the GFA-R subscale scores were added to the analysis, the model was again significant, $F(3, 176) = 90.11$, $P < .001$, and $R^2 = .606$. Furthermore, the R^2 increase of .083 was statistically significant ($P < .001$). Both the SOGS, $\beta = .544$, $P < .001$, and the GFA-R escape subscale scores, $\beta = .278$, $P < .001$, were significant predictors of PGSI scores, but GFA-R positive reinforcement subscale scores were not, $\beta = .100$, $P = .073$. When this analysis was repeated excluding the female participants who scored 0 on the GFA-R, identical results were observed. The initial model was significant, $F(1, 136) = 148.82$, $P < .001$, and $R^2 = .523$, and SOGS scores were a significant predictor of PGSI scores, $\beta = .723$, $P < .001$. When the GFA-R subscale scores were added, the model was again significant, $F(3, 134) = 62.93$, $P < .001$, and $R^2 = .585$, and the R^2 increase of .062 was statistically significant ($P < .001$). SOGS, $\beta = .572$, $P < .001$, and GFA-R escape subscale scores, $\beta = .262$, $P < .001$, were significant predictors of PGSI scores, but GFA-R positive reinforcement subscale scores were not, $\beta = .063$, $P = .301$.

Analysis of the data from the male participants produced different results. When data from all male participants were analyzed, the initial model was significant, $F(1, 66) = 32.68$, $P < .001$, and $R^2 = .331$, and SOGS scores were significant predictors of PGSI scores, $\beta = .575$, $P < .001$. When the GFA-R subscale scores were added, the model was again significant, $F(3, 64 = 16.61$, $P < .001$, and $R^2 = .438$. The R^2 increase of .107 was statistically significant ($P = .004$), and SOGS scores were again significant predictors, $\beta = .470$, $P < .001$. However, GFA-R positive reinforcement subscale scores, $\beta = .321$, $P = .004$, and not GFA-R escape subscale scores, $\beta = .042$, $P = .717$, were significant predictors of PGSI scores. Likewise, when data from male participants scoring 0 on the GFA-R were analyzed, the initial model was again significant, $F(1, 61) = 29.07$, $P < .001$, and $R^2 = .323$, and SOGS scores were again significant predictors of PGSI scores, $\beta = .568$, $P < .001$. When the GFA-R subscale scores were added, the model was again significant, $F(3, 59) = 13.29$, $P < .001$, $R^2 = .403$, and the R^2 increase of .081 was statistically significant ($P = .024$). SOGS, $\beta = .480$, $P < .001$, and GFA-R positive reinforcement subscale scores, $\beta = .278$, $P = .014$, were significant predictors of PGSI scores, but GFA-R escape subscale scores were not, $\beta = .042$, $P = .724$.

Thus, for both female and male participants, the GFA-R subscales accounted for a significant amount of the variance in PGSI scores above and beyond that accounted for by SOGS scores. However, which subscale accounted for that increase varied as a function of sex. For females, it was endorsing gambling as an escape. For males, it was endorsing gambling for positive reinforcement.

4. Discussion

Previous research on the GFA-R has suggested that respondents typically endorse gambling for positive reinforcement to a greater extent that they endorse gambling as an escape, but that endorsing gambling as an escape is more strongly related to potential pathology, as measured by the SOGS, than is endorsing gambling for positive reinforcement. Results from the present study replicated the former finding; both female and male participants endorsed gambling for positive reinforcement to a significantly greater extent than they did gambling as an escape. Likewise, endorsing gambling as an escape was strongly related to potential pathology, as measured by the SOGS, for respondents of both sexes. However, endorsing gambling as an escape was only significantly more correlated with SOGS scores than endorsing gambling for positive reinforcement for the female participants.

One potential criticism of previous research is that conclusions about the GFA-R have been drawn by comparing GFA-R scores to SOGS scores. The present study, therefore, had participants complete a widely used measure designed to study potential gambling problems in the general population (i.e., the PGSI). As with the comparisons to the SOGS, GFA-R subscale scores were strongly correlated with PGSI scores. Also as with the SOGS comparisons, endorsing gambling as an escape was a significantly more correlated with PGSI scores than was endorsing gambling for positive reinforcement, but only for the female participants. In fact, for males, endorsing gambling for positive reinforcement was more predictive of PGSI scores than was endorsing gambling as an escape.

Although created to measure somewhat different things in different populations, the SOGS and PGSI scores were, not surprisingly, highly correlated. Furthermore, SOGS scores were significant predictors of PGSI scores. However, the GFA-R subscale scores accounted for a significant amount of the variance in PGSI scores above and beyond that accounted for by SOGS scores. Which GFA-R subscale accounted for that variance varied by sex. For females, endorsing gambling as an escape was the significant predictor. For males, endorsing gambling for positive reinforcement was the significant predictor. These results lead to two conclusions. First, although the GFA-R and SOGS are strongly correlated, the GFA-R is measuring something beyond what is measured by the SOGS. Second, there appears to be a significant relationship between the contingencies maintaining gambling behavior and the display of gambling problems in a university sample of participants. However, the contingency of interest appears to differ between females and males.

One might argue that given the fact that males suffer from pathological gambling significantly more frequently than females (see [1]), the results from the male participants might be most important. Before taking that tack, however, it should be noted that the display of gambling problems as measured by either the SOGS or PGSI was relatively similar for both female and male participants (see Table 1). Finding that the GFA-R was predictive of gambling problems above and beyond scores on the SOGS and that the different GFA-R subscales were differentially predictive of gambling problems between the two sexes should indicate two things to researchers and practitioners. First, there is additional information about a person's gambling behavior that can be gained by measuring the function of the behavior rather

than only whether the behavior is problematic. Second, different functions of the behavior might be more indicative of gambling problems depending on the sex of the individual.

One could also argue that the sex differences reported here are consistent with the broader research. That is, research indicates that men tend to be more sensation seeking than women [23], which is consistent with the present finding that endorsing gambling for positive reinforcement was a predictor of gambling problems for male respondents. Likewise, females tend to suffer from certain disorders, such as eating disorders, more frequently than men, and those disorders have been linked to the contingencies of escape (e.g., [24, 25]). Thus, although the present results should be generalized with caution because they require replication, there does appear to be convergent validity for them within the research literature.

There are, in fact, numerous reasons to be cautious in generalizing the present results. First, the participants were all university students from the upper Midwest of the United States and were relatively young even relative to the legal age to gamble in many states. It is, for instance, possible that university students gamble for different reasons than individuals in the general population. Thus, future research should attempt to collect data from a more diverse sample. Next, the present procedure particularly targeted a largely nonpathological sample using a measure of gambling problems (i.e., the PGSI) that is the best at identifying moderate, rather than severe, gambling problems (see [18]). Thus, one cannot assume that similar results would be observed if the present procedure was conducted using a clinical sample. In fact, one might argue that a major limitation of the present study was the lack of focus on pathological gamblers. One potential counter to that argument is that identifying predictor variables of gambling problems in individuals who have yet to be diagnosed as pathological allows for the potential development of preventative measures. Then again, one cannot assume that any of the present participants will eventually become pathological gamblers.

One could also criticize the present analyses because P values were not adjusted to accommodate the multiple analyses that were conducted on the same data. However, it should be noted that, had such adjustments been made, the conclusions would not have changed. In the vast majority of cases, the outcomes that were statistically significant were significant at $P < .001$ and would have remained statistically significant had the threshold been raised to be more conservative.

5. Conclusions

The present results are largely consistent with prior findings that endorsing gambling as an escape might be indicative of the respondent experiencing gambling problems. For both sexes, endorsing gambling as an escape appears to be a strong predictor of the potential presence of problem or pathological gambling as measured by the SOGS. However, when using a more general measure of gambling problems (i.e., the PGSI), there appear to be sex differences in whether endorsing gambling for positive reinforcement (males) or as an escape (females) is more predictive of those problems. This finding is augmented by the fact that scores on the GFA-R subscales accounted for a significant amount of the variance in PGSI scores beyond that accounted for by SOGS scores. Thus, the present results lead to the conclusions that the function of one's gambling is potentially predictive of whether one might be prone to experience gambling problems. This finding is of potential importance to both practitioners and researchers. Further, finding that gambling to get something versus to get away from something might be differentially predictive of gambling problems depending on the sex of the individual highlights the need for more theoretical and empirical research in this area. It may be possible that the current results can be incorporated into existing theories of pathological gambling (e.g., [15]). Then again, new theories might be required.

References

[1] N. M. Petry, *Pathological Gambling: Etiology, Comorbidity, and Treatment*, American Psychological Association, Washington , DC, USA, 2005.

[2] H. R. Lesieur and S. B. Blume, "The South Oaks Gambling Screen (SOGS): a new instrument for the identification of Pathological gamblers," *American Journal of Psychiatry*, vol. 144, no. 9, pp. 1184–1188, 1987.

[3] D. R. Gerstein, R. A. Volberg, M. T. Toce, H. Harwood, A. Palmer, and R. Johsnon, *Gambling Impact and Behavior Study: Report to the National Gambling Impact Study Commission*, University of Chicago, National Opinion Center, Chicago, Ill, USA, 1999.

[4] J. Ferris and H. Wynne, *The Canadian Problem Gambling Index: Final report*, Canadian Center on Substance Abuse, Ottawa, ON, Canada, 2001.

[5] J. Ferris, H. Wynne, and E. Single, *Measuring Problem Gambling in Canada: Draft Final Report*, Canadian Centre on Substance Abuse, Ottawa, ON, Canada, 1999.

[6] M. R. Dixon and T. E. Johnson, "The gambling functional assessment (GFA): an assessment device for identification of the maintaining variables of pathological gambling," *Analysis of Gambling Behavior*, vol. 1, pp. 44–49, 2007.

[7] V. M. Durand and D. B. Crimmins, "Identifying the variables maintaining self-injurious behavior," *Journal of Autism and Developmental Disorders*, vol. 18, no. 1, pp. 99–117, 1988.

[8] J. C. Miller, E. Meier, J. Muehlenkamp, and J. N. Weatherly, "Testing the construct validity of dixon and Johnson's (2007) gambling functional assessment," *Behavior Modification*, vol. 33, no. 2, pp. 156–174, 2009.

[9] J. N. Weatherly, J. C. Miller, and H. K. Terrell, "Testing the construct validity of the gambling functional assessment—Revised (GFA-R)," *Behavior Modification*, vol. 35, pp. 553–569, 2011.

[10] J. N. Weatherly, J. C. Miller, K. S. Montes, and C. Rost, "Assessing the reliability of the gambling functional assessment," *Journal of Gambling Studies*, vol. 28, pp. 217–223, 2012.

[11] J. C. Miller, M. R. Dixon, A. Parker, A. M. Kulland, and J. N. Weatherly, "Concurrent validity of the gambling function assessment (GFA): correlations with the South Oaks Screen (SOGS) and indicators of diagnostic efficiency," *Analysis of Gambling Behavior*, vol. 4, pp. 61–75, 2010.

[12] J. N. Weatherly and A. Derenne, "Investigating the relationship between the contingencies that maintain gambling and probability discounting of gains and losses," *European Journal of Behavior Analysis*, vol. 13, pp. 39–46, 2012.

[13] J. N. Weatherly and K. B. Miller, "Exploring the factors related to endorsing gambling as an escape," *International Gambling Studies*. In press.

[14] American Psychiatric Association, *Diagnostic and Statistical Manual of Mental Disorders*, American Psychiatric Association, Washington, DC, SA, 4th edition, 2003.

[15] A. Blaszczynski and L. Nower, "A pathways model of problem and pathological gambling," *Addiction*, vol. 97, no. 5, pp. 487–499, 2002.

[16] B. Gambino, "The correction for bias in prevalence estimation with screening tests," *Journal of Gambling Studies*, vol. 13, no. 4, pp. 343–351, 1997.

[17] R. Stinchfield, "Reliability, validity, and classification accuracy of the South Oaks Gambling Screen (SOGS)," *Addictive Behaviors*, vol. 27, no. 1, pp. 1–19, 2002.

[18] J. M. Boldero and R. C. Bell, "An evaluation of the factor structure of the problem gambling severity index," *International Gambling Studies*, vol. 12, pp. 89–110, 2012.

[19] T. Holtgraves, "Evaluating the problem gambling severity index," *Journal of Gambling Studies*, vol. 25, no. 1, pp. 105–120, 2009.

[20] R. Stinchfield, "Reliability, validity, and classification accuracy of a measure of DSM-IV diagnostic criteria for pathological gambling," *American Journal of Psychiatry*, vol. 160, no. 1, pp. 180–182, 2003.

[21] J. McMillen and M. Wenzel, "Measuring problem gambling: assessement of three prevalence screens," *International Gambling Studies*, vol. 6, pp. 147–174, 2006.

[22] D. C. Howell, *Statistical Methods for Psychology*, Cengage Wadsworth, Belmont, Calif, USA, 7th edition, 2010.

[23] C. P. Cross, L. T. Copping, and A. Campbell, "Sex differences in impulsivity: a meta-analysis," *Psychological Bulletin*, vol. 137, no. 1, pp. 97–130, 2011.

[24] K. H. Gordon, J. M. Holm-Donoma, W. Troop-Gordan, and E. Sand, "Rumination and body dissatisfaction interact to predict concurrent binge eating," *Body Image*, vol. 9, pp. 352–357, 2012.

[25] T. F. Heatherton and R. F. Baumeister, "Binge eating as escape from self-awareness," *Psychological Bulletin*, vol. 110, no. 1, pp. 86–108, 1991.

An Association between Emotional Responsiveness and Smoking Behavior

Robert D. Keeley[1,2] **and Margaret Driscoll**[3]

[1] Division of Community Health Services, Denver Health Medical Center, Denver, CO 80204, USA
[2] Department of Family Medicine, University of Colorado at Denver Health Sciences Center, Aurora, CO 80045-0508, USA
[3] Driscoll Consulting, 866 Paragon Dr., Boulder, CO 80303, USA

Correspondence should be addressed to Robert D. Keeley; robert.keeley@dhha.org

Academic Editor: Michael Joseph Zvolensky

Introduction. Emotional responsiveness (ER) has been theorized to play a protective role in pathways to tobacco initiation, regular use, and dependence, yet a possible association between ER and smoking behavior has not been studied. Our aim was to test whether measuring ER to a neutral stimulus was associated with decreased odds of current smoking. *Methods.* We measured ER and smoking status (current, former, and never) in two datasets: a cross-sectional dataset of persons with diabetes ($n = 127$) and a prospective dataset of depressed patients ($n = 107$) from an urban primary care system. Because there were few former smokers in the datasets, smoking status was dichotomized (current versus former/never) and measured at baseline (cross-sectional dataset) or at 36 weeks after-baseline (prospective dataset). ER was ascertained with response to a neutral facial expression (any ER versus none). *Results.* Compared to their nonresponsive counterparts, adjusted odds of current smoking were lower among participants endorsing emotional responsiveness in both the cross-sectional and prospective datasets (ORs = .29 and .32, P's < .02, resp.). *Discussion.* ER may be protective against current smoking behavior. Further research investigating the association between ER and decreased smoking may hold potential to inform treatment approaches to improve smoking prevalence.

1. Introduction

In the United States about 20% of persons aged 16 and older report smoking, and smoking rates are higher among persons from lower socioeconomic strata [1]. While a range of treatments exist to help smokers quit, among persons from lower socioeconomic groups the evidence that interventions increase cessation is sparse [2]. Elucidation of novel factors associated with smoking behavior holds potential to substantively improve understanding of who experiments with tobacco, who becomes a regular user, or who successfully quits. Moreover, uncovering such person-level factors may inform adjustments to treatment approaches that prevent initiation, decrease prevalence of regular tobacco use, and support cessation.

Person-level characteristics associated with smoking behavior are generally classified as psychopathology, personality, or gene related. Depressive symptoms, anxiety, psychosis, anger, social alienation, impulsivity, sensation seeking tendency, and attentional dysfunction have all been associated with current smoking [3]. Neurotic, extraverted, and open personality characteristics are associated with lifetime tobacco use [4]. Genetic variations in the nicotinic and dopamine receptors have been associated weakly with variation in nicotine dependence [5, 6]. Yet the generally weak associations between psychological states, personality traits, or receptor gene variations and smoking phenotype [7] raise some questions about clinical significance [8, 9].

Even small improvements in understanding pathways to regular smoking and dependence would hold potential to positively impact outcomes at the population level. The incremental PRIME model of addiction, which compiles extant demonstrated and proposed pathways to smoking phenotype, posits potentially important novel factors, perception, and response, as components of a hierarchical model of tobacco addiction [10]. Unfortunately, perception and response are conceptualized in PRIME as events occurring under specific circumstances that may be difficult to measure.

Moreover, response has not been studied to our knowledge as a correlate of smoking behavior. To address these limitations, we have begun developing a general measure of an individual's tendency toward emotional responsiveness and have demonstrated evidence of a possible association between responsiveness and two other outcomes, blunted adherence to antidepressant adherence and decreased coronary heart disease risk [11, 12].

Evolutionary biologists have established evidence that emotional responses evolved to guide behavioral responses to an array of environmental challenges, thus maximizing the individual's chance of meeting survival-related goals [13, 14]. In addition, it is theorized that some mental health and possibly substance abuse disorders may be viewed through the lens of evolution and may in some cases provide short-term survival benefit to the afflicted person. For instance, nicotine in cigarettes may function to provide enhanced emotional responsiveness for individuals who are otherwise less responsive emotionally than their nonsmoking counterparts, thereby possibly enhancing social function and some short-term fitness.

Measuring emotional responsiveness to relatively neutral stimuli is a practical approach to beginning to ascertain an individual's tendency toward emotional responsiveness [11]. Persons manifesting greater emotional responsiveness to relatively neutral stimuli may have a lower threshold to respond emotionally to a range of environmental stimuli, for example, public health admonishments against smoking, than their less responsive counterparts, and to exhibit subsequent behaviors protective against tobacco initiation and addiction.

Thus, we examined how demonstrating a low threshold for responsiveness, ascertained by self-report of emotional responsiveness to a neutral facial expression (ER-NFE) [15], was associated with current smoking. We hypothesized ER-NFE would be associated with decreased odds of current smoking in nonoverlapping cross-sectional and prospective datasets.

2. Method

2.1. Sample and Study Design. Study participants were persons with diabetes attending seven primary care clinics at an urban community health system in the midwestern United States. The cross-sectional sample of persons with diabetes was recruited in waiting rooms, and by telephone from a diabetic registry. Baseline data were collected between May 2008 and March 2009. Subjects for the prospective dataset were screened by telephone for probable depression 2 days prior to a primary care visit, and those screening positive were recruited from the waiting room. Baseline data were collected from April 2009 to October 2011. Patients who were less than 18 years of age, were not English-speaking, were pregnant or breastfeeding, did not have a smoking status noted currently or within the previous 3 months, or were not able to answer survey questions requiring 30-day recall were excluded. In the prospective dataset, those not having major depressive disorder, or with bipolar disorder by diagnostic schedule, were disqualified. Both studies were approved by the Colorado Multiple Institutional Review Board (*COMIRB protocols no. 07-1180 and no. 08-1282*).

2.2. Outcome

2.2.1. Smoking Behavior. For the cross-sectional dataset, self-reported smoking status was assessed at baseline from the electronic medical record, which categorized tobacco use as "current," "former," or "never." We dichotomized smoking behavior as "current" versus "former" or "never." In the prospective dataset, current smoking status (*yes/no*) was collected at 36 weeks by self-report. Self-reported smoking status is reliable and valid [16].

2.3. Independent Variables

2.3.1. Factor of Interest: Emotional Responsiveness. Emotional responsiveness was ascertained using grey-scaled normalized Ekman neutral facial expressions (*NFEs*) [15]. We assessed response by asking: "What emotion best describes how you feel when viewing this picture?" Likert anchors were "fear," disgust," "anger," "sadness," "surprise," "happiness," or "no emotion." For the cross-sectional study, a female NFE monograph, no. C2-3, was presented, and for the prospective dataset the no. C2-3 monograph and a second male NFE monograph, no. EM2-4, were also rated. For analytical purposes ER was dichotomized as any versus no response to the NFE(s) [14].

ER was associated with medication taking in a previous study, demonstrating face validity regarding associations with health-related behavior [11]. Discriminant validity appears good, as assessment of emotional responsiveness was not associated with educational attainment (*Pearson r* = .02), depressive symptom severity (*r* = .09), age (*r* = .08), gender (*r* = −.05), or race/ethnicity (*non-Hispanic black* (*r* = .13), *non-Hispanic white* (*r* = −.09), *and Hispanic* (*r* = −.05) *race/ ethnicity*) in the prospective dataset. No significant associations between emotional responsiveness and personality traits identified by the 5-factor model were noted (*r's* < .15) [17], and 3-month test-retest reliability was good at .79.

As a theoretical framework for this study, we synthesized theories from Paul Ekman, Mary Phillips, Richard Nesse, and others developed over the last 4 decades. In the 1970s Ekman described how perception of a neutral facial expression varied, with substantial numbers of persons rating the face as revealing negative or positive emotion. Neurobiological research uncovered pathways from general perception of the environment to emotional responsiveness and then to subsequent behaviors. In fact, evolutionary biologists have established evidence that emotions evolved to guide behavioral responses to an array of perceived environmental challenges, thus maximizing the individual's chance of meeting survival-related goals [18]. In perceiving and judging their environment, persons will often have a measurable emotional responsiveness that drives subsequent behavior. According to this resultant theory of emotional perception, response, and health-promoting behavior (Figure 1), we theorized that persistent smoking behavior would be more prevalent among

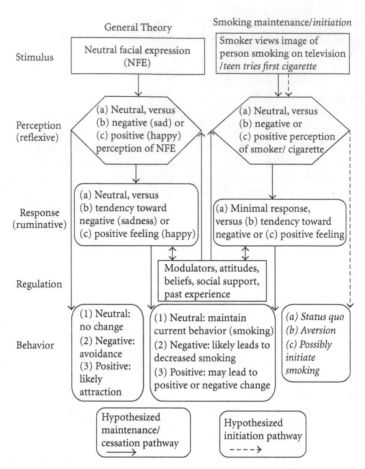

FIGURE 1: Theory of emotional perception, response, and health-promoting behavior applied to tobacco use.

persons with relatively blunted emotional responsiveness when presented with neutral stimuli.

Moreover, sensitivity toward perceiving emotion varies by mood state and personality [19]. Neutrally valenced expressions may tend to elicit less ER than positively or negatively valenced facial expressions [20]. Thus, perception of and emotional responsiveness to a NFE may represent a simple way to ascertain subtle differences in activation thresholds for ER [11, 21]. Persons exhibiting emotional responsiveness to a neutral facial expression may more likely respond emotionally to a range of environmental stimuli, for example, public health admonishments against smoking, than their less responsive counterparts. Consistent with this theoretical framework, we theorized that emotional non-responsiveness to NFE would be associated with increased smoking behavior, while emotional responsiveness to NFE would be associated with smoking abstinence.

2.3.2. Possible Confounders. Based upon literature review and theoretical plausibility, possible confounders of an association between ER and current smoking were selected and determined at baseline from electronic medical record review, pharmacy refill records, and self-report (Table 1).

Demographic factors included age, educational attainment, race/ethnicity (Hispanic, non-Hispanic (NH) White,

and NH Black), gender, unadjusted income, and insurance status. Educational attainment was dichotomized as less than high school versus a high school equivalent education or higher. Insurance was categorized as public, including Medicare and Medicaid, a partial coverage program for otherwise uninsured indigent persons, or private.

Psychosocial variables were measured through a series of survey questions. A collaborative relationship with the primary care clinician was assessed with a 3-item scale from the Helping Alliance Questionnaire [22].

Self-efficacy [23] was ascertained with the first question from the General Self-Efficacy scale. A single question assessment has been used before in tobacco studies [24].

Social support was assessed by self-report of number of household members, and social function with a question from the Short-Form 36 instrument (*SF-36*) assessing the extent to which mental or physical health problems affect social activities [25].

Comorbid measures included a measure of probable depressive disorder as measured by the Patient Health Questionnaire-2 (*PHQ-2*) [26]. A score of 3 or higher was considered to represent probable major depressive disorder. Depression often precedes smoking initiation and experimentation [27]. Lifetime generalized anxiety disorder was assessed with a diagnostic schedule,

TABLE 1: Study populations.

Characteristic	n (cross-sectional dataset)	Mean (95% CI; range) or frequencies	n (prospective dataset)	Mean (95% CI; range) or frequencies
Demographic				
Age (years)	127	51.3 (49.5–53.2; 26–77)	107	50.9 (48.4–53.5; 18–66)
Gender	127	52.0% female	107	71.0% female
Race-ethnicity	127	40.2% NH White 26.8% NH Black 33.1% Hispanic	107	21.5% NH White 32.7% NH Black 35.5% Hispanic 2.8% NH Native American 7.5% NH other
Educational attainment (years)		NA	100	24.0% < high school 76.0% high school or greater
Income (US dollars)	115	$10,309; (7598.5–12,919.2; $0–$40,086)		NA
Insurance	127	51.2% no insurance 48.8% public (Medicaid or Medicare) or private		NA
Smoking status	127	40.9% current 9.5% former 49.6% never	107	34.6% current 65.4% former/never
Psychosocial				
Collaborative patient-clinician relationship	125	15.6 or "moderately good" (15.2, 16.0; 4–18)		NA
Self-efficacy	123	3.2 or "good" (3.0, 3.4; 1–4)		NA
Social				
Health interference	122	2.8 or "moderate interference" (2.5, 3.0; 1–5)		NA
No. of household members	127	1.5 (1.4, 1.7; 1–6)		NA
Comorbid				
Probable depressive disorder (PHQ-2 ≥ 3: or PHQ-9 depressive symptoms score[†])	127	31.7%	107	16.0[†] (15.2, 16.8; 10–23)
Generalized anxiety disorder		NA	107	24.2%
No. of physical comorbidities (0–10)	107	NA		2.6 (2.2–2.9; 0–7)
Functional				
Bodily pain	124	6.8 or "moderate" (6.3, 7.4; 2–13)		NA
Body mass index	126	0.8% underweight 12.7% normal 23.0% overweight 63.5% obese	107	0% underweight 18.7% normal 26.2% overweight 55.1% obese
Medical care				
No. of primary care visits/previous year	126	4.9 (4.4, 5.5; 0–16)		NA
Current narcotic use	126	35.7%		NA
Factor of interest				
Emotional response to neutral facial expression(s)[§]	127	36.2%	107	70.1%[§]

[§] Any emotional response to one of two neutral Ekman monographs; NH: non-Hispanic; [†]PHQ: Patient Health Questionnaire-9 depressive symptoms score (range 0–27).

Functional assessments were also included in the study. Smoking is associated with chronic pain [28], and bodily pain was determined from the sum of two questions from the SF-36 [25]. Body mass index (BMI) was measured both as a continuous variable and as a categorical variable (*per National Heart Lung and Blood Institute criteria*) [29].

Because visiting a primary care office may increase the odds of receiving a smoking intervention, the number of primary care visits over the previous 12 months at the urban health care system was ascertained from the EMR. Current narcotic use has been associated with smoking and was defined as filling a monthly prescription for narcotics at least two times in the previous 4 months as determined from automated pharmacy refill records.

2.4. Analytical Approach. For both cross-sectional and prospective models, we assessed for univariate associations between the factor of interest, possible confounders, and current smoking. We selected those variables associated at $P < .10$ (*Spearman's correlation*) for further analysis. We conducted a multivariate logistic regression analysis with the dependent variable current smoking and the independent variable ER, entered possible confounders in blocks by domain (*demographic, psychosocial, comorbid, etc.*), and retained those variables associated with smoking at $P < .10$ for the final model.

2.4.1. Size of the Clinical Association. For dichotomous risk factors, nonparametric methodology generates the "area under the curve" (AUC) size of the clinical association (ES). An AUC = .56 is equivalent to a small association (*Cohen's d = .2*), while AUC = .64 and AUC = .71 are equivalent to medium and large associations (*Cohen's d = .5 and .8, resp.*) [30].

We used SAS 9.2 (SAS, Cary, NC) with PROC SUR-VEYMEANS and SURVEYLOGISTIC nested by clinic site for descriptive and multivariate analyses. Alpha was set at $P < .05$ for multivariate analyses.

3. Results

3.1. Characteristics of the Participants (Table 1). For the cross-sectional dataset, we recruited 129 persons with diabetes for inclusion in the study. Of these, 127 with complete information regarding the primary outcome smoking status were included in the current study. For the prospective dataset, we included 107 subjects with available 36-week smoking status.

A relatively high proportion of the cross-sectional sample reported current smoking (52/127, 40.9%). About half reported never smoking (63/127, 49.6%), and 9.5% (12/127) were former smokers. In the prospective dataset, 34.6% (37/107) were current smokers.

3.2. Hypothesized Correlate: Emotional Responsiveness. In the cross-sectional dataset we found that 36.2% (46/127) of the subjects endorsed a non-neutral ER-NFE (e.g., sadness, fear, anger, happiness, and surprise). In the prospective dataset,

70.1% (75/107) gave a non-neutral response to at least one of two NFEs. The rate was higher in the prospective dataset because the respondent only had to provide an emotional response to one of two NFEs, while in the cross-sectional dataset only one NFE was rated.

In the cross-sectional dataset, over twice as many non-smokers (46.7% (35/75)), including never and former smokers, reported emotional responsiveness as current smokers (21.2% (11/52)). In this dataset, almost half of never smokers endorsed emotional responsiveness to the neutral facial expression (49.2% (31/63)), in contrast with former smokers of whom only 33.3% (4/12) appeared responsive. Overall, current smokers were significantly less likely than never smokers to report ER-NFE (*Chi-square = 8.2, P = .004*). Former smokers did not demonstrate significantly different rates of ER-NFE than current (*Chi-square = .81, P = .47*) or never smokers (*Fisher's Exact test P = .36*).

In the prospective dataset, 77.1% (54/70) of non-smokers reported ER-NFE, compared with 56.8% of current smokers (21/37).

3.3. Multivariate Logistic Regression Analyses (Table 2)

3.3.1. Cross-Sectional. The adjusted odds for smoking were over three times lower for patients reporting ER-NFE relative to their less responsive counterparts (OR = .29, 95% CI .11, .72, $P = .008$). The multivariate model was adjusted for age, current narcotic medication use, and self-efficacy. Increasing age was associated with lower odds of smoking in this cohort (OR = .57, 95% CI .36, .89, $P = .014$, *for 1 SD (10.8 years) increase from median age (50.0 years)*). Self-efficacy was associated with lower probability of current smoking (OR = .17, 95% CI .05, .66, $P = .01$). Current use of narcotic pain medication appeared to be associated with increased odds of smoking (OR = 2.50, 95% CI 1.08, 5.81, $P = .033$). The model *c*-statistic was .76.

3.3.2. Prospective. Patients endorsing ER-NFE were over 3 times less likely to smoke than their nonresponsive counterparts (OR = .32, 95% CI .13, .82, $P = .018$). The multivariate model was adjusted for educational level and BMI. The *c*-statistic was .71.

3.4. Clinical Association between ER-NFE and Current Smoking. In the cross-sectional and prospective datasets, the AUC clinical associations for ER-NFE comparing current to non-smokers were .63 and .61, respectively. These would be considered small associations equivalent to Cohen's *d*'s of .43 and .41. The size of the association was medium when comparing current to never smokers in the cross-sectional dataset (AUC ES = .64, Cohen's *d* = .51).

4. Discussion

This is the first study of which we are aware to demonstrate that a measure of emotional responsiveness to neutral facial expression was robustly associated with not smoking in two nonoverlapping samples of urban-dwelling primary

TABLE 2: Multivariate logistic regression models.

	Estimate (SE)	Adjusted odds ratio (95% CI)	Pr (> |t|)
(A) *Cross-sectional dataset* ($n = 122$)°			
Dependent variable = current			
smoking at baseline ($n = 49$)			
Intercept	.83 (.56)		.13
Self-efficacy	−1.75 (.68)	.17* (.05, .66)	.01
Narcotic pain medication use	.46 (.22)	2.50 (1.08, 5.81)	.033
Emotional responsiveness	−.62 (.24)	.29 (.11, .72)	.008
Age	−.56 (.23)	.57* (.36, .89)	.014
c-statistic = .76			
(B) *Prospective dataset* ($n = 100^{\Omega}$)			
Outcome = current smoking at 36			
weeks after baseline ($n = 44$)			
Intercept	−1.02 (.74)		.17
At least 12 years education	−.56 (.26)	.33 (.12, .90)	.03
Emotional responsiveness	−.57 (.24)	.32 (.13, .82)	.018
Categorical body mass index	.54 (.29)	1.72 (.98, 3.03)	.058
c-statistic = .71			

°$n − 5$ with missing educational attainment data; *odds of smoking for each 1 SD increase from median score.
$^{\Omega}n = 7$ with missing self-efficacy (4) or use of narcotic pain medication (1) data.

care patients. In adjusted analyses, current smoking was over 3 times less likely for persons endorsing emotional responsiveness relative to their nonresponsive counterparts. The extent of the clinical association was more than twice a recommended threshold for association between independent factors and current smoking, demonstrating a robust level of clinical significance [9, 31]. Emotional responsiveness was not related to a range of potential confounders including depressive symptoms, general anxiety disorder, and personality domains. Thus, our findings signify that the measure of emotional responsiveness appears to represent a novel, positive correlate of tobacco use behavior.

Other potentially modifiable correlates of smoking behavior in the cross-sectional dataset included self-efficacy and narcotic use. Self-efficacy appeared protective against current smoking, and previous studies have suggested possible associations between self-efficacy and decreased current smoking [2]. Narcotic use has been positively associated with current smoking [32]. In one study, persons receiving prescription narcotic pain medication were over twice as likely to smoke as their peers who did not receive narcotic pain relievers. On the one hand, tobacco users are more likely to develop chronic pain than persons who do not smoke, thereby increasing likelihood of narcotic treatment for pain. On the other hand, the finding may be explained in part because tendency toward addiction to one substance (e.g., tobacco) has been associated with addictions to other substances (e.g., narcotic medications).

In the prospective multivariate analysis of patients with probable depression, greater than 12 years education was associated with decreased odds of smoking, consistent with previous research [33], while increasing BMI was associated with higher odds of smoking. The latter observation is not surprising, as both tobacco use and obesity are more prevalent among depressed persons, relative to their nondepressed counterparts [29]. The samples had high rates of smoking, likely because they were drawn from patients of mostly low socioeconomic status attending an urban public health care system.

4.1. Strengths and Limitations. Strengths of the study include the theory-driven hypothesis, the adjustment for a broad set of possible confounders, and confirmation of the cross-sectional findings in a second prospective analysis in a nonoverlapping dataset. It is possible that the association between a neutral response to NFEs and current smoking was explained by a nicotine-related influence; that is, nicotine may suppress emotional responsiveness. However, this explanation is unlikely because former and current smokers in the cross-sectional study had lower rates of ER-NFE than never smokers. Threats to external validity include two relatively small samples of lower SES individuals from one health system. Validity would be improved by demonstrating associations between ER-NFE and other measures of emotional responsiveness such as electrophysiological correlates of facial expression processing [20].

5. Conclusion

The study appears to demonstrate a robust association between emotional responsiveness to neutral facial expression and decreased odds of current smoking. As even modestly improved understanding of tobacco use holds potential to inform improvements to prevention and treatment approaches, we recommend further research to confirm and further explore this initial description of a relationship between ER-NFE and current smoking in other study populations.

Conflict of Interests

Neither author has a connection to the tobacco, alcohol, pharmaceutical or gaming industries or anybody substantially funded by one of these organizations.

Acknowledgments

The authors would like to express gratitude to Lucy Loomis, M.D., and the Division of Community Health Services for funding the data collection for the cross-sectional dataset. This study was funded in part by a Grant from the National Institute of Mental Health (K23 MH082997) to R. Keeley.

References

[1] J. Sargeant, M. Valli, S. Ferrier, and H. MacLeod, "Lifestyle counseling in primary care: opportunities and challenges for changing practice," *Medical Teacher*, vol. 30, no. 2, pp. 185–191, 2008.

[2] R. Hiscock, L. Bauld, A. Amos, J. A. Fidler, and M. Munafò, "Socioeconomic status and smoking: a review," *Annals of the New York Academy of Sciences*, vol. 1248, no. 1, pp. 107–123, 2012.

[3] D. G. Gilbert and B. O. Gilbert, "Personality, psychopathology, and nicotine response as mediators of the genetics of smoking," *Behavior Genetics*, vol. 25, no. 2, pp. 133–147, 1995.

[4] C. W. Kahler, A. M. Leventhal, S. B. Daughters et al., "Relationships of personality and psychiatric disorders to multiple domains of smoking motives and dependence in middle-aged adults," *Nicotine and Tobacco Research*, vol. 12, no. 4, pp. 381–389, 2010.

[5] L. J. Bierut, "Nicotine dependence and genetic variation in the nicotinic receptors," *Drug and Alcohol Dependence*, vol. 104, supplement 1, pp. S64–S69, 2009.

[6] A. M. Leventhal, S. P. David, M. Brightman et al., "Dopamine D4 receptor gene variation moderates the efficacy of bupropion for smoking cessation," *Pharmacogenomics Journal*, vol. 12, pp. 86–92, 2010.

[7] S. P. David, E. C. Johnstone, M. Churchman, P. Aveyard, M. F. G. Murphy, and M. R. Munafò, "Pharmacogenetics of smoking cessation in general practice: results from the Patch II and Patch in Practice trials," *Nicotine and Tobacco Research*, vol. 13, no. 3, pp. 157–167, 2011.

[8] C. W. Kahler, S. B. Daughters, A. M. Leventhal et al., "Personality, psychiatric disorders, and smoking in middle-aged adults," *Nicotine and Tobacco Research*, vol. 11, no. 7, pp. 833–841, 2009.

[9] M. R. Munafò, J. I. Zetteler, and T. G. Clark, "Personality and smoking status: a meta-analysis," *Nicotine and Tobacco Research*, vol. 9, no. 3, pp. 405–413, 2007.

[10] R. West and A. Hardy, *Theory of Addiction*, Blackwell, Oxford, UK, 2006.

[11] R. D. Keeley, A. J. Davidson, L. A. Crane, B. Matthews, and W. Pace, "An association between negatively biased response to neutral stimuli and antidepressant nonadherence," *Journal of Psychosomatic Research*, vol. 62, no. 5, pp. 535–544, 2007.

[12] J. Lee, R. Keeley, and A. Reiter, "Novel correlates of coronary heart disease risk," *Journal of Bioscience and Medicine*, vol. 2, no. 3, pp. 1–10, 2012.

[13] M. L. Phillips, W. C. Drevets, S. L. Rauch, and R. Lane, "Neurobiology of emotion perception II: implications for major psychiatric disorders," *Biological Psychiatry*, vol. 54, no. 5, pp. 515–528, 2003.

[14] R. M. Nesse and P. C. Ellsworth, "Evolution, emotions, and emotional disorders," *American Psychologist*, vol. 64, no. 2, pp. 129–139, 2009.

[15] P. Ekman and W. V. Friesen, *Emotion in the Human Face*, Pergamon, Elmsford, NY, USA, 1972.

[16] D. L. Patrick, A. Cheadle, D. C. Thompson, P. Diehr, T. Koepsell, and S. Kinne, "The validity of self-reported smoking: a review and meta-analysis," *American Journal of Public Health*, vol. 84, no. 7, pp. 1086–1093, 1994.

[17] O. P. John and E. M. Donahue, *The Big Five Inventory: Construction and Validation*, Institute of Personality and Social Research, Berkeley, Calif, USA, 1998.

[18] M. L. Phillips, W. C. Drevets, S. L. Rauch, and R. Lane, "Neurobiology of emotion perception I: the neural basis of normal emotion perception," *Biological Psychiatry*, vol. 54, no. 5, pp. 504–514, 2003.

[19] J. M. Leppänen, M. Milders, J. S. Bell, E. Terriere, and J. K. Hietanen, "Depression biases the recognition of emotionally neutral faces," *Psychiatry Research*, vol. 128, no. 2, pp. 123–133, 2004.

[20] W. Luo, W. Feng, W. He, N. Y. Wang, and Y. J. Luo, "Three stages of facial expression processing: ERP study with rapid serial visual presentation," *Neuroimage*, vol. 49, no. 2, pp. 1857–1867, 2010.

[21] J. Joormann, K. Gilbert, and I. H. Gotlib, "Emotion identification in girls at high risk for depression," *Journal of Child Psychology and Psychiatry and Allied Disciplines*, vol. 51, no. 5, pp. 575–582, 2010.

[22] G. H. De Weert-Van Oene, C. A. J. De Jong, F. Jörg, and G. J. P. Schrijvers, "The helping alliance questionnaire: psychometric properties in patients with substance dependence," *Substance Use and Misuse*, vol. 34, no. 11, pp. 1549–1569, 1999.

[23] M. Jerusalem and R. Schwarzer, "Self-efficacy as a resource factor in stress appraisal processes," in *Self-Efficacy: Thought Control of Action*, R. Schwarzer, Ed., pp. 195–213, Hemisphere, Washington, DC, USA, 1992.

[24] S. Schneider, M. Gadinger, and A. Fischer, "Does the effect go up in smoke? A randomized controlled trial of pictorial warnings on cigarette packaging," *Patient Education and Counseling*, vol. 86, no. 1, pp. 77–83, 2012.

[25] C. A. McHorney, J. E. Ware, J. F. Lu, and C. D. Sherbourne, "The MOS 36-item Short-Form Health Survey (SF-36): III. Tests of data quality, scaling assumptions, and reliability across diverse patient groups," *Medical Care*, vol. 32, no. 1, pp. 40–66, 1994.

[26] B. Löwe, K. Kroenke, and K. Gräfe, "Detecting and monitoring depression with a two-item questionnaire (PHQ-2)," *Journal of Psychosomatic Research*, vol. 58, no. 2, pp. 163–171, 2005.

[27] J. D. Kassel, L. R. Stroud, and C. A. Paronis, "Smoking, stress, and negative affect: correlation, causation, and context across stages of smoking," *Psychological Bulletin*, vol. 129, no. 2, pp. 270–304, 2003.

[28] T. N. Weingarten, Y. Shi, C. B. Mantilla, W. M. Hooten, and D. O. Warner, "Smoking and chronic pain: a real-but-puzzling relationship," *Minnesota Medicine*, vol. 94, no. 3, pp. 35–37, 2011.

[29] T. W. Strine, A. H. Mokdad, S. R. Dube et al., "The association of depression and anxiety with obesity and unhealthy behaviors among community-dwelling US adults," *General Hospital Psychiatry*, vol. 30, no. 2, pp. 127–137, 2008.

[30] H. C. Kraemer and D. J. Kupfer, "Size of treatment effects and their importance to clinical research and practice," *Biological Psychiatry*, vol. 59, no. 11, pp. 990–996, 2006.

[31] B. Chapman, K. Fiscella, P. Duberstein, and I. Kawachi, "Education and smoking: confounding or effect modification by phenotypic personality traits?" *Annals of Behavioral Medicine*, vol. 38, no. 3, pp. 237–248, 2009.

[32] Y. Shi, T. N. Weingarten, C. B. Mantilla, W. M. Hooten, and D. O. Warner, "Smoking and pain: pathophysiology and clinical implications," *Anesthesiology*, vol. 113, no. 4, pp. 977–992, 2010.

[33] L. G. Escobedo, R. F. Anda, P. F. Smith, P. L. Remington, and E. E. Mast, "Sociodemographic characteristics of cigarette smoking initiation in the United States: implications for smoking prevention policy," *Journal of the American Medical Association*, vol. 264, no. 12, pp. 1550–1555, 1990.

3

An Exploration of Responses to Drug Conditioned Stimuli during Treatment for Substance Dependence

Benjamin Goddard, Leanne S. Son Hing, and Francesco Leri

Department of Psychology, University of Guelph, 50 Stone Road East, Guelph, ON, Canada N1G 2W1

Correspondence should be addressed to Francesco Leri; fleri@uoguelph.ca

Academic Editor: Ingmar Franken

Although it is well established that drug conditioned stimuli produce a variety of conditioned responses, it is not known whether such stimuli can also reinforce an arbitrary operant response and thus serve as conditioned reinforcers. Volunteers (n = 39) recruited from a residential treatment center for substance dependence were tested on a task in which presses on computer keys activated images of drugs/drug paraphernalia on a progressive ratio schedule of reinforcement. They also completed a personalized craving questionnaire and a personalized Implicit Association Test. A significant bias in responding was found for images of preferred drugs/route of drug administration. Craving, however, was low and the images generated negative evaluative reactions. Two additional studies were performed to ascertain the generalizability of the effects to a different population of drug-using individuals (i.e., students who drink) and to incentive stimuli of a different nature (i.e., sexual). The additional studies partially replicated and extended the central findings of the main study. Therefore, although these data should be considered preliminary in light of small group sizes, it is concluded that cue specificity and availability of the unconditioned stimuli (drugs and sex) plays a role in modulating responding maintained by conditioned reinforcers.

1. Introduction

Drug conditioned stimuli, which can be discrete (i.e., a syringe) and/or environmental (i.e., a room), acquire the ability to activate drug-oriented behaviors because they are repeatedly perceived in conjunction with the unconditioned effects of drugs of abuse [1–3]. Hence, through Pavlovian conditioning, drug conditioned stimuli become wanted [4] and preferred [5], grab attention [6–8], and produce a variety of physiological and psychological responses [9–15].

The current study had two primary objectives. The first was to establish whether drug conditioned stimuli (i.e., images of drugs and drug paraphernalia) can serve as conditioned reinforcers. Conditioned reinforcing stimuli, unlike primary reinforcing stimuli, strengthen behavioral responses in virtue of their learned value. Therefore, the objective of this study was to determine whether the occurrence of stimuli associated with the effects of drugs can maintain an arbitrary operant response (i.e., pressing a computer key) in the absence of drugs [16]. This is of interest because it is possible that the assessment of the reinforcing value of

drug conditioned stimuli could complement other measures of "cue reactivity" such as self-reported craving [17, 18], and thus help predict clinical outcomes [19, 20].

To determine whether drug conditioned stimuli would reinforce arbitrary operant responses, subjects were recruited from Stonehenge Therapeutic Community, a long-term (6 months) residential treatment facility designed for chronic and relapsing substance dependence. Therefore, these individuals were likely to have experienced substantial conditioning as a result of excessive exposure to various drugs of abuse. Although the selection of this population precluded manipulation of important variables such as availability of the unconditioned stimuli (i.e., drugs), it allowed the exploration of whether this novel putative index of cue-reactivity could be related to self-reported drug cravings, and predictive of treatment completion, which is typically low in therapeutic communities [21].

The second objective was to study the relationship between explicit behavioral reactivity (i.e., operant responding) and automatic evaluative processes elicited by drug conditioned stimuli. Using the Implicit Association Test

(IAT), for example, it has been established that words such as beer, wine, whisky, and rum generate significant automatic negative responses in heavy drinking individuals who do not try to abstain [22]. That is, subjects are faster at categorizing alcohol-associated words with negative concepts such as "bad" or "disgust," than with positive concepts such as "good" or "pleasant." In light of leading neurobiological theories of addiction predicting dissociations between what people do when they are exposed to drug associated stimuli compared to how they feel [23, 24], the IAT was used to assess automatic responses to drug conditioned stimuli within the context of their conditioned reinforcing effect. It was hypothesized that the two measures would reveal independent aspects of cue reactivity.

Studies performed in clinical populations, however, can have limited generalizability. That is, it can often be questioned whether the results apply to other clinical populations, or if they can help understand basic psychological processes that play a role in the behavior of nonclinical samples. Because the third objective of this research was to explore the relationship between basic psychological processes, two additional studies were performed. These studies were specifically implemented in nonmatched groups to ascertain whether significant relationships could be observed between cravings for incentives, behavioral responses to stimuli-associated with these incentives, and automatic evaluative processes elicited by these stimuli.

Therefore, one study investigated whether drug conditioned stimuli can reinforce operant behavior also in individuals who regularly consume drugs, but are not dependent and not in treatment for excessive use. Therefore, volunteers were recruited from the population of undergraduate students at the University of Guelph on the basis of self-reported levels of alcohol consumption. The focus on this particular drug was constrained by the selection of the sample: undergraduate students in this University rarely report the use of other drugs, including cannabis.

The second study investigated whether only stimuli paired with drugs of abuse can function as conditioned reinforcers. Therefore, always in undergraduate students, it was tested whether images of sexy attractive models in swimsuits could support operant responding. Sexual stimuli were selected because: (1) it is fairly intuitive to predict the gender of the reinforcing stimulus in heterosexual individuals; (2) it is known that sexual stimuli can act as conditioned reinforcers in animals [25]; and (3) it is clear that responses to sexual stimuli can be observed in the absence of sexual "addiction" [26]. Similar methodologies were employed in the three studies to allow for meaningful comparisons across findings.

2. Methods

2.1. Participants

2.1.1. Stonehenge Therapeutic Community Study. The sample consisted of 28 males and 11 females, aged (mean ± standard error of the mean; sem) 36.8 ± 1.5 and 37.5 ± 3.9, respectively,

primarily Caucasian (87%), with education below university level (98%). The power calculation was performed using the effect size estimated using the *Cohen's d* model, although subsequent analyses required to split the sample in subgroups (see below). The vast majority (92%) of subjects had received previous treatment; 38% reported one, and 54% reported 2 or more treatment attempts in different programs. All subjects were poly-drug users. Excluding tobacco (because almost all smoked cigarettes), the drug most often used (more than 15 days) in the 30 days prior to treatment admission was crack/cocaine (77% of subjects). Volunteering participants were eligible only if they had completed at least two weeks of treatment. The average (±sem) number of days in treatment at the time of study interview was 70 ± 5.5. Typical duration of the entire program is between 120 and 180 days. The Research Ethics Board of the University of Guelph approved the study.

2.1.2. Additional Studies

Alcohol Study. The study of responses to alcohol-related stimuli included 49 participants (17 males and 32 females, aged 19.1 ± 0.2 and 19.2 ± 0.2, resp.). *Sex Study.* The study of responses to sexual stimuli included 106 heterosexual participants (43 males and 63 females, aged 18.6 ± 0.2 and 18.3 ± 0.1, resp.). All participants were undergraduate students at the University of Guelph, recruited by mass-testing questions about drinking and sexual behavior (see below). The Research Ethics Board of the University of Guelph approved both studies.

2.2. Measures and Procedures

2.2.1. Stonehenge Therapeutic Community Study. First, a brief survey assessed drug use in the 30 days prior to arrival at the community, as well as drug of choice and preferred route of administration.

Second, participants completed a questionnaire about craving for their drug of choice. This questionnaire included 10 questions about desire for the drug (i.e., "I have an urge for_____") and 10 questions about anticipated drug effects (i.e., "Using _____ right now would make me feel less tired"). The experimenter completed the blank for each item with the particular participant's drug of choice. The questions were derived from items common to half of 12 validated questionnaires assessing craving for alcohol, cocaine, speed, heroin, or tobacco [27–37]. This "composite" questionnaire was created because participants drug of choice was not known prior to the initial survey, and thus there was a need for questions that would apply regardless of the name of the drug that was used to fill the blanks. Answers were provided on a visual analog scale ranging from 0 to 10. Therefore, the maximal total craving score on this questionnaire was 200. The Cronbach's alpha of this composite craving questionnaire was 0.91.

Third, volunteers were asked to perform the Conditioned Reinforcement Task (CRT). This was an adaptation of a conditioned reinforcement procedure [38–41] in which operant behavior is reinforced by stimuli previously associated with the effects of drugs of abuse. In the current study, participants responded to keys generating pictures (see Figure 1) of drug look-alike substances (i.e., white powder, crystals), of actual drugs (i.e., bottles of different alcoholic beverages), of simulated drug taking behavior (i.e., snorting, smoking, injecting, drinking), and of drug paraphernalia (i.e., syringe, needle, crack pipe). Six keys were linked to 6 categories of images, and each category included 40 images. Four categories were created to represent drugs of choice commonly reported by individuals in treatment at Stonehenge: cocaine/crack, heroin, alcohol, and marijuana. Two additional categories were created for control purposes and included pictures of buildings, and random colours. These categories were selected because buildings are recognizable visual stimuli with neutral motivational value, and random colors can have motivational value but do not represent identifiable objects. All images were equalized for contrast and luminance.

Pressing any of the 6 keys activated a single image of a specific category for 1 second according to a progressive ratio schedule of reinforcement. The computer randomly determined the order of image presentation within each category/key. The progressive ratio schedule has been employed in animal [42] and humans [43, 44] to measure motivation to self-administer drugs when the response requirement for each subsequent administration progressively increases within the session [45]. Of course, in the current study, no drug was provided after completion of each response ratio.

Participants were not informed about the association between keys and image categories prior to the beginning of testing, no practice trials were given, and there was no time limit to perform the task. The test began after the following instructions were read:

> *"Pressing the keys D, F, G, H, J, and K will produce pictures on the screen. Some of these will be drug-related and some will not. Pressing the same key twice will produce another picture and so on. Presses required will go up after each picture. You have complete choice as to which keys you choose to press. There is no requirement and you may stop at any time. Please press any key to begin."*

Fourth, after a short break, all participants completed a personalized IAT [46–49] to assess automatic responses to drugs generated by exposure to the same drug-associated images employed in the CRT task. Unlike the traditional IAT that includes general attribute categories such as "good" and "bad," the personalized IAT requires a categorization of test items into attributes that are specific to the individual being tested: "I like" and "I dislike." This particular version was selected because it reduces extrapersonal automatic contamination [46, 50, 51] and thus better taps into personal automatic associations with drug (and nondrug) stimuli.

Therefore, participants were asked to categorize 40 drug associated images of their drug of choice, 40 control images (building images), 6 positive words (i.e., joy, happy), and 6 negative words (i.e., rotten, disgust) into one of four categories: two concept categories ("drugs" and "buildings"), and two attribute categories ("I like" and "I dislike").

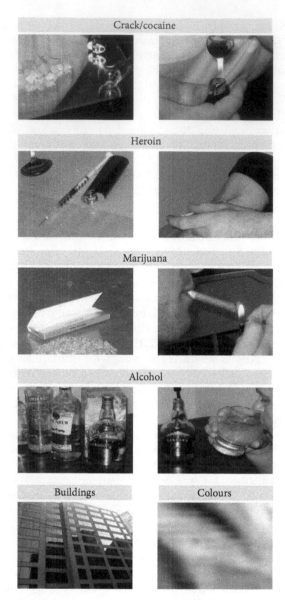

FIGURE 1: Examples of images (in black and white) employed in the CRT task.

The IAT consisted of 5 blocks of trials. For each trial, participants were required to sort a target word or a target picture that appeared in the middle of the screen into a category that appeared at the top left or the top right of the screen using respective computer keys. In the first practice block, participants sorted drug and control images into the concept category "buildings" on the left or "drugs" on the right. In the next practice block, participants sorted positive and negative words into the attribute category "I like" on the left, or "I dislike" on the right. The third block was a test block: the earlier tasks were combined and now participants sorted both picture and word targets in categories "buildings" combined with "I like" that appeared on the left of the screen, or categories "drugs" combined with "I dislike" that appeared on the right side of the screen. In the final two test blocks, the concept and attribute categories matches were reversed.

Therefore, in the next practice block, target images were sorted into either "drugs" on the left, or "buildings" on the right side of the screen. And, in the final test block, stimuli were sorted into either categories "drugs" combined with "I like" that appeared on the left, or categories "buildings" combined with "I dislike" that appeared on the right side of the screen. The dependent measure in this task is time (msec) required to assign target words and pictures to the matched concept/attribute categories on test two blocks. Faster reaction times reflect dominant automatic associations between concept and attribute categories that share a side of the computer screen. The interesting comparison was between reaction times displayed on the test blocks when "drugs" and "I dislike" shared a side of the screen versus when the side was shared by "drugs" and "I like."

2.2.2. Additional Studies. The measures and procedure employed in the two additional studies differed from the main study in three ways.

First, in the Alcohol study, student participants completed the alcohol dependency scale (ADS), in which a score of 9 or greater indicates potential problematic drinking [52]. They also (1) self-reported drinking in the 30 days prior to study interview (days of drinking and number of times they drank 0–4, 5–9, or 10+ standard drinks on each of those occasions); (2) completed the timeline follow-back measure (TFM) [53]; and (3) completed the questionnaire about craving with the word "alcohol" included in each question. In the Sex study, participants answered a questionnaire about aspects of sexual behavior in the 30 days prior to study interview (sexual relationship status, frequency of intercourse, and number of partners), and completed the questionnaire about craving employed in the other studies with the spaces for drug names (i.e., cocaine, alcohol) filled by the word "sex."

Second, in the Sex study, the images of drugs/drug use/drug paraphernalia employed in the CRT task were replaced by pictures of sexy, attractive models (women and men) in swimsuits taken from magazines such as Maxim, FHM, and GQ. Previously, the pictures were ranked on sexiness by a focus group, and the top 40 were selected for the study. Two additional control categories were included representing stimuli likely to have motivational value in undergraduate students: "junk" food (McDonald's, pizza) and snack food (chocolate, potato chips). As in the study at Stonehenge Therapeutic Community, there were also control pictures of building and random colours. The stimuli used in the Stonehenge study and in the Alcohol study were identical.

Finally, in the *Alcohol study*, participants categorized the images of alcoholic beverages and drinking (from the CRT), control images (buildings), positive words (i.e., joy, happy), and negative words (i.e., rotten, disgust), into one of four categories: two concept categories ("alcohol" and "buildings") and two attribute categories ("I like" and "I dislike"). Similarly, in the *Sex study*, participants categorized the sexy images of opposite sex models (from the CRT), control images (buildings), positive words (i.e., joy, happy), and negative words (i.e., rotten, disgust) into one of four categories: two concept categories ("sex" and "buildings"), and two attribute categories ("I like" and "I dislike").

2.3. Data Analysis. For the CRT, one-, two-, and three-factor repeated measure ANOVAs were used to compare total responding across the various keys. When data were not normally distributed, the analysis was performed using the Friedman repeated measures ANOVA on ranks. In case of significant interactions or significant main effects, multiple comparisons were performed using the Student-Newman-Keuls method to identify individual mean differences (α = 0.05).

For IAT the data, mean response latencies to categorize stimuli in the critical test blocks were computed and compared using paired t-tests. If they were not normally distributed, the data were analyzed using the Wilcoxon signed rank test. Furthermore, an IAT Difference score was calculated for each individual with lower scores reflecting more negative-automatic attitudes toward drugs/alcohol/sex [54]. Pearson correlations were employed to explore relationships between IAT Difference scores and other variables. For all analyses, the specific values of nonsignificant findings are not reported.

For analyses presented below, subgroups were created on the basis of drug of choice and preferred route of administration. Unfortunately, for the heroin- and alcohol/oral administration-based groupings, the sample sizes were too small for statistical analyses. Therefore, data for these subgroups are reported in descriptive terms only.

3. Results

3.1. Stonehenge Therapeutic Community Study. From the admission survey, it was determined that 31, 4, and 4 subjects identified crack/cocaine, heroin, and alcohol as their drug of choice, respectively. As a result, these three groups of subjects were employed for analysis. The overall average (±sem) level of self-reported craving was low (47± 6.3), with no significant differences between the groups.

Time spent on the CRT task varied between approximately 3 and 5 minutes. From a conditioning perspective, it was predicted that specific images of drugs/drug paraphernalia/drug-taking behavior would serve as reinforcers primarily in those subjects who identified that drug as their drug of choice. The results of the CRT partially supported this prediction. In fact, the crack/cocaine group emitted significantly more responses on the keys generating images of crack/cocaine and heroin (in comparison to control images—Figure 2(a); $[X^2(5) = 25.04, P = 0.0001]$), the heroin group emitted more responses on the key generating heroin images (in comparison to control images—Figure 2(b)), but the alcohol group showed no apparent response bias (Figure 2(c)).

When considering the interpretations of these results, it was noted that many subjects who reported crack/cocaine as drug of choice also reported intravenous use, and that images of needles and injection/injection rituals were included only

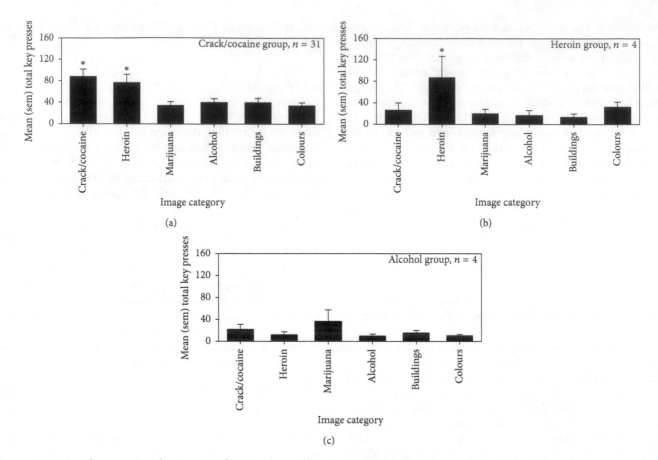

FIGURE 2: CRT performance in volunteers tested at Stonehenge Therapeutic Community. Mean and sem total number of responses made on computer keys by groups created on the basis of drug of choice ((a) = crack/cocaine, $n = 31$; (b) = heroin, $n = 4$; and (c) = alcohol, $n = 4$). A progressive ratio schedule of reinforcement controlled the relationship between responses on the keys and a 1 sec activation of pictures. Four different keys generated images of cocaine/crack, heroin, marijuana, or alcohol look-alike substances use, and paraphernalia. Two additional keys generated control images of buildings and random colors. The * indicates a significant difference, within group, between responding a specific key and all other keys. In (a) responses to the crack/cocaine and heroin keys were not significantly different from each other.

in the "heroin" category. Therefore, the subjects were regrouped on the basis of preferred route of administration: nonintravenous (smoked and snorted), $n = 19$; intravenous, $n = 16$; and oral (drank alcohol), $n = 4$, and the analysis of responses was repeated. It was found that the non-intravenous group responded significantly more to the key generating images of powder/crack smoking and snorting paraphernalia in comparison to control images ("crack/cocaine" category in Figure 3(a); $[X^2(5) = 20.79, P = 0.0008]$). By contrast, the intravenous group responded significantly more to the key generating images of needle paraphernalia and intravenous usage in comparison to control images ("heroin" category in Figure 3(b); $[X^2(5) = 13.74, P = 0.017]$). Level of operant responding of the third group (oral) was already represented in Figure 2(c) (alcohol), and no differences were apparent.

On the IAT, it was found that reaction times were quicker when the categories "drugs" and "I dislike" shared the same side of the computer screen, in comparison to when the same side of the screen was shared by the categories "drugs" and "I like." This effect was equivalent when groups were created by drug of choice (Figure 4(a): crack/cocaine group

$[t(30) = 3.85, P = 0.0006]$; heroin (Figure 4(b)) and alcohol (Figure 4(c)) groups: trend in the same direction) or by preferred route of administration (Figure 4(d): nonintravenous group $[t(17) = -3.12, P = 0.006]$; Figure 4(e): intravenous group $[W = 74.00, Z = 2.90, P = 0.001]$; (Figure 4(c)) oral group: trend in the same direction). Thus, overall, the IAT D scores were negative.

There were no significant correlations between craving scores, responding on the preferred key in the CRT (regardless of grouping), and IAT D scores. However, in the nonintravenous group, there was a significant negative correlation between days in treatment and responding on the key generating powder/crack smoking and snorting paraphernalia $[r = -0.59, P = 0.0068$; corrected $\alpha = 0.016]$. Finally, when treatment completers (87%) and noncompleters (13%) were compared, no significant differences were found in responding to the preferred key in the CRT (regardless of grouping), craving scores, or IAT D scores.

3.2. Alcohol Study. From the TFM questionnaire, it was established that the average number of days on which drinking occurred in the 30 days previous to the interview

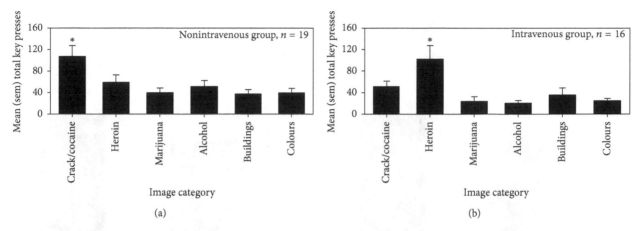

FIGURE 3: CRT performance of volunteers tested at Stonehenge Therapeutic Community. Mean and sem total number of responses made on computer keys by groups created on the basis of route of administration ((a) = nonintravenous (smoking/snorting), $n = 19$; (b) = intravenous, $n = 16$). The * indicates a significant difference, within group, between responding a specific key and all other keys.

was 5.6 ± 0.5. In spite of infrequent drinking, more than half of the subjects had an ADS score equal or greater than 9 (see Table 1) and, overall, there was a significant positive correlation between ADS score and self-reported craving for alcohol ($r = 0.40$, $P = 0.004$).

Unlike in participants tested at Stonehenge, the undergraduates in this study did not display a significant response bias on the CRT (time spent on the CRT task varied between approximately 3 and 4 minutes), regardless of the ADS score (see Table 1). However, as in the study at Stonehenge, reaction times on the IAT were significantly quicker when the categories "alcohol" and "I dislike" shared the same side on the screen (Table 2; <9 group: [$t(41) = -2.96$, $P = 0.007$]; ≥ 9 group: [$t(26) = -2.67$, $P = 0.013$]). Although there were no overall significant correlations between the IAT D scores and ADS scores, craving scores, or responding on the CRT, it was noted that 65% of the participants were females, and when ADS scores were correlated to IAT D scores and craving scores separately in females and males, it was found that, in males, higher ADS scores were associated with more positive automatic attitudes ($r = 0.66$, $P = 0.005$) and with higher craving scores ($r = 0.49$, $P = 0.051$).

3.3. Sex Study. From the questionnaires about sexual behavior and sexual craving, it was noted that although males and females did not differ on craving (97.7 ± 4.1 and 92.7 ± 4.2), there was a significant modulation by relationship status. In fact, craving for sex was significantly higher in both males [$t(41) = 2.39$, $P = 0.021$] and females [$t(61) = 2.49$, $P = 0.015$] that were actively involved in a relationship at the time of testing (Table 2). This suggested that regular access to a sexual partner could play an important role in modulating performance on the CRT and IAT. Therefore, for analyses of performance on these tests, both males and females were further subdivided in those involved or not involved in a relationship (Table 2).

On the CRT, both males and females responded significantly more to the key generating images of sexy women or men, compared to all other keys, respectively (Table 2;

significant main effect of Key [$F(5, 510) = 11.02$, $P < 0.0001$] and significant interaction between Gender and Key [$F(5, 510) = 29.53$, $P < 0.0001$]; statement above based on the results of multiple comparisons). Time spent on the CRT task varied between approximately 3 and 4 minutes. Furthermore, within both males and females, those involved in relationships responded significantly more to activate images of models of the opposite sex (significant main effect of relationship status [$F(1, 102) = 11.97$, $P = 0.0008$], significant interaction between relationship status, and key [$F(5, 510) = 3.61$, $P = 0.003$], and significant interaction between gender, relationship status, and key [$F(5, 510) = 4.51$, $P = 0.0005$]; statement above based on the results of multiple comparisons). Finally, there was a significant correlation between responses to view images of models of the opposite sex and craving scores (males and females combined; $r = 0.43$, $P = 0.001$), but only for those involved in a relationship.

The analysis of IAT data revealed that both males and females were slower to respond when the categories "sex" and "I dislike" shared the same side of the screen, and this effect was not significantly altered by relationship status (males: main effect of category [$F(1, 39) = 9.99$, $P = 0.003$]; females: main effect of category [$F(1, 54) = 12.74$, $P = 0.0008$]). There were no significant correlations between the IAT D scores and craving scores or responding to the CRT.

4. Discussion

The principal finding of this study is that individuals in long-term residential treatment for substance dependence emitted a significant number of operant responses (i.e., presses on a computer key) to view images of drugs, drug use, and drug paraphernalia. Responding was selective to images of drug of choice and of paraphernalia associated with participants' preferred route of administration. In fact, those reporting crack cocaine as their drug of choice responded significantly more on the key activating images of crack cocaine and crack cocaine use/pipes. And, when groups were re-established on

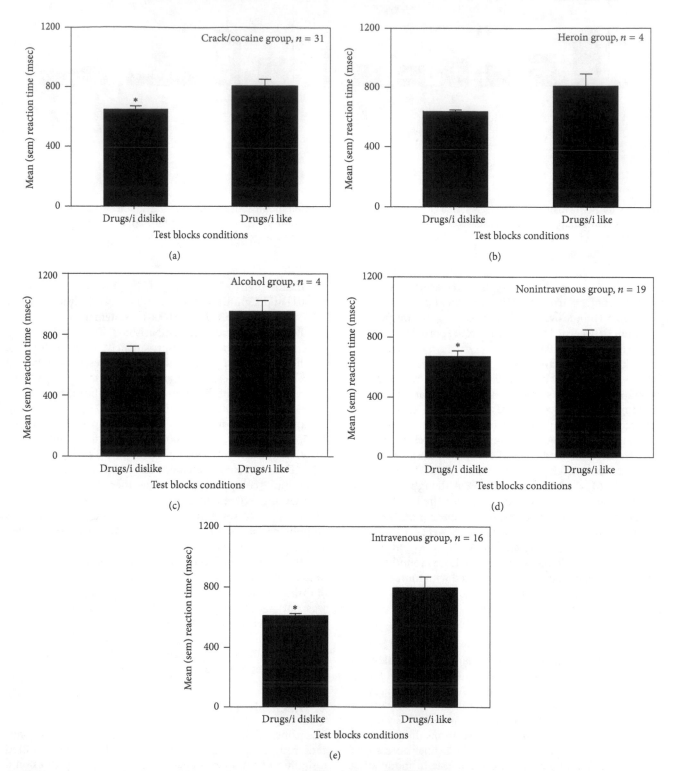

FIGURE 4: IAT performance of volunteers tested at Stonehenge Therapeutic Community. Mean and sem reaction times (msec) on test trials comparing "drugs" and "I dislike" versus "drugs" and "I like" in groups created on the basis of drug of choice or preferred route of administration ((a) = crack/cocaine, (b) = heroin, (c) = alcohol, (d) = non intravenous; and (e) = intravenous). The * indicates a significant difference within group.

TABLE 1: Groups, sample size, craving score, and performance on the CRT and IAT in subjects tested in the *Alcohol study*.

ADS score	n	Craving	CRT						IAT	
			Crack/cocaine	Heroin	Marijuana	Alcohol	Buildings	Colors	Alcohol/I dislike	Alcohol/I like
<9	22	31.6 (4.1)	13.5 (3.4)	11.7 (2.8)	10.4 (2.1)	22.7 (6.8)	17.8 (3)	20.1 (4.1)	581.8 (19.8)*	676.1 (27)
≥9	27	42.8 (4.7)	14.5 (2.8)	11.2 (3)	14.7 (2.8)	18 (2.4)	17.1 (2.4)	23.4 (4.7)	567.6 (23)*	640.7 (23.4)

The first two columns include sample size and scores on the alcohol craving questionnaire in subjects scoring below, or equal to and above, 9 (i.e., threshold of potential problematic drinking) on the ADS. The next six columns include performance on the CRT (mean (sem) responses on each key). The last two columns include performance on the IAT (mean (sem) reaction time in msec). The * indicates a significant difference within group.

TABLE 2: Groups, sample size, craving score, and performance on the CRT and IAT in subjects tested in the *Sex study*.

	n	Craving	CRT						IAT	
			Male model	Female model	"Junk" food	Snacks	Buildings	Colors	Sex/I dislike	Sex/I like
Males Involved	20	108 (6.5)*	7 (3.3)	429 (84.8)*#	70.5 (20.2)	62.6 (16.6)	51.3 (15.7)	75.3 (18.6)	624 (32.1)	555.1 (25.1)*
Males not involved	23	89 (4.7)	4.5 (1.1)	155.3 (46.3)*	57.3 (13.6)	69 (20)	28.3 (8.4)	51.6 (15.1)	605.2 (25)	545.3 (21.3)*
Females involved	36	102 (5.4)*	265.3 (92)*#	34.2 (13.6)	38.5 (9.5)	64.1 (11.7)	30.8 (8.8)	93 (23.7)	590.2 (16.8)	543.7 (13.1)*
Females not involved	27	81 (6.2)	165.8 (41)*	11.7 (3.2)	22.7 (4.3)	51.4 (11.3)	17.6 (3.4)	48.7 (11.2)	716.1 (49.3)	604 (23)*

The first two columns include sample size and scores on the sexual craving questionnaire. The * indicates a significant difference, within gender, between those involved and those not involved in a relationship. The next six columns include performance on the CRT (mean (sem) responses on each key). The * indicates a significant difference, within group, between responding a specific key and all other keys; the # indicates a significant difference in response on the same key, within gender, between those involved and not involved in a relationship. The last two columns include performance on the IAT (mean (sem) reaction time in msec). The * indicates a significant difference within group.

the basis of typical route of administration, it was found that injectors responded preferentially to the key generating images of needles and associated paraphernalia/use, and smokers/inhalers responded preferentially to the key generating images of white power, crystals, and associated paraphernalia/use.

It is widely believed that selective attention to drug related stimuli is critical for the experience of cravings and the maintenance of addictive behaviors, and it is known that users display attention biases for drug related words, scenes, and images [5, 7, 55]. For example, Moeller et al. [56] found that the choice of cocaine-related picture correlated with subjects' concurrent cocaine and other drug use, and predicted cocaine and other drug use over a period of 6 months. The results of the conditioned reinforcement task in abstinent participants corroborate and expand these findings. Not only did subjects voluntarily select the key(s) generating images of drug/route of choice while in treatment, but also responded more to these keys (versus other keys) in spite of progressively escalating response requirements.

The primary interpretation of this finding is based on classical learning theory, which suggests that drug associated stimuli acquire conditioned reinforcing properties through association with the effects of drugs [57], and hence gain the ability to reinforce behavior in the absence of drugs [16]. However, there are possible alternative interpretations. For example, subjects may have been bored, and thus willing to respond to any novel image. That said, participants' responding was significantly greater on keys generating images directly associated with their drug of choice or preferred route of administration. Alternatively, the images of drugs and drug paraphernalia might have been very appealing, and thus capable of promoting responding independent of prior learning. However, this seems unlikely given that undergraduate students selected on the basis of alcohol use (Alcohol study) responded very little to keys generating images of powders, needles, crack pipes, or burning spoons. Finally, the conditioning interpretation is further supported by the findings of the sex study. In fact, participants' magnitude of responding to view pictures of sexy opposite-sex models was significantly modulated by the frequency of sexual behavior. Hence, more frequent contact with the unconditioned stimulus (in this case sexual partner) increased responses to stimuli predictive of sexual behavior (sexy models; conditioned stimuli). Therefore, although the alcohol and the sex studies were not performed in subjects that were matched to subjects in the Stonehenge studies for age, gender, race, and education, they provided important results about basic psychological processes activated by the exposure to learned incentive stimuli.

Interestingly, a different pattern of responding was observed in abstinent alcoholics in treatment at Stonehenge, who did not preferentially respond to the key generating images of beer, wine, spirits, and consumption of these beverages. Although it is possible that this was due to a low-sample size (*n* = 4), it should be noted that low response to these images was also observed in undergraduate students who scored above 9 on the ADS (see results of Alcohol study). The discrepancy between findings with alcohol and other drugs/sexual images is difficult to explain.

It could be that there is something peculiar about alcohol or alcoholics [58, 59], although it is more likely that the images of alcohol/drinking were not specific enough [60] (i.e., preferred drink or brand). Such possibility could be tested by recruiting a larger sample and by presenting subjects with keys generating images of specific alcoholic beverages and then determine whether key selection is related to beverage of choice.

In the study at Stonehenge, the lack of correlation between responding to the CRT and score on the drug craving questionnaire could imply that the psychological constructs assessed by these tasks are independent. Although it is possible that subjects may have not been willing to disclose their craving because of the therapeutic setting in which testing was conducted, it is more likely that the low craving scores may have resulted from perceived "nonavailability" of drugs [61–63]. Such interpretation is supported by the Sex study, in which it was found that self-reported levels of craving for sex were significantly higher in those in active relationships, and frequency of sexual behavior was significantly associated with responding to the CRT. Furthermore, in a separate pilot study ($n = 18$) also performed at the Stonehenge Therapeutic Community, craving was assessed before and after performance on the CRT, and the pre- and post-CRT craving scores were virtually identical. Therefore, it is likely that within the context of long-term treatment centers, craving may be a psychological dimension of substance dependence that is more difficult to assess using a questionnaire and/or manipulate by exposure to drug-associated stimuli. This is consistent with low levels of spontaneous craving described within inpatient addiction units for alcohol and cocaine dependence (see [64] for review).

Also, in the study at Stonehenge, it was found that the drug images employed in the CRT elicited significant negative automatic associations assessed by the personalized IAT. It is important to note that the IAT does not measure attitudes toward the exemplars (i.e., a specific picture of cocaine) but rather the concepts primed by the exemplars [65]. Furthermore, the specific task employed in the current study has been found to assess personal evaluative associations independent from cultural norms [46]. Therefore, this pattern of results suggests that conditioned stimuli can reinforce operant responding independently from their automatic valence, and that they retain the ability to generate these responses in abstinent individuals.

Previous studies of automatic evaluations of alcohol using the personalized IAT revealed mixed findings. One study of light drinkers found significant negative implicit attitudes [66] and one study of heavy drinkers found a nonsignificant trend toward positive implicit attitudes [50]. Because negative implicit associations were also observed in student drinkers tested in the Alcohol study, it is possible that the image-based version of the personalized IAT does not explore the same automatic concepts that are generated by words (i.e., beer, wine). But, other explanations exist. First, students completing the image-based sex IAT generated scores reflective of positive automatic attitudes toward sex. Therefore, exposure to images can indeed activate positive evaluative reactions. Second, the personalized IAT has never been administered

to substance dependent individuals recovering from cocaine and opiate addiction, and it is very likely that implicit attitudes toward these drugs change during the development of dependence. Finally, in the Alcohol study, ADS scores were associated with more positive automatic attitudes ($r = 0.66$, $P = 0.005$) and with higher craving scores ($r = 0.49$, $P = 0.051$), but in males only. The reason for the discrepancy between males and females in not clear, although it is fairly well established that there are significant sexual differences in psychological and physiological responses to alcohol [67–69].

Somewhat disappointing was the lack of significant relationship between performance on the CRT and treatment completion, even though duration in treatment was negatively correlated to amount of responding on the crack/cocaine key. Clearly, this issue should be addressed more systematically by additional studies that could administer the CRT at multiple times during treatment. And, it may be premature to dismiss the predictive clinical value of the CRT because it is also possible that self-selection bias played an important confounding role. In fact, approximately 87% of the individuals who volunteered for this study completed the program, and this is at odds with typical retention rates at Stonehenge of 40%–50%, which are in line with those of other therapeutic communities [70].

In conclusion, although the data should be considered preliminary in light of small group sizes, this paper reports that substance dependent individuals in a long-term residential treatment program who did not report significant cravings for drugs voluntarily responded to view images of preferred drugs/drug use or preferred route of administration. Although the predictive clinical utility of the CRT is yet to be fully validated, current treatment approaches based on cue-exposure and extinction [71] could profit from assessing behavioral responses to drug conditioned stimuli when self-reports of drug craving are uninformative.

Acknowledgments

The authors wish to thank Ms. Heather Kerr, Executive Director of Stonehenge Therapeutic Community, for supporting the implementation of this study. They also wish to thank Dr. Martin Zack (Center for Addiction and Mental Health, Toronto) for the thoughtful commentary and feedback on previous versions of the manuscript. This study was supported by a Discovery Grant from the Natural Sciences and Engineering Research Council of Canada (NSERC).

References

[1] J. Stewart, "Conditioned and unconditioned drug effects in relapse to opiate and stimulant drug self-administration," *Progress in Neuro-Psychopharmacology and Biological Psychiatry*, vol. 7, no. 4–6, pp. 591–597, 1983.

[2] J. Stewart, H. de Wit, and R. Eikelboom, "Role of unconditioned and conditioned drug effects in the self-administration of opiates and stimulants," *Psychological Review*, vol. 91, no. 2, pp. 251–268, 1984.

[3] A. R. Childress, R. Ehrman, D. J. Rohsenow et al., "Classically conditioned factors in drug dependence. Substance abuse: a comprehensive textbook," *Baltimore*, pp. 56–69, 1992.

[4] T. E. Robinson and K. C. Berridge, "The neural basis of drug craving: an incentive-sensitization theory of addiction," *Brain Research Reviews*, vol. 18, no. 3, pp. 247–291, 1993.

[5] S. J. Moeller, T. Maloney, M. A. Parvaz et al., "Enhanced choice for viewing cocaine pictures in cocaine addiction," *Biological Psychiatry*, vol. 66, no. 2, pp. 169–176, 2009.

[6] I. H. A. Franken, "Drug craving and addiction: integrating psychological and neuropsychopharmacological approaches," *Progress in Neuro-Psychopharmacology and Biological Psychiatry*, vol. 27, no. 4, pp. 563–579, 2003.

[7] M. Field and W. M. Cox, "Attentional bias in addictive behaviors: a review of its development, causes, and consequences," *Drug and Alcohol Dependence*, vol. 97, no. 1-2, pp. 1–20, 2008.

[8] D. I. Lubman, L. A. Peters, K. Mogg, B. P. Bradley, and J. F. W. Deakin, "Attentional bias for drug cues in opiate dependence," *Psychological Medicine*, vol. 30, no. 1, pp. 169–175, 2000.

[9] C. P. O'Brien, T. Testa, T. J. O'Brien, and R. Greenstein, "Conditioning in human opiate addicts," *Pavlovian Journal of Biological Science*, vol. 11, no. 4, pp. 195–202, 1976.

[10] C. P. O'Brien, A. R. Childress, A. T. McLellan, R. Ehrman, and J. W. Ternes, "Types of conditioning found in drug-dependent humans," *NIDA Research Monograph Series*, no. 84, pp. 44–61, 1988.

[11] A. R. Childress, P. D. Mozley, W. McElgin, J. Fitzgerald, M. Reivich, and C. P. O'Brien, "Limbic activation during cue-induced cocaine craving," *American Journal of Psychiatry*, vol. 156, no. 1, pp. 11–18, 1999.

[12] N. D. Volkow, G.-J. Wang, F. Telang et al., "Cocaine cues and dopamine in dorsal striatum: mechanism of craving in cocaine addiction," *Journal of Neuroscience*, vol. 26, no. 24, pp. 6583–6588, 2006.

[13] B. L. Carter and S. T. Tiffany, "Meta-analysis of cue-reactivity in addiction research," *Addiction*, vol. 94, no. 3, pp. 327–340, 1999.

[14] M. D. Skinner and H.-J. Aubin, "Craving's place in addiction theory: contributions of the major models," *Neuroscience and Biobehavioral Reviews*, vol. 34, no. 4, pp. 606–623, 2010.

[15] R. Sinha, T. Fuse, L.-R. Aubin, and S. S. O'Malley, "Psychological stress, drug-related cues and cocaine craving," *Psychopharmacology*, vol. 152, no. 2, pp. 140–148, 2000.

[16] W. M. Davis and S. G. Smith, "Role of conditioned reinforcers in the initiation, maintenance and extinction of drug seeking behavior," *Pavlovian Journal of Biological Science*, vol. 11, no. 4, pp. 222–236, 1976.

[17] M. A. Sayette, S. Shiffman, S. T. Tiffany, R. S. Niaura, C. S. Martin, and W. G. Schadel, "The measurement of drug craving," *Addiction*, vol. 95, supplement 2, pp. S189–S210, 2000.

[18] D. C. Drummond, R. Z. Litten, C. Lowman, and W. A. Hunt, "Craving research: future directions," *Addiction*, vol. 95, supplement 2, pp. S247–S255, 2000.

[19] D. C. Drummond, "What does cue-reactivity have to offer clinical research?" *Addiction*, vol. 95, supplement 2, pp. S129–S144, 2000.

[20] S. T. Tiffany and J. M. Wray, "The clinical significance of drug craving," *Annals of the New York Academy of Sciences*, vol. 1248, no. 1, pp. 1–17, 2012.

[21] G. Leon, "Therapeutic communities," in *Textbook of Substance Abuse Treatment*, M. K. Galanter and D. De Herbert, Eds., American Psychiatric Press, Washington, DC, USA, 2nd edition, 1999.

[22] R. W. Wiers, N. Van Woerden, F. T. Y. Smulders, and P. J. de Jong, "Implicit and explicit alcohol-related cognitions in heavy and light drinkers," *Journal of Abnormal Psychology*, vol. 111, no. 4, pp. 648–658, 2002.

[23] S. T. Tiffany, "A cognitive model of drug urges and drug-use behavior: role of automatic and nonautomatic processes," *Psychological Review*, vol. 97, no. 2, pp. 147–168, 1990.

[24] T. E. Robinson and K. C. Berridge, "Addiction," *Annual Review of Psychology*, vol. 13, pp. 155–162, 2003.

[25] J. G. Pfaus, T. E. Kippin, and S. Centeno, "Conditioning and sexual behavior: a review," *Hormones and Behavior*, vol. 40, no. 2, pp. 291–321, 2001.

[26] F. D. Garcia and F. Thibaut, "Sexual addictions," *American Journal of Drug and Alcohol Abuse*, vol. 36, no. 5, pp. 254–260, 2010.

[27] A. Love, D. James, and P. Willner, "A comparison of two alcohol craving questionnaires," *Addiction*, vol. 93, no. 7, pp. 1091–1102, 1998.

[28] M. J. Bohn, D. D. Krahn, and B. A. Staehler, "Development and initial validation of a measure of drinking urges in abstinent alcoholics," *Alcoholism*, vol. 19, no. 3, pp. 600–606, 1995.

[29] B. D. Sussner, D. A. Smelson, S. Rodrigues, A. Kline, M. Losonczy, and D. Ziedonis, "The validity and reliability of a brief measure of cocaine craving," *Drug and Alcohol Dependence*, vol. 83, no. 3, pp. 233–237, 2006.

[30] S. T. Tiffany, E. Singleton, C. A. Haertzen, and J. E. Henningfield, "The development of a cocaine craving questionnaire," *Drug and Alcohol Dependence*, vol. 34, no. 1, pp. 19–28, 1993.

[31] I. H. A. Franken, V. M. Hendriks, and W. van den Brink, "Initial validation of two opiate craving questionnaires: the Obsessive Compulsive Drug Use Scale and the Desires for Drug Questionnaire," *Addictive Behaviors*, vol. 27, no. 5, pp. 675–685, 2002.

[32] D. James, G. Davies, and P. Willner, "The development and initial validation of a questionnaire to measure craving for amphetamine," *Addiction*, vol. 99, no. 9, pp. 1181–1188, 2004.

[33] A. J. Heinz, D. H. Epstein, J. R. Schroeder, E. G. Singleton, S. J. Heishman, and K. L. Preston, "Heroin and cocaine craving and use during treatment: measurement validation and potential relationships," *Journal of Substance Abuse Treatment*, vol. 31, no. 4, pp. 355–364, 2006.

[34] W. Ooteman, M. W. J. Koeter, R. Vserheul, G. M. Schippers, and W. Van Den Brink, "Measuring craving: an attempt to connect subjective craving with cue reactivity," *Alcoholism*, vol. 30, no. 1, pp. 57–69, 2006.

[35] S. J. Heishman, E. G. Singleton, and A. Liguori, "Marijuana Craving Questionnaire: development and initial validation of a self-report instrument," *Addiction*, vol. 96, no. 7, pp. 1023–1034, 2001.

[36] L. S. Cox, S. T. Tiffany, and A. G. Christen, "Evaluation of the brief questionnaire of smoking urges (QSU-brief) in laboratory and clinical settings," *Nicotine and Tobacco Research*, vol. 3, no. 1, pp. 7–16, 2001.

[37] S. J. Heishman, E. G. Singleton, and E. T. Moolchan, "Tobacco Craving Questionnaire: reliability and validity of a new multifactorial instrument," *Nicotine and Tobacco Research*, vol. 5, no. 5, pp. 645–654, 2003.

[38] P. Di Ciano and B. J. Everitt, "Differential control over drug-seeking behavior by drug-associated conditioned reinforcers and discriminative stimuli predictive of drug availability," *Behavioral Neuroscience*, vol. 117, no. 5, pp. 952–960, 2003.

[39] P. Di Ciano and B. J. Everitt, "Conditioned reinforcing properties of stimuli paired with self-administered cocaine, heroin or sucrose: implications for the persistence of addictive behaviour," *Neuropharmacology*, vol. 47, supplement 1, pp. 202–213, 2004.

[40] B. Goddard and F. Leri, "Reinstatement of conditioned reinforcing properties of cocaine-conditioned stimuli," *Pharmacology Biochemistry and Behavior*, vol. 83, no. 4, pp. 540–546, 2006.

[41] S. L. Grella, A. Levy, A. Campbell et al., "Oxycodone dose-dependently imparts conditioned reinforcing properties to discrete sensory stimuli in rats," *Pharmacological Research*, vol. 64, no. 4, pp. 364–370, 2011.

[42] E. L. Gardner, "What we have learned about addiction from animal models of drug self-administration," *American Journal on Addictions*, vol. 9, no. 4, pp. 285–313, 2000.

[43] S. C. Sigmon, J. W. Tidey, G. J. Badger, and S. T. Higgins, "Acute effects of D-amphetamine on progressive-ratio performance maintained by cigarette smoking and money," *Psychopharmacology*, vol. 167, no. 4, pp. 393–402, 2003.

[44] W. W. Stoops, A. R. Vansickel, J. A. Lile, and C. R. Rush, "Acute d-amphetamine pretreatment does not alter stimulant self-administration in humans," *Pharmacology Biochemistry and Behavior*, vol. 87, no. 1, pp. 20–29, 2007.

[45] D. C. S. Roberts and S. A. L. Bennett, "Heroin self-administration in rats under a progressive ratio schedule of reinforcement," *Psychopharmacology*, vol. 111, no. 2, pp. 215–218, 1993.

[46] M. A. Olson and R. H. Fazio, "Reducing the influence of extrapersonal associations on the implicit association test: personalizing the IAT," *Journal of Personality and Social Psychology*, vol. 86, no. 5, pp. 653–667, 2004.

[47] J. E. S. Swanson, L. A. Rudman, and A. G. Greenwald, "Using the implicit association test to investigate attitude-behaviour consistency for stigmatised behaviour," *Cognition and Emotion*, vol. 15, no. 2, pp. 207–230, 2001.

[48] R. W. Wiers, A. W. Stacy, S. L. Ames et al., "Implicit and explicit alcohol-related cognitions," *Alcoholism*, vol. 26, no. 1, pp. 129–137, 2002.

[49] M. Field, K. Mogg, and B. P. Bradley, "Cognitive bias and drug craving in recreational cannabis users," *Drug and Alcohol Dependence*, vol. 74, no. 1, pp. 105–111, 2004.

[50] K. Houben and R. W. Wiers, "Are drinkers implicitly positive about drinking alcohol? Personalizing the alcohol-IAT to reduce negative extrapersonal contamination," *Alcohol and Alcoholism*, vol. 42, no. 4, pp. 301–307, 2007.

[51] J. De Houwer, R. Custers, and A. De Clercq, "Do smokers have a negative implicit attitude toward smoking?" *Cognition and Emotion*, vol. 20, no. 8, pp. 1274–1284, 2006.

[52] H. E. Ross, D. R. Gavin, and H. A. Skinner, "Diagnostic validity of the MAST and the alcohol dependence scale in the assessment of DSM-III alcohol disorders," *Journal of Studies on Alcohol*, vol. 51, no. 6, pp. 506–513, 1990.

[53] L. C. Sobell, J. Brown, G. I. Leo, and M. B. Sobell, "The reliability of the Alcohol Timeline Followback when administered by telephone and by computer," *Drug and Alcohol Dependence*, vol. 42, no. 1, pp. 49–54, 1996.

[54] A. G. Greenwald, B. A. Nosek, and M. R. Banaji, "Understanding and using the implicit association Test: I. An improved scoring algorithm," *Journal of Personality and Social Psychology*, vol. 85, no. 2, pp. 197–216, 2003.

[55] I. H. Franken, "Drug craving and addiction: integrating psychological and neuropsychopharmacological approaches," *Progress in Neuro-Psychopharmacology & Biological Psychiatry*, vol. 27, pp. 563–579, 2003.

[56] S. J. Moeller, N. Beebe-Wang, P. A. Woicik, A. B. Konova, T. Maloney, and R. Z. Goldstein, "Choice to view cocaine images predicts concurrent and prospective drug use in cocaine addiction," *Drug and Alcohol Dependence*, vol. 130, no. 1–3, pp. 178–185, 2012.

[57] C. P. O'Brien, A. R. Childress, R. Ehrman, and S. J. Robbins, "Conditioning factors in drug abuse: can they explain compulsion?" *Journal of Psychopharmacology*, vol. 12, no. 1, pp. 15–22, 1998.

[58] J. M. Townshend and T. Duka, "Attentional bias associated with alcohol cues: differences between heavy and occasional social drinkers," *Psychopharmacology*, vol. 157, no. 1, pp. 67–74, 2001.

[59] K. M. Stormark, N. P. Field, K. Hugdahl, and M. Horowitz, "Selective processing of visual alcohol cues in abstinent alcoholics: an approach-avoidance conflict?" *Addictive Behaviors*, vol. 22, no. 4, pp. 509–519, 1997.

[60] C. A. Conklin, K. A. Perkins, N. Robin, F. J. McClernon, and R. P. Salkeld, "Bringing the real world into the laboratory: personal smoking and nonsmoking environments," *Drug and Alcohol Dependence*, vol. 111, no. 1-2, pp. 58–63, 2010.

[61] R. E. Meyer and S. M. Mirin, *The Heroin Stimulus, Implications for a Theory of Addiction*, Plenum, New York, NY, USA, 1979.

[62] S. R. Bailey, K. C. Goedeker, and S. T. Tiffany, "The impact of cigarette deprivation and cigarette availability on cue-reactivity in smokers," *Addiction*, vol. 105, no. 2, pp. 364–372, 2010.

[63] D. McBride, S. P. Barrett, J. T. Kelly, A. Aw, and A. Dagher, "Effects of expectancy and abstinence on the neural response to smoking cues in cigarette smokers: an fMRI study," *Neuropsychopharmacology*, vol. 31, no. 12, pp. 2728–2738, 2006.

[64] J. P. De Los Cobos, N. Siñol, J. Trujols, E. Bañuls, F. Batlle, and A. Tejero, "Drug-dependent inpatients reporting continuous absence of spontaneous drug craving for the main substance throughout detoxification treatment," *Drug and Alcohol Review*, vol. 30, no. 4, pp. 403–410, 2011.

[65] J. De Houwer, "A structural and process analysis of the Implicit Association Test," *Journal of Experimental Social Psychology*, vol. 37, no. 6, pp. 443–451, 2001.

[66] K. Houben and R. W. Wiers, "Personalizing the alcohol-IAT with individualized stimuli: relationship with drinking behavior and drinking-related problems," *Addictive Behaviors*, vol. 32, no. 12, pp. 2852–2864, 2007.

[67] L. J. Beckman, "Women alcoholics. A review of social and psychological studies," *Journal of Studies on Alcohol*, vol. 36, no. 7, pp. 797–824, 1975.

[68] R. S. Brienza and M. D. Stein, "Alcohol use disorders in primary care: do gender-specific differences exist?" *Journal of General Internal Medicine*, vol. 17, no. 5, pp. 387–397, 2002.

[69] S. Nolen-Hoeksema, "Gender differences in risk factors and consequences for alcohol use and problems," *Clinical Psychology Review*, vol. 24, no. 8, pp. 981–1010, 2004.

[70] G. De Leon, J. Hawke, N. Jainchill, and G. Melnick, "Therapeutic communities: enhancing retention in treatment using "Senior Professor" staff," *Journal of Substance Abuse Treatment*, vol. 19, no. 4, pp. 375–382, 2000.

[71] Y.-X. Xue, Y.-X. Luo, P. Wu et al., "A memory retrieval-extinction procedure to prevent drug craving and relapse," *Science*, vol. 336, no. 6078, pp. 241–245, 2012.

Association between Acculturation and Binge Drinking among Asian-Americans: Results from the California Health Interview Survey

Monideepa B. Becerra,[1] Patti Herring,[1] Helen Hopp Marshak,[1] and Jim E. Banta[2]

[1] Department of Health Promotion and Education, School of Public Health, Loma Linda University, 24951 North Circle Drive, Loma Linda, CA 92350, USA
[2] Department of Health Policy and Management, School of Public Health, Loma Linda University, 24951 North Circle Drive, Loma Linda, CA 92350, USA

Correspondence should be addressed to Monideepa B. Becerra; mbecerra@llu.edu

Academic Editor: Monica H. Swahn

Objective. Evaluate the association between acculturation and binge drinking among six Asian-American subgroups. *Methods*. A cross-sectional analysis of public access adult portion of 2007, 2009, and 2011/2012 California Health Interview Survey data was conducted. Univariate and multivariable logistic regression analyses were utilized with any binge drinking in the past year as the outcome variable and language spoken at home and time in USA as proxy measures of acculturation. *Results*. A total of 1,631 Asian-Americans ($N = 665,195$) were identified as binge drinkers. Binge drinking was positively associated with being first generation South Asian (OR = 3.05, 95% CI = 1.55, 5.98) and monolingual (English only) Vietnamese (OR = 3.00; 95% CI = 1.58, 5.70), especially among females. Other factors associated with increased binge drinking were being female (Chinese only), not being current married (South Asian only), and being an ever smoker (all subgroups except South Asians). *Conclusion*. First generation South Asians and linguistically acculturated Vietnamese, especially females, are at an increased risk of binge drinking. Future studies and preventive measures should address the cultural basis of such health risk behaviors among Asian-American adults.

1. Background

The Asian-American racial group is comprised of those having origins or immigrated from the Far East, Southeast East, or the Indian Subcontinent, thus consisting of a vast range of nationalities and reflective of a heterogeneous population. According to the US Census Bureau's 2010 Census Brief [1], a total of 10.2 million Asian-Americans (excluding those in combination with other races) were reported in 2000 and increased to 14.7 million by 2010, a 43.3% change. Of the Asian-American subgroups with at least one million responses were Chinese, Filipino, Asian-Indian, Vietnamese, Korean, and Japanese, with Asian-Indians experiencing the largest growth. Current estimates further report that by 2050, Asian-Americans are expected to comprise 9% of the entire

US population, a rise of 4% compared to 2005 [2]. Such trends are indicative of an urgent need for research and health promotion measures to address the needs of a growing population.

The Asian-American population also varies in their socioeconomic status. For example, Asian-Indians are more likely to have a Bachelor's degree or higher compared to those who are Vietnamese. Similarly median household income can vary among Asian-Americans, ranging from $53,887 among Koreans to that of $90,528 among Asian-Indians [3]. Assessment of the National Health Interview Survey 2004–2006 further demonstrated that more than 75% of Japanese, Filipino, and Asian-Indian adults had incomes at or above 200% of the federal poverty level. On the other hand, Vietnamese, Koreans, and Chinese adults are twice as likely as Filipinos to at or below the poverty level [4], further demonstrating the heterogeneity among various Asian-American subgroups.

Similar to the aforementioned heterogeneous characteristics, cardiovascular disease (CVD) risk and behavioral patterns are also diverse among Asian-American subgroups. While the majority of current studies collapse the heterogeneous population into one, a few that have independently evaluated Asian-Americans demonstrated that certain sectors of the population, such as Asian-Indians and Filipinos, are at a greater risk of various CVDs than the general US population [4, 5]. For example, Barnes and colleagues [4] reported that Asian-Indian adults were twice as likely, as compared to Koreans to have ever been told to have heart disease.

Additionally, risk for hospitalization due to ischemic heart disease was significantly higher among Filipinos and South Asians, as compared to the referent group of Chinese adults [5]. Prevalence of type 2 diabetes mellitus, a risk factor for CVD, has also been reported to differ among Asian-Americans [6–9]. For example, diabetes prevalence was shown to be twice as high among Asian-Indians, as compared to Chinese and Japanese adults [4]. Using a nationally representative database, Ye and colleagues [9] also showed that, compared to Whites, Asian-Indians were 130% more likely to have diabetes.Despite such growing trends in the population and associated cardiovascular health outcomes, little research exists on elucidating the various health risk behaviors among the heterogeneous population, especially disaggregated by subgroups. This study examines the association between acculturation and binge drinking among six major Asian-American subgroups utilizing the California Health Interview Survey (CHIS), a population-based survey.

It is imperative to address current binge drinking behaviors as it is associated with significant negative health and socioeconomic consequences, including increased risk of cardiovascular diseases, motor vehicle accidents, violence, homicide, suicide, and loss of productivity [10–17]. Some researchers have suggested that moderate drinking could have cardioprotective effect [18], while others have highlighted that such potential cardioprotective role of moderate drinking could be overestimated due to lack of adequate adjustment for confounders [13]. Regardless of the debate whether light or moderate alcohol consumption can be a cardioprotective factor, several researchers have shown that at-risk drinking (binge or heavy) is associated with increased risk of CVD. Binge drinking is usually defined as 5 or more drinks for men and 4 or more drinks for women per occasion [19]. According to the Centers for Disease Control and Prevention, at least 15% of Americans report binge drinking in the past 30 days and currently 4 million binge drinking episodes occur each day [20]. Reducing binge drinking among US adults is one of the leading objectives of the Healthy People initiative [21] and given the increasing trends in binge drinking [22] and associated health outcomes, understanding the determinants of such behaviors is critical.

In recent years, a plethora of studies have highlighted the role of acculturation, the process by which immigrants adopt the views, attitudes, culture, and ways of the host nation [23, 24], in influencing various health behaviors, including alcohol consumption [25–28]. For example, Akins et al. [25] reported that acculturation was significantly associated with increased binge drinking with acculturated Hispanics reporting twice as much binge drinking as their nonacculturated counterparts. Similarly, high acculturation has been shown to increase drinking behavior among Hispanic women [26]. Zemore [28], in evaluating the 1995 National Alcohol Survey, demonstrated that acculturation was a significant predictor of various alcohol outcomes including drinking versus abstinence and average volume of drinks among drinkers.

The majority of such studies, however, have been conducted among the Hispanic population with limited research among Asian-Americans disaggregated by subgroups. Of the few studies among Asian-American subgroups, results remain limited in generalizability due to samples being limited to adolescent or college students [29–32]. Gomez and colleagues [33] assessed various health outcomes and behaviors among adult Asian-Americans by subgroup (Filipino, Chinese, and Japanese) including that of alcohol consumption. Results demonstrated that having a foreign language preference, thus low acculturation, was associated with lower odds of drinking. Despite highlighting the importance of acculturation, such results lack generalizability due to sample recruitment from a managed care setting and low sample size of some Asian-American subgroups, leading to collapsing such groups as "other Asian." Given the heterogeneity of Asian-Americans it is critical to assess the determinants of such behaviors by distinct subgroup analysis to identify high-risk groups and thus the need for larger population-based studies, as further indicated by the authors themselves. Thus, utilizing CHIS, the largest state population-based survey in the nation, to evaluate the role of acculturation on binge drinking among adult Asian-Americans, disaggregated by subgroups (Chinese, Filipino, South Asian, Japanese, Korean, or Vietnamese), this study not only adds to the current limited body of literature but further highlights high-risk populations in need of health promotion measures.

2. Methods

2.1. Data Source. CHIS is a biennial population-based survey utilizing a random-digit-dial sample, including telephone and cellphones. Starting 2011, CHIS researchers released 2011/2012 combined data for public use. It is conducted in several languages, such as English, Spanish, Cantonese, Mandarin, Korean, and Vietnamese. Adults, who had a California address and telephone number, were at least 18 years of age or older, and completed ≥80% of the questionnaire, were included in the adult CHIS surveys. Those incarcerated, institutionalized, under 18 years of age, or residing in group quarters (dwelling where nine or more unrelated individuals lived together) were excluded. The mean ages of 2007, 2009, and 2001/2012 participants for CHIS were 53.8 years (standard deviation (SD) = 17.3), 55.7 years (SD = 17.3), and 55.1 years (SD = 18.0), respectively.

2.2. Sample. Data from adult respondents (18 years of age or older) who self-reported as one of the six Asian-American subgroups (Chinese, Filipino, South Asian, Japanese, Korean, or Vietnamese) in CHIS surveys were included in the study. This resulted in a total sample (n) of 12,839 participants for a population estimate (N) of 3,407,420 Asian-Americans in California.

2.3. Measures. The outcome variable for the study was any reported binge drinking (yes or no to binge drinking in the past 12 months), created from a CHIS-provided binge drinking variable. CHIS defined binge drinking as 5 or more drinks for men and 4 or more drinks for women per occasion. Due to lack of CHIS questionnaire on volume and types of drinks, further detailed analyses of other alcohol outcomes could not be included.

The exposure variable for this study was the latent construct of acculturation. Given that proxy measures of acculturation in current studies of the Asian-American population are varied, ranging from generation level [34] to country of birth [35], comparison across results remains difficult [36, 37]. To address such a limitation in the literature, this study included two proxies of acculturation: generation level and language spoken at home. Generation level was defined as zero (born outside USA), first (born in USA with both parents born outside USA), and second or more (born in USA and at least one parent born in USA). Language spoken at home was recoded from CHIS-provided variable to English only, English and another language, and a non-English language only. While CHIS assessed language of entertainment and language spoken with friends, such questions were also asked to a subset of the population. Moreover, variables such as language of interview and English language proficiency demonstrated strong multicolinearity with language spoken at home and thus only one was utilized. Similarly, variables such as citizenship status, country of birth, and years in USA had strong multicolinearity with generation level and thus only one was utilized.

Several studies have discussed the "alcohol income puzzle" where moderate and even heavy drinking have been associated with higher wages [38–40], a proxy for higher socioeconomic status. On the other hand, rates of alcohol abuse and associated outcomes have been associated with lower educational attainment [41, 42]. As a result, both education attainment (Bachelor's degree or more versus Associate degree or less) and poverty (at or above 200% federal poverty level versus below 200%) were utilized as covariates in the present study. Federal poverty level (FPL) takes into account both annual household income and size.

Our analyses further included smoking (ever versus never) as a potential covariate. The literature has consistently shown alcohol use and smoking to be strongly correlated, with some demonstrating tobacco use as a predictor of heavy alcohol use [43–45]. Moreover, in both men and women, poor health status has been associated with episodic heavy drinking [46] or frequent binge drinking [47]. Similarly, mental health status has been strongly associated with substance abuse, including alcohol [48, 49]. As a result, health status

(poor versus good) was included in the study. Reporting at least one of the following was defined as poor health status: self-rated general health as poor, at least one chronic disease (diabetes, hypertension, heart disease, and congestive heart failure), Kessler 6-scale score of 13 or more indicating poor mental health [50, 51], and body mass index (BMI) of $23 \, kg/m^2$ or more, based on Asian-American BMI categories [52, 53].

Additionally, demographics, such as age, gender, and marital status, were further included. Finally, given that our study utilized several years of CHIS data, the year was included as a covariate to adjust for potential differences in sample size.

2.4. Statistical Analysis. Descriptive analyses were conducted to determine distribution of sociodemographics and other characteristics of each Asian-American subgroup in the study sample. Next, univariate analyses were performed using survey linear regression for continuous variable of age and Pearson's test, using design-based F values, for categorical variables, to assess if there were statistically significant differences between sociodemographics and other characteristics for Asian-Americans reporting binge drinking in the past 12 months. Multivariable logistic regression analyses were conducted, upon checking for assumptions, independently for each Asian-American subgroup with binge drinking as the dependent variable. Variables included in regression modeling were proxy measures of acculturation (language spoken at home and time in USA) along with covariates of age, gender, education level, poverty level, smoking behavior, health status, and survey year. A jackknife approach was utilized to adequately compute standard errors due to the survey's multistage complex sampling design, as in previous studies [54, 55]. Given that the literature has demonstrated acculturation to be gender specific [56, 57], interactions between each proxy measure of acculturation with gender, education, and poverty were further assessed using separate regression analyses after controlling for covariates. The criterion α for statistical significance was set at 0.05. Bonferroni adjustments were further conducted to reduce probability of type I error during each regression analysis by dividing 0.05 by the total number of independent variables. All statistical analyses were conducted using SAS 9.3 (SAS Institute, Inc., Cary, NC). The study was approved by Loma Linda University Institutional Review Board.

3. Results

3.1. Univariate Analyses. Table 1 demonstrates the sample size, population estimates, sociodemographics, and other characteristics of binge drinkers compared to nonbinge drinkers for each Asian-American subgroup. The largest population estimates of binge drinkers were Filipinos ($N = 246,050$) while the smallest group were Japanese ($N = 42,899$). The mean age was significantly different among each subgroup ($P < 0.0001$), with the youngest binge drinkers being South Asians. Except for gender and marital status, significant differences were further noted for each characteristic across Asian-American subgroups.

3.2. Multivariable Analyses. Table 2 displays the results from multivariable logistic regression analyses with binge drinking as the outcome variable among six independent subgroups. Upon testing assumptions of logistic regression, age was non-linear for several subgroups and thus a polynomial term was utilized. After adjusting for covariates, higher odds of binge drinking were associated with speaking only English at home among Vietnamese and being first generation among South Asians. South Asians reporting being currently unmarried were also more likely to binge drinks. Other characteristics associated with higher odds of binge drinking were being an ever smoker among all Asian-American subgroups except for South Asians. On the other hand, being female was significantly associated with lower binge drinking among Chinese subgroup. For all regression analyses presented in Table 2 Bonferroni adjustment resulted in criterion for $P \leq 0.004$.

Significant interaction was obtained for gender and language spoken at home among Vietnamese subgroup only. While interactions of each acculturation proxy with poverty and education were assessed, no significant results (Bonferroni adjustment criterion of $P \leq 0.003$) were obtained (data not shown). Independent regression analyses, upon adjusting for potential covariates (as in previous models), demonstrated that odds of binge drinking were significantly higher among bilingual Vietnamese females (adjusted odds ratio = 15.24; 95% confidence interval: 4.70, 49.45).

4. Discussion

Currently, much of the empirical evidence on Asian-American health behaviors relies on collapsing the heterogeneous population as one group [30, 38]. By utilizing CHIS, a population-based survey, we were able to provide independent evaluation of six major Asian-American subgroups in California and further evaluate the association between acculturation and binge drinking behavior among such groups.

Our results highlight specific Asian-American subgroups, first generation South Asians, and monolingual (English only) Vietnamese, specifically females, as high-risk of binge drinking. The results from our study are partially consistent with previous studies on acculturation and cardiovascular behaviors. For example, Klonoff and Landrine [58] evaluated the role of acculturation on drinking behavior among African-Americans and demonstrated that abstainers were more likely to be traditional while the more acculturated ones were drinkers. In our study, a similar trend was observed among specific subgroups. Similarly, Zemore [28] also demonstrated that increased acculturation among Mexican-Americans was associated with drinking versus abstinence, though younger age was a higher predictor of frequency of drunkenness. While similar studies among Asian-American adults are limited, some have shown similar results. Gomez and colleagues [33] reported that among Asian-Americans

lower odds of alcohol consumption were associated with a preference for foreign language, thus less acculturated. Similar to our results, the authors also noted that females were less likely to drink while not being currently married was associated with higher odds of drinking, though our results were specific to certain subgroups only.

Our study also showed that acculturation was not a significant predictor of binge drinking behavior among several Asian-American subgroups (Chinese, Filipinos, Japanese, and Koreans). While studies among adult Asian-Americans are limited, results from research among adolescent and college students may provide insight into such results. For example, Hahm et al. [29] noted that social factors, such as best friend's behavior, were a significant predictor of alcohol and tobacco use among Asian-American adolescents. On the other hand, Hendershot and colleagues [30] noted that acculturation was associated with decreased drinking behavior among college students. One of the potential explanations for such inconsistent results could be our disaggregation of Asian-Americans by subgroup thus leading to Simpson's paradox; where acculturation could be associated with drinking among all Asian-Americans collapsed as on group, but such a trend disappears upon subgroup analyses. Moreover, researchers have argued that acculturation can be either protective or negative based on an immigrant's native country [59]. For example, if a behavior, such as binge drinking, is likely to be high in the host nation, an acculturated immigrant is likely to increase such a behavior among immigration, resulting in the healthy immigrant paradox. Such a theory can partially explain the results of this study. For example, current epidemiologic data demonstrate that lifetime abstinence from alcohol is higher in Vietnam and India, immigrants of which nation are the majority of South Asians in the USA, as compared to the USA Thus, as expected immigrants from such nations are more likely to drink in the host nation. However, similar trends among Chinese and Filipinos were not observed, despite China and Philippines having higher abstinence rate than USA Due to significant association with smoking, prospective studies could potentially evaluate whether smoking behavior is a stronger predictor of alcohol consumption among such subgroups. Some studies have demonstrated that genetic variation, particularly the ALDH2*2 allele involved in alcohol metabolism, is diverse among the Asian population, with higher rates noted among Chinese [60]. Partly, the differences in binge drinking rate could be attributed to this. However, researchers have further noted that ethnicity, particularly Korean, is associated with drinking, independent of ALDH2 status [61].

Consistent with the literature on the association between alcohol consumption and cigarette smoking [43, 44, 62, 63], our results also show a strong positive relationship between binge drinking and smoking among Asian-Americans, except for South Asians. The co-occurrence of two addictive behaviors should be a tremendous public health concern due to the negative health outcomes associated with both [64–66]. As a result, both alcohol abuse and tobacco prevention measures must address Asian-Americans with higher rates of both addictive behaviors in order to lower the associated morbidities and mortalities.

TABLE 1: Sociodemographic and other characteristics of Asian American binge drinkers versus nonbinge drinkers by subgroup.

(a)

	Chinese		Filipino		South Asian	
	Binge	Nonbinge	Binge	Nonbinge	Binge	Nonbinge
Total sample size (n)	311	3265	310	1328	163	1189
Average annual population estimate of binge drinkers (N)	130,357	921,453	246,050	654,662	83,462	384,216
Mean age (95% CI)	32.89 (31.12, 34.66)	45.70 (44.84, 46.57)	34.24 (32.20, 36.27)	46.40 (45.27, 47.54)	32.17 (29.94, 34.41)	39.40 (38.44, 40.37)
Female (%)	32.91	56.26	38.98	60.54	32.18	46.09
Currently married (%)	36.76	63.09	42.42	62.00	36.74	74.07
Bachelor's degree or higher (%)	62.11	55.25	39.53	55.30	81.40	76.01
Less than 200% FPL (%)	21.14	31.71	18.68	26.46	11.38	18.07
Language spoken at home (%)						
Non-English only	38.99	44.54	3.71	13.00	5.69	14.37
English and another	42.49	39.46	47.90	52.60	65.16	71.47
English only	18.51	16.00	48.39	34.40	29.15	14.15
Generation level (%)						
Zero	60.92	77.24	49.07	75.44	57.97	88.72
First	31.58	17.31	36.97	17.96	41.17	9.83
Second or more	7.49	5.45	13.96	6.60	0.86	1.44
Ever smoker (%)	30.38	16.38	48.58	23.94	23.14	12.60
Poor health status (%)	36.99	44.03	17.04	24.17	40.59	37.37

(b)

	Japanese		Korean		Vietnamese		P value	
	Binge	Nonbinge	Binge	Nonbinge	Binge	Nonbinge	Binge	Nonbinge
Total sample size (n)	151	1024	391	1907	305	2495		
Average annual population estimate of binge drinkers (N)	42,899	179,492	90,729	249,920	71,700	352,484		
Mean age (95% CI)	41.51 (37.94, 45.09)	57.26 (55.45, 59.08)	36.46 (33.66, 39.26)	46.07 (44.39, 47.75)	32.91 (29.55, 36.27)	45.01 (43.80, 46.22)	0.0002	<.0001
Female (%)	49.98	60.42	51.25	68.95	38.21	53.34	0.1578	<.0001
Currently married (%)	48.11	65.75	47.76	59.50	33.95	64.60	0.3804	.0005
Bachelor's degree or higher (%)	59.77	51.64	55.55	57.33	43.95	28.93	<.0001	<.0001
Less than 200% FPL (%)	16.02	13.29	22.10	35.90	34.86	56.18	0.0205	<.0001
Language spoken at home (%)								
Non-English only	6.54	3.83	36.60	52.06	16.75	52.35	<.0001	<.0001
English and another	28.98	25.12	46.36	37.24	73.81	40.40		
English only	64.48	71.05	17.04	10.70	9.43	7.25		
Generation level (%)								
Zero	32.58	25.72	67.21	81.13	53.01	90.04	<.0001	<.0001
First	7.77	20.28	31.59	17.00	46.67	9.54		
Second or more	59.65	53.99	1.20	1.87	0.32	0.42		
Ever smoker (%)	47.31	30.47	50.74	27.39	52.94	24.36	<.0001	<.0001
Poor health status (%)	33.49	23.98	43.89	42.83	51.48	43.33	<.0001	<.0001

CI: confidence interval; FPL: federal poverty level.

TABLE 2: Multivariable logistic regression odds ratio (and 95% confidence interval) for binge drinking among adult Asian-Americans.

	Chinese	Filipino	South Asian	Japanese	Korean	Vietnamese
Acculturation						
Language spoken at home						
Non-English only (ref.)						
English and another	0.98 (0.55, 1.74)	1.99 (0.83, 4.77)	2.12 (0.85, 5.33)	0.56 (0.19, 1.61)	1.32 (0.58, 2.99)	1.62 (0.51, 5.22)
English only	0.83 (0.52, 1.33)	2.91 (1.21, 6.96)	1.54 (0.72, 3.27)	0.52 (0.17, 1.59)	0.98 (0.59, 1.63)	3.00 (1.58, 5.70)*
Generation level						
Zero (ref.)						
First	0.97 (0.59, 1.60)	1.50 (0.88, 2.55)	3.05 (1.55, 5.98)*	0.35 (0.08, 1.57)	1.70 (0.73, 3.96)	3.34 (0.67, 16.65)
Second or more	1.50 (0.74, 3.05)	2.25 (0.76, 6.68)	0.72 (0.11, 4.60)	0.57 (0.28, 1.16)	0.38 (0.04, 3.64)	0.92 (0.10, 8.68)
Gender						
Male (ref.)						
Female	0.49 (0.33, 0.74)*	0.75 (0.47, 1.20)	0.75 (0.40, 1.41)	0.66 (0.38, 1.16)	0.49 (0.27, 0.90)	0.86 (0.40, 1.84)
Marital status						
Currently married (ref.)						
Not currently married	1.44 (0.83, 2.50)	1.55 (0.96, 2.51)	3.99 (1.95, 8.16)*	2.21 (1.16, 4.22)	1.19 (0.57, 2.51)	1.79 (0.97, 3.30)
Education level						
Associate degree or less (ref.)						
Bachelor's degree or higher	1.46 (0.92, 2.33)	0.70 (0.46, 1.08)	2.05 (0.88, 4.81)	1.64 (0.90, 3.00)	0.65 (0.38, 1.11)	1.94 (1.04, 3.63)
Poverty level						
<200% FPL (ref.)						
≥200% FPL	1.41 (0.82, 2.42)	1.87 (1.14, 3.09)	1.51 (0.69, 3.29)	1.20 (0.50, 2.91)	1.66 (0.89, 3.08)	1.13 (0.60, 2.13)
Health status						
Good (ref.)						
Poor	1.62 (1.00, 2.65)	1.83 (0.99, 3.38)	1.53 (0.90, 2.59)	0.63 (0.32, 1.23)	1.21 (0.70, 2.08)	1.22 (0.70, 2.13)
Smoking status						
Never smoker (ref.)						
Ever smoker	2.86 (1.89, 4.33)*	3.21 (2.05, 5.05)*	1.89 (0.95, 3.75)	4.26 (2.38, 7.64)*	2.70 (1.44, 5.07)*	8.43 (3.73, 19.06)*
Survey year						
2007 (ref.)						
2009	1.77 (1.00, 3.14)	0.96 (0.59, 1.58)	1.31 (0.63, 2.70)	1.16 (0.60, 2.25)	1.16 (0.63, 2.14)	1.06 (0.48, 2.34)
2011/2012	2.13 (1.39, 3.25)*	1.04 (0.71, 1.54)	0.92 (0.47, 1.80)	3.04 (1.52, 6.07)*	0.97 (0.51, 1.83)	1.28 (0.57, 2.87)

FPL: federal poverty level.
* Bonferroni adjustment criterion of $P < 0.004$.

Additionally, Asian-Americans have often been considered a model minority due to socioeconomic achievements and low rates of alcohol consumption [67, 68]. Such a concept, however, has been consistently shown to be a myth based on recent empirical evidence demonstrating the heterogeneity among the population and specific high-risk groups [69–71]. Our study further adds to the literature by highlighting such high-risk Asian-American subgroups (Vietnamese and South Asians) and thus the need for binge drinking preventive measures. Based on our results, an average annual estimate of 665,195 Asian-Americans in California are binge drinkers, with the highest among Filipinos followed by the Chinese. Moreover, a recent study [72] utilizing CHIS 2005 data showed the heterogeneity in various health behaviors among Asian-American subgroups, though South Asians were excluded from such analysis. In our study, an annual population estimate of 83,462 South Asians reported being binge drinkers and given that our results show that first generation South Asians are at an increased risk of binge drinking, the need for further research among such a growing population [73] is imperative.

The results from this study should be interpreted with caution due to certain limitations. The cross-sectional design limits assessment of causality and demands further longitudinal studies. The self-reported data of CHIS is also susceptible to recall and social desirability biases. Moreover, due to lack of questionnaire in all Asian-American languages (especially South Asian languages) those with limited English proficiency are less likely to participate. The South Asian population in this study is also an aggregated group of various nationalities from the Indian Subcontinent. Generally South Asians have national origins from various countries, such as Bangladesh, Bhutan, India, Nepal, Pakistan, and Sri Lanka. As a result, while disaggregation of specific Asian-American subgroups is a critical component of this study, further analysis by specific South Asian groups is necessary. Additionally, other population based surveys, such as Behavioral Risk Factor Surveillance System, assess binge drinking in the past 30 days while starting 2007 the CHIS assessed binge drinking in the past 12 months, making such results difficult to be compared with other population-based surveys. Additionally, due to lack of questions on volume and types of drinks, more rigorous analysis of alcohol consumption behaviors among Asian-American subgroups could not be conducted.

The literature also suggests that current proxy measures of acculturation, including language and generation, may not adequately address all domains of acculturation [74]. Researchers have noted that language may only serve as an indirect measure of acculturation which further includes factors such as values and beliefs [75]. While lack of other domains of acculturation can be a limitation of the study, other researchers [76] have also acknowledged that other factors, such as values, customs, are often embedded in language and thus such a measure can adequately serve as a proxy for acculturation in population-based studies. Since CHIS lacks assessment of such domains, the acculturation proxies utilized in this study may not provide a comprehensive assessment of acculturation among Asian-Americans. Finally, due to the limitation of state samples, results from this study may not be generalizable to Asian-Americans residing outside of California.

Despite such limitations, the present study provides a significant contribution to the literature. CHIS is a population-based survey utilizing random-digit-dial system, thus reducing selection bias. The statistical adjustments in the study, including sample weights, further minimize selection biases and make results generalizable to Asian-Americans in California. Given that, based on Census 2010 [1], California reports 4,861,007 Asian-alone groups, the highest among all other states and Puerto Rico, CHIS provides an ideal scope of evaluation of health behaviors and determinants of such outcomes among the population.

5. Conclusion

The Healthy People 2020 initiative provides science-based, 10-year national benchmarks for improving the health and quality of life for all Americans. An integral component of this national initiative is to improve the nation's cardiovascular health by 20% [77]. This study provides critical empirical evidence of binge drinking, a cardiovascular health risk behavior, among Asian-American subgroups in California. The positive association between acculturation and binge drinking among specific Asian-American subgroups, as demonstrated in this study, can further provide health educators the foundations for setting preventive strategies. Some studies have suggested that traditional view towards alcohol could be a factor associated with drinking behavior. For example, a study [78] noted that while Pakistani young adults (in the UK) maintained similar views against alcohol as their parents', they further recognized that increased levels of drinking among their population are often unrecognized by the community leading to as the authors described "generational dislocation," a potential phenomenon noted in our study with higher binge drinking among first generation South Asians. Moreover, given the importance of acculturation highlighted in this study, further evaluation of the role of such a latent construct on other cardiovascular health behaviors, such as diet, physical activity, and smoking, among Asian-American subgroups, is warranted.

Conflict of Interests

The authors declare no conflict of interests.

Acknowledgments

The authors would like to thank UCLA Center for Health Policy Research and their collaborators for making the California Health Interview Survey publically available. The authors would also like to thank Benjamin Becerra for his editorial and statistical support. This project was partially funded by Center for Health Research Dissertation Award at Loma Linda University.

References

[1] E. M. Hoeffel, S. Rastogi, M. O. Kim, and H. Shahid, *2010 Census*, U.S. Census Bureau, 2012, http://www.census.gov/prod/cen2010/briefs/c2010br-11.pdf.

[2] J. Passel and D. Cohn, *U.S. Population Projections: 2005–2050*, Pew Hispanic Center, 2008, http://www.pewhispanic.org/2008/02/11/us-population-projections-2005-2050/.

[3] L. P. Palaniappan, M. R. G. Araneta, T. L. Assimes et al., "Call to action: cardiovascular disease in Asian Americans: a science advisory from the American Heart Association," *Circulation*, vol. 122, no. 12, pp. 1242–1252, 2010.

[4] P. M. Barnes, P. F. Adams, and E. Powell-Griner, "Health characteristics of the Asian adult population: United States, 2004–2006," *Advance Data*, no. 394, pp. 1–22, 2008.

[5] A. L. Klatsky, I. Tekawa, M. A. Armstrong, and S. Sidney, "The risk of hospitalization for ischemic heart disease among Asian Americans in Northern California," *American Journal of Public Health*, vol. 84, no. 10, pp. 1672–1675, 1994.

[6] E. A. Enas, V. Mohan, M. Deepa, S. Farooq, S. Pazhoor, and H. Chennikkara, "The metabolic syndrome and dyslipidemia among Asian Indians: a population with high rates of diabetes and premature coronary artery disease," *Journal of the Cardiometabolic Syndrome*, vol. 2, no. 4, pp. 267–275, 2007.

[7] J. W. R. Lee, F. L. Brancati, and H.-C. Yeh, "Trends in the prevalence of type 2 diabetes in Asians versus whites: results from the United States National Health Interview Survey, 1997–2008," *Diabetes Care*, vol. 34, no. 2, pp. 353–357, 2011.

[8] R. Oza-Frank, M. K. Ali, V. Vaccarino, and K. M. V. Narayan, "Asian Americans: diabetes prevalence across U.S. and World Health Organization weight classifications," *Diabetes Care*, vol. 32, no. 9, pp. 1644–1646, 2009.

[9] J. Ye, G. Rust, P. Baltrus, and E. Daniels, "Cardiovascular risk factors among Asian Americans: results from a National Health Survey," *Annals of Epidemiology*, vol. 19, no. 10, pp. 718–723, 2009.

[10] S. Malyutina, M. Bobak, S. Kurilovitch et al., "Relation between heavy and binge drinking and all-cause and cardiovascular mortality in Novosibirsk, Russia: a prospective cohort study," *The Lancet*, vol. 360, no. 9344, pp. 1448–1454, 2002.

[11] K. J. Mukamal, M. Maclure, J. E. Muller, and M. A. Mittleman, "Binge drinking and mortality after acute myocardial infarction," *Circulation*, vol. 112, no. 25, pp. 3839–3845, 2005.

[12] M. J. Pletcher, P. Varosy, C. I. Kiefe, C. E. Lewis, S. Sidney, and S. B. Hulley, "Alcohol consumption, binge drinking, and early coronary calcification: findings from the Coronary Artery Risk Development in Young Adults (CARDIA) Study," *American Journal of Epidemiology*, vol. 161, no. 5, pp. 423–433, 2005.

[13] I. B. Puddey and L. J. Beilin, "Alcohol is bad for blood pressure," *Clinical and Experimental Pharmacology and Physiology*, vol. 33, no. 9, pp. 847–852, 2006.

[14] H. Wechsler, A. Davenport, G. Dowdall, B. Moeykens, and S. Castillo, "Health and behavioral consequences of binge drinking in college: a national survey of students at 140 campuses," *The Journal of the American Medical Association*, vol. 272, no. 21, pp. 1672–1677, 1994.

[15] R. D. Brewer and M. H. Swahn, "Binge drinking and violence," *The Journal of the American Medical Association*, vol. 294, no. 5, pp. 616–618, 2005.

[16] M. Schaffer, E. J. Jeglic, and B. Stanley, "The relationship between suicidal behavior, ideation, and binge drinking among college students," *Archives of Suicide Research*, vol. 12, no. 2, pp. 124–132, 2008.

[17] T. S. Naimi, R. D. Brewer, A. Mokdad, C. Denny, M. K. Serdula, and J. S. Marks, "Binge drinking among US adults," *The Journal of the American Medical Association*, vol. 289, no. 1, pp. 70–75, 2003.

[18] R. L. Sacco, M. Elkind, B. Boden-Albala et al., "The protective effect of moderate alcohol consumption on ischemic stroke," *The Journal of the American Medical Association*, vol. 281, no. 1, pp. 53–60, 1999.

[19] National Institute of Alcohol Abuse and Alcoholism, *NIAAA Newsletter*, no. 3, 2004, http://pubs.niaaa.nih.gov/publications/Newsletter/winter2004/Newsletter_Number3.pdf.

[20] CDC, "Excessive Alcohol Use," 2011, http://www.cdc.gov/chronicdisease/resources/publications/aag/alcohol.htm.

[21] US Department of Health and Human Services, "Healthy People 2020. Substance Abuse," 2013, http://www.healthypeople.gov/2020/topicsobjectives2020/objectiveslist.aspx?topicid=40.

[22] T. S. Naimi, R. D. Brewer, A. Mokdad, C. Denny, M. K. Serdula, and J. S. Marks, "Binge drinking among US adults," *The Journal of the American Medical Association*, vol. 289, no. 1, pp. 70–75, 2003.

[23] J. W. Berry, "Conceptual approaches to acculturation," in *Acculturation: Advances in Theory, Measurement and Applied Research*, K. M. Chun, P. Balls, and G. Mar, Eds., pp. 17–37, American Psychological Association, Washington, DC, USA, 2003.

[24] V. S. Castro, *Acculturation and Psychological Adaptation*, Praeger Publishers/Greenwood Publishing Group, Westport, Conn, USA, 2003.

[25] S. Akins, C. Mosher, C. L. Smith, and J. F. Gauthier, "The effect of acculturation on patterns of Hispanic substance use in Washington State," *Journal of Drug Issues*, vol. 38, no. 1, pp. 103–118, 2008.

[26] P. A. C. Vaeth, R. Caetano, and L. A. Rodriguez, "The Hispanic Americans Baseline Alcohol Survey (HABLAS): the association between acculturation, birthplace and alcohol consumption across Hispanic national groups," *Addictive Behaviors*, vol. 37, no. 9, pp. 1029–1037, 2012.

[27] R. Otero-Sabogal, F. Sabogal, E. J. Pérez-Stable, and R. A. Hiatt, "Dietary practices, alcohol consumption, and smoking behavior: ethnic, sex, and acculturation differences," *Journal of the National Cancer Institute. Monographs*, no. 18, pp. 73–82, 1995.

[28] S. E. Zemore, "Acculturation and alcohol among Latino adults in the United States: a comprehensive review," *Alcoholism: Clinical and Experimental Research*, vol. 31, no. 12, pp. 1968–1990, 2007.

[29] H. C. Hahm, M. Lahiff, and N. B. Guterman, "Asian American adolescents' acculturation, binge drinking, and alcohol- and tobacco-using peers," *Journal of Community Psychology*, vol. 32, no. 3, pp. 295–308, 2004.

[30] C. S. Hendershot, T. M. Dillworth, C. Neighbors, and W. H. George, "Differential effects of acculturation on drinking behavior in Chinese- and Korean-American college students," *Journal of Studies on Alcohol and Drugs*, vol. 69, no. 1, pp. 121–128, 2008.

[31] C. Lum, H. L. Corliss, V. M. Mays, S. D. Cochran, and C. K. Lui, "Differences in the drinking behaviors of Chinese, Filipino, Korean, and Vietnamese college students," *Journal of Studies on Alcohol and Drugs*, vol. 70, no. 4, pp. 568–574, 2009.

[32] D. Iwamoto, S. Takamatsu, and J. Castellanos, "Binge drinking and alcohol-related problems among U.S.-born Asian Americans," *Cultural Diversity & Ethnic Minority Psychology*, vol. 18, no. 3, pp. 219–227, 2012.

[33] S. L. Gomez, J. L. Kelsey, S. L. Glaser, M. M. Lee, and S. Sidney, "Immigration and acculturation in relation to health and health-related risk factors among specific Asian subgroups in a health maintenance organization," *American Journal of Public Health*, vol. 94, no. 11, pp. 1977–1984, 2004.

[34] N. R. Ghai, S. J. Jacobsen, S. K. van den Eeden et al., "A comparison of lifestyle and behavioral cardiovascular disease risk factors between Asian Indian and White non-Hispanic men," *Ethnicity & Disease*, vol. 22, no. 2, pp. 168–174, 2012.

[35] D. H. Chae, A. R. Gavin, and D. T. Takeuchi, "Smoking prevalence among Asian Americans: findings from the National Latino and Asian American Study (NLAAS)," *Public Health Reports*, vol. 121, no. 6, pp. 755–763, 2006.

[36] T. Salant and D. S. Lauderdale, "Measuring culture: a critical review of acculturation and health in Asian immigrant populations," *Social Science and Medicine*, vol. 57, no. 1, pp. 71–90, 2003.

[37] L. P. Palaniappan, M. R. G. Araneta, T. L. Assimes et al., "Call to action: cardiovascular disease in Asian Americans: a science advisory from the American Heart Association," *Circulation*, vol. 122, no. 12, pp. 1242–1252, 2010.

[38] M. T. French, "Is moderate alcohol use related to wages? Evidence from four worksites," *Journal of Health Economics*, vol. 14, no. 3, pp. 319–344, 1995.

[39] D. M. Heien, "Do drinkers earn less?" *Southern Economic Journal*, vol. 63, no. 1, pp. 60–68, 1996.

[40] M. C. Berger and J. P. Leigh, "The effect of alcohol use on wages," *Applied Economics*, vol. 20, no. 10, pp. 1343–1351, 1988.

[41] R. M. Crum, J. E. Helzer, and J. C. Anthony, "Level of education and alcohol abuse and dependence in adulthood: a further inquiry," *American Journal of Public Health*, vol. 83, no. 6, pp. 830–837, 1993.

[42] R. M. Crum and J. C. Anthony, "Educational level and risk for alcohol abuse and dependence: differences by race-ethnicity," *Ethnicity and Disease*, vol. 10, no. 1, pp. 39–52, 2000.

[43] T. J. Craig and P. A. van Natta, "The association of smoking and drinking habits in a community sample," *Journal of Studies on Alcohol*, vol. 38, no. 7, pp. 1434–1439, 1977.

[44] M. K. Jensen, T. I. A. Sørensen, A. T. Andersen et al., "A prospective study of the association between smoking and later alcohol drinking in the general population," *Addiction*, vol. 98, no. 3, pp. 355–363, 2003.

[45] C. S. Morgen, K. B. Bové, K. S. Larsen, S. K. Kjaer, and M. Grønbaek, "Association between smoking and the risk of heavy drinking among young women: a prospective study," *Alcohol and Alcoholism*, vol. 43, no. 3, pp. 371–375, 2008.

[46] I. S. Okosun, J. P. Seale, J. B. Daniel, and M. P. Eriksen, "Poor health is associated with episodic heavy alcohol use: evidence from a National Survey," *Public Health*, vol. 119, no. 6, pp. 509–517, 2005.

[47] J. L. Valencia-Martín, I. Galán, and F. Rodríguez-Artalejo, "Alcohol and self-rated health in a Mediterranean country: the role of average volume, drinking pattern, and alcohol dependence," *Alcoholism: Clinical and Experimental Research*, vol. 33, no. 2, pp. 240–246, 2009.

[48] D. A. Regier, M. E. Farmer, D. S. Rae et al., "Comorbidity of mental disorders with alcohol and other drug abuse. Results from the epidemiologic catchment area (ECA) study," *The Journal of the American Medical Association*, vol. 264, no. 19, pp. 2511–2518, 1990.

[49] T. Weaver, P. Madden, V. Charles et al., "Comorbidity of substance misuse and mental illness in community mental health and substance misuse services," *British Journal of Psychiatry*, vol. 183, no. 4, pp. 304–313, 2003.

[50] R. C. Kessler, G. Andrews, L. J. Colpe et al., "Short screening scales to monitor population prevalences and trends in non-specific psychological distress," *Psychological Medicine*, vol. 32, no. 6, pp. 959–976, 2002.

[51] R. C. Kessler, O. Demler, R. G. Frank et al., "Prevalence and treatment of mental disorders, 1990 to 2003," *The New England Journal of Medicine*, vol. 352, no. 24, pp. 2515–2523, 2005.

[52] F. F. Samaha, "New international measuring stick for defining obesity in non-Europeans," *Circulation*, vol. 115, no. 16, pp. 2089–2090, 2007.

[53] WHO Expert Consultation, "Appropriate body-mass index for Asian populations and its implications for policy and intervention strategies," *The Lancet*, vol. 363, no. 9403, pp. 157–163, 2004.

[54] J. E. Banta, S. James, M. G. Haviland, and R. M. Andersen, "Race/ethnicity, parent-identified emotional difficulties, and mental health visits among California children," *The Journal of Behavioral Health Services & Research*, vol. 40, no. 1, pp. 5–19, 2013.

[55] J. E. Banta, P. Przekop, M. G. Haviland, and M. Pereau, "Binge drinking among California adults: results from the 2005 California health interview survey," *American Journal of Drug and Alcohol Abuse*, vol. 34, no. 6, pp. 801–809, 2008.

[56] M. L. Alaniz, A. J. Treno, and R. F. Saltz, "Gender, acculturation, and alcohol consumption among Mexican Americans," *Substance Use & Misuse*, vol. 34, no. 10, pp. 1407–1426, 1999.

[57] L. Lopez-Gonzalez, V. C. Aravena, and R. A. Hummer, "Immigrant acculturation, gender and health behavior: a research note," *Social Forces*, vol. 84, no. 1, pp. 581–593, 2005.

[58] E. A. Klonoff and H. Landrine, "Acculturation and alcohol use among Blacks: the benefits of remaining culturally traditional," *The Western Journal of Black Studies*, vol. 23, no. 4, pp. 211–216, 1999.

[59] A. F. Abraído-Lanza, M. T. Chao, and K. R. Flórez, "Do healthy behaviors decline with greater acculturation?: implications for the Latino mortality paradox," *Social Science and Medicine*, vol. 61, no. 6, pp. 1243–1255, 2005.

[60] T. L. Wall, "Genetic associations of alcohol and aldehyde dehydrogenase with alcohol dependence and their mechanisms of action," *Therapeutic Drug Monitoring*, vol. 27, no. 6, pp. 700–703, 2005.

[61] S. E. Luczak, T. L. Wall, S. H. Shea, S. M. Byun, and L. G. Carr, "Binge drinking in Chinese, Korean, and White college students: genetic and ethnic group differences," *Psychology of Addictive Behaviors*, vol. 15, no. 4, pp. 306–309, 2001.

[62] A. C. King and A. M. Epstein, "Alcohol dose-dependent increases in smoking urge in light smokers," *Alcoholism: Clinical and Experimental Research*, vol. 29, no. 4, pp. 547–552, 2005.

[63] M. B. Reed, R. Wang, A. M. Shillington, J. D. Clapp, and J. E. Lange, "The relationship between alcohol use and cigarette smoking in a sample of undergraduate college students," *Addictive Behaviors*, vol. 32, no. 3, pp. 449–464, 2007.

[64] J. M. Elwood, J. C. G. Pearson, D. H. Skippen, and S. M. Jackson, "Alcohol, smoking, social and occupational factors in the aetiology of cancer of the oral cavity, pharynx and larynx," *International Journal of Cancer*, vol. 34, no. 5, pp. 603–612, 1984.

[65] S. J. Smith, J. M. Deacon, C. E. D. Chilvers et al., "Alcohol, smoking, passive smoking and caffeine in relation to breast cancer risk in young women. UK National Case-Control Study Group," *British Journal of Cancer*, vol. 70, no. 1, pp. 112–119, 1994.

[66] W. J. Blot, J. K. McLaughlin, D. M. Winn et al., "Smoking and drinking in relation to oral and pharyngeal cancer," *Cancer Research*, vol. 48, no. 11, pp. 3282–3287, 1988.

[67] R. Caetano, C. L. Clark, and T. Tam, "Alcohol consumption among racial/ethnic minorities: theory and research," *Alcohol Health and Research World*, vol. 22, no. 4, pp. 233–238, 1998.

[68] K.-Y. Lee and S.-H. Joo, "The portrayal of Asian Americans in mainstream magazine ads: an update," *Journalism and Mass Communication Quarterly*, vol. 82, no. 3, pp. 654–671, 2005.

[69] M. M. Chao, C.-Y. Chiu, and J. S. Lee, "Asians as the model minority: implications for US Government's policies," *Asian Journal of Social Psychology*, vol. 13, no. 1, pp. 44–52, 2010.

[70] T. Yu, "Challenging the politics of the "model minority" stereotype: a case for educational equality," *Equity & Excellence in Education*, vol. 39, no. 4, pp. 325–333, 2006.

[71] S. Sue, D. W. Sue, L. Sue, and D. T. Takeuchi, "Psychopathology among Asian Americans: a model minority?" *Cultural Diversity and Mental Health*, vol. 1, no. 1, pp. 39–51, 1995.

[72] A. E. Maxwell, C. M. Crespi, R. E. Alano, M. Sudan, and R. Bastani, "Health risk behaviors among five Asian American subgroups in California: identifying intervention priorities," *Journal of Immigrant and Minority Health*, vol. 14, no. 5, pp. 890–894, 2012.

[73] SAALT, "About the South Asian Community," 2012, http://saalt.org/pages/About-the-South-Asian-Community.html.

[74] J. W. Berry, "Immigration, acculturation, and adaptation," *Applied Psychology*, vol. 46, no. 1, pp. 5–34, 1997.

[75] L. J. Cabassa, "Measuring acculturation: where we are and where we need to go," *Hispanic Journal of Behavioral Sciences*, vol. 25, no. 2, pp. 127–146, 2003.

[76] W. A. Vega and A. G. Gil, *Drug Use and Ethnicity in Early Adolescence*, Springer, New York, NY, USA, 1998.

[77] Healthy People 2020, "Heart Disease and Stroke—Healthy People," 2012, http://www.healthypeople.gov/2020/topicsobjectives2020/objectiveslist.aspx?topicId=21.

[78] D. Heim, S. C. Hunter, A. J. Ross et al., "Alcohol consumption, perceptions of community responses and attitudes to service provision: results from a survey of Indian, Chinese and Pakistani young people in Greater Glasgow, Scotland, UK," *Alcohol and Alcoholism*, vol. 39, no. 3, pp. 220–226, 2004.

5

Receipt of Prescribed Controlled Substances by Adolescents and Young Adults Prior to Presenting for Opiate Dependence Treatment

Steven C. Matson,[1,2] Cathleen Bentley,[3] Vicki Hughes Dughman,[3] and Andrea E. Bonny[1,2]

[1] Department of Pediatrics, The Ohio State University College of Medicine, Columbus, OH, USA
[2] Division of Adolescent Medicine, Nationwide Children's Hospital, 700 Children's Drive,
  G353 Timken Hall, Columbus, OH 43205-2664, USA
[3] Department of Clinical Services and Care Coordination, Nationwide Children's Hospital, Columbus, OH, USA

Correspondence should be addressed to Steven C. Matson; steven.matson@nationwidechildrens.org

Academic Editor: James Zacny

Purpose. The objective of this study was to document the number of controlled substance prescriptions filled by adolescents and young adult patients in the 2 years prior to presentation for opiate dependence treatment. *Methods.* Opiate-dependent youth ($N = 125$) presenting to our Medication-Assisted Treatment for Addiction program from January 1, 2008 to June 30, 2010 were identified via electronic medical record. Subjects were further classified based on their opiate use as dependent to heroin-only, prescription (Rx) opiate-only, or combined heroin + Rx opiate only. The Ohio Automated Rx Reporting System (OARRS) was used to identify each subject's controlled substance prescription history. Negative binomial regression was used to examine the relationships between patient characteristics and the total number of prescriptions filled. *Results.* Twenty-five percent of subjects had filled ≥ 6 prescriptions, and 15% had filled ≥ 11 prescriptions. The mean number of prescriptions filled was 5 (range: 0–59). Thirteen percent had filled ≥ 6 opiate/narcotic prescriptions, and 8% had filled ≥ 11 prescriptions. *Conclusions.* A subset of opiate-dependent youth had filled multiple opiate/narcotic prescriptions providing some evidence that physician-provided prescriptions may be a source of opiate abuse or diversion for a minority of opiate-dependent adolescents and young adults.

1. Introduction

The nonmedical use of Rx opiates and other controlled drugs by adolescents and young adults has surpassed all illicit drugs except marijuana [1]. A recent report found that, for youth, the peak risk in nonmedical use of prescription pain relievers occurred at the age of 16 years, not during the postsecondary school years as previously suspected [2]. According to the Monitoring the Future Study, the nonmedical use of several prescription medications by 12th graders in the United States is at its highest level in the past 15 years [3].

Concurrently, prescriptions by healthcare providers for controlled substances have also increased. A recent review of over 2.3 million visits by adolescents and young adults found that controlled medications were prescribed for an increasing proportion of adolescent (6.4 versus 11.2%) and young adult visits (8.3 versus 16.1%) between 1994 and 2007, respectively [4]. McCabe et al. found that the estimated prevalence of lifetime medical use of prescription opioids among US high school seniors was 17.6% while the estimated prevalence of lifetime nonmedical use was 12.9% [5]. McCabe has also demonstrated that the prevalence of medical misuse of controlled medication classes (pain, stimulant, sleeping, and anxiety) in adolescents was 18% and was higher among female versus male adolescents (20.8% versus 15.1%). Finally, medical misusers of controlled medications had a higher prevalence of all substance use and abuse behaviors than medical users who took their medications appropriately [6].

The precise role that legitimate prescriptions play in adolescent and young adult opiate dependence is not known. This study was specifically interested in examining the quantity of controlled medications prescribed by healthcare providers and filled by adolescents and young adults who later presented for opiate dependence treatment. The objective of this study was to document, utilizing a statewide database, the number of controlled substance prescriptions that adolescent and young adult patients filled in the two years prior to presentation for opiate dependence treatment.

2. Methods

2.1. Subjects. The study sample consisted of all adolescents and young adults, aged from 15 to 21 years, who presented to our Medication-Assisted Treatment for Addiction (MATA) clinic for outpatient treatment of opiate dependence from January 1, 2008 to June 30, 2010. The insurance mix of our MATA clinic is private insurance 35%, Medicaid 49%, and uninsured 16%. Although the General Adolescent Clinic which runs out of the same location sees a racially diverse patient population, patients who have presented to the MATA clinic to date have been predominantly Caucasian. Reasons for this are not entirely known but seem to reflect the demographics of the opiate-dependent population in our community. Data were extracted from the institution's electronic medical records database. There were no exclusionary criteria applied to the overall patient cohort except presentation to the MATA clinic for treatment of opiate dependence during the study period. The study protocol was reviewed and approved by the Institutional Review Board of the participating institution.

2.2. Data Collection. At each patient's initial visit to the MATA clinic a diagnosis of opiate dependence was confirmed using DSM IV-R criteria [7]. We then reviewed each subject's initial visit to the MATA clinic and obtained information on specific opiates used, gender, and age. Subjects were further classified based on their opiates use as (a) heroin-only dependent, (b) prescription (Rx) opiate-only dependent, or (c) combined heroin + Rx opiate dependent.

As part of routine care in the MATA clinic, a patient's controlled substance prescription history for the two years prior to their intake visit was obtained utilizing the Ohio Automated Rx Reporting System (OARRS). The OARRS Prescription History Report provides information on the number and type of prescriptions for controlled substances filled by a patient during a specific time period. OARRS was established in 2006 as a tool to assist healthcare professionals in providing better treatment for patients with medical needs while quickly identifying drug seeking behaviors. Reports include all controlled substance prescriptions that were filled back until 2008 when complete reporting was available. Information includes the name of medications, the number of pills/capsules/films delivered, the prescribing physician, and the pharmacy that filled the prescription. An OARRS Prescription History Report can assist in assuring that a patient is getting the appropriate drug therapy and is taking medication as prescribed.

We reviewed the OARRS Prescription History Report obtained on each subject at initial visit and collected the following information: (1) total number of prescriptions for controlled substances filled in the two years prior to presentation; (2) total number of pills for controlled substances obtained during the two years prior to presentation; and (3) specific type of controlled substances filled. Controlled substances filled by each subject were further categorized as belonging to one of the four following classes: (1) opiate/narcotic, (2) other analgesic (e.g., tramadol), (3) benzodiazepine, or (4) stimulant. We considered excluding stimulants from our data analyses since our clinical experience indicates that regular prescriptions for this class of medications are more common than for the other drug classes. However, we opted to keep stimulants in the analyses for the following reasons: (1) indications for receipt of controlled substance prescription were not known for any drug class, as such, speculation as to the indications of a prescription, stimulant or not, was not warranted; (2) a full picture of the controlled substances filled by our patients prior to presenting for opiate dependence treatment was desired; and (3) associations between stimulant prescriptions with gender and age were distinct from those seen for other drug classes and, hence, provided a meaningful contrast for interpretation of our study results.

2.3. Data Analysis. Data analysis was conducted using SAS statistical software, version 6.12 (SAS Institute Inc., Cary, NC, USA). The main outcome measure was the total number of prescriptions for controlled substances filled in the two years prior to presentation to the MATA clinic. Secondary outcomes examined included the total number of pills for controlled substances filled in the two years prior to presentation and receipt of drugs from specific drug classes.

Descriptive statistics included means, standard deviations, and range for continuous variables and percentages and counts for categorical variables. As appropriate for count data, negative binomial regression was used to examine the relationships between subject characteristics with the total number of prescriptions, total number of pills, and receipt of prescriptions from specific drug classes. The negative binomial dispersion parameter was estimated by maximum likelihood. Total number of prescriptions and total number of pills were highly correlated and as such demonstrated identical associations. Since the total number of prescriptions filled was our primary outcome of interest, final analyses focused on this outcome. Backward elimination negative binomial regression was used to build our final multivariate model. Eligible covariates for the multivariate model included gender, age, and type of opiate dependence.

3. Results

A total of 125 adolescents and young adults presented to the MATA clinic for treatment of opiate dependence from January 1, 2008 to June 30, 2010. The mean age of the study subjects was 18.5 ± 1.5 years. All subjects were Caucasian,

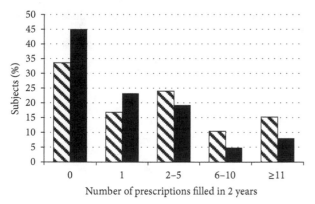

FIGURE 1: Distribution of total number of prescriptions for all controlled medications and opiate/narcotics filled in the 2 years prior to presentation for outpatient medication-assisted treatment for opioid dependence.

and 59% were female. Forty-two percent of subjects were identified as heroin-only dependent, 37% as Rx opiate-only dependent, and 22% as combined heroin + Rx opiate dependent. Mean age and gender distribution were similar for all three opiate-dependent groups: heroin-only dependent (mean age 18.5 (±1.3); 60% female); Rx-opiate only dependent (mean age 18.5 (±1.7); 57% female); and combined heroin + Rx opiate dependent (mean age 18.5 (±1.4); 63% female).

Two out of three patients had filled at least one prescription for controlled substances in the 2 years prior to intake, 25% had filled ≥6 prescriptions, and 15% had filled ≥11 prescriptions (Figure 1). The mean number of prescriptions filled was 5.3 (range: 0–59). The average number of pills or capsules dispensed was 194 pills (range: 0–2269). Examination of specific drug classes found that 54% of the subjects had filled a prescription for an opiate/narcotic, 13% had filled ≥6 opiate/narcotic prescriptions, and 8% had filled ≥11 prescriptions (Figure 1). Among opiate/narcotic prescriptions, specific medications prescribed to our study sample were as follows: hydrocodone/acetaminophen (43% of subjects); oxycodone (19% of subjects); codeine/acetaminophen (17% of subjects); codeine/cough formulation (3% of subjects); and meperidine (2% of subjects). Twenty-five percent of subjects filled a prescription for an analgesic, 18% for a benzodiazepine, and 13% for a stimulant.

In bivariate analyses, gender, age, and type of opiate dependence were all significantly associated with total number of prescriptions filled. Females filled on average 6.9 prescriptions versus 3.0 for males (P = 0.006). Subjects with Rx opiates-only dependence filled on average 8.7 prescriptions as compared to 3.3 for subjects with heroin-only dependence (P = 0.002) and 3.4 for subjects with heroin + Rx opiate dependence (P = 0.02). Increasing age was associated with a higher total number of prescriptions filled (maximum likelihood parameter estimate = 0.214; P = 0.02). In multivariate modeling, gender and type of opiate

dependence remained independently associated with total number of prescriptions filled (Table 1).

Examination of prescriptions by specific drug classes showed some differences across gender, type of opiate dependence, and age (Table 2). Females were significantly more likely than males to have filled a prescription for benzodiazepines 24% versus 10%, respectively (P = 0.04). Although not statistically significant, filled opiate prescriptions were more common among subjects with Rx opiate-only dependence. Sixty-seven percent of patients with Rx opiate-only dependence had filled an opiate prescription, as compared to 46% of those with heroin-only dependence and 48% of those with combined heroin + Rx opiate dependence (P = 0.08). Mean age was significantly higher among patients who had filled an opiate (P = 0.004) or other analgesic (P = 0.001) prescription as compared to those who had not. In contrast, mean age was significantly lower for those who had filled a stimulant prescription as compared to those who had not (P = 0.001).

4. Discussion

This study found that the majority of adolescents and young adults presenting for opiate dependence treatment had filled at least one prescription for controlled medications in the preceding two years. Fifty-four percent had filled at least 1 prescription for opiate/narcotics. This percent is higher than that reported among the general adolescent and young adult population [4, 5]. Thirteen percent of our subjects had filled ≥6 prescriptions for opiate/narcotics in the two years prior to presentation. The high number of prescriptions filled by this subset of subjects suggests that physician-provided prescriptions may be a source of abuse or diversion for this subset of these opiate-dependent youths.

We have noted three distinct opiate-dependent subtypes in our treatment program: patients dependent on Rx opiates only, those dependent on heroin only, and those dependent on both. Among these opiate-dependent subtypes, we found variation in both the total number of filled prescriptions for controlled substances and the number of filled prescriptions from specific drug classes. Subjects with heroin-only dependence and those with both heroin + Rx opiate dependence showed a similar profile which was distinct from subjects with Rx opiates-only dependence. Those with Rx opiates-only dependence filled almost three times as many prescriptions for controlled substances as compared to the other two groups. Opiate prescriptions accounted for the largest difference in total number of prescriptions among these three groups.

Among our study subjects, females filled on average twice as many prescriptions for controlled substances as compared to males. Similarly, McCabe et al. found that females were more likely to have filled a prescription for a controlled medication as compared to male adolescents (56.4% versus 40.2%; P ≤ 0.001) [8]. Females are also significantly more likely than males to report nonmedical use of pain medication (22.2% versus 12.3%) [3]. The reasons behind these gender differences are not entirely clear. They

TABLE 1: Multivariate[a] negative binomial regression predicting the total number of prescriptions for controlled substances filled in the 2 years prior to presenting for outpatient medication-assisted treatment for opiate dependence.

Parameter	Parameter estimate[b]	95% confidence interval		P value
Intercept	1.638	1.053	2.224	<0.0001
Type of opiate dependence				
Heroin only	−0.900	−1.522	−0.278	0.005
Heroin + Rx opiate	−0.866	−1.613	−0.119	0.023
Rx opiate only	Reference	—	—	
Gender				
Female	0.711	0.143	1.278	0.014
Male	Reference	—	—	
Dispersion	2.204	1.627	2.986	

[a] Eligible covariates included age, gender, and type of opiate dependence.

[b] The negative binominal dispersion parameter was estimated by maximum likelihood.

TABLE 2: Likelihood of filling prescriptions for specific drug classes by gender, type of opiate dependence, and age.

Characteristic	Opiate	Other analgesic	Benzodiazepine	Stimulant
Gender:				
% of females who filled each drug class	58.1	29.7	24.3[a]	10.8
% of males who filled each drug class	49.0	17.6	9.8[a]	15.7
Type of opiate dependence:				
% of Rx opiate-only dependents who filled each drug class	67.4	21.7	23.9	17.4
% of heroin + Rx opiate dependents who filled each drug class	48.2	37.0	18.5	3.7
% of heroin-only dependents who filled each drug class	46.2	21.2	13.5	13.5
Mean age by receipt of specific drug class:				
Yes	18.8[b]	19.3[b]	18.9	17.2[b]
No	18.1[b]	18.2[b]	18.4	18.7[b]

[a] Comparison significant at $P < 0.05$.

[b] Comparison significant at $P < 0.01$.

could represent differences in patient behavior such as female adolescents asking for controlled substances with higher frequency or communicating symptoms in a distinct manner. In addition, they could represent provider differences in their approach to male and female patients.

Limitations of our current study include lack of racial diversity in our study sample and lack of information on receipt of controlled medications for nonmedical use from other sources such as peers. In addition, concurrent information on the number of prescriptions for controlled substances filled by adolescents without a diagnosis of substance abuse or dependence is not available. However, based on previously published data we expect that the past-year medical use of controlled medications by adolescents by medication class is as follows: 14.2% for pain medication, 2.2% for antianxiety medication, 1.6% for sleeping medication, and 3.5% for stimulant medication [6]. We also do not know the reasons why controlled medications were prescribed and filled by our subjects. Our clinical experience suggests that indications for opiates, other analgesics, and benzodiazepines in a general adolescent population are limited, and, except for the rare patient, multiple prescriptions for these controlled medications are not generally warranted. Regular prescriptions for stimulants, on the other hand, may in fact be indicated for some adolescent patients, and we considered removing stimulants from the current analyses. However, to get a complete picture of the controlled medications provided to our adolescent opiate-dependent patients, we opted to retain stimulants in our analyses. Interestingly, stimulants demonstrated a different relationship with both gender and age as compared to the other drug classes. Since stimulants were more prevalent in males and younger subjects, their effect on our final multivariate model would be to minimize the effect of female gender and increasing age on total number of prescriptions filled. Finally, information on concurrent psychiatric or substance abuse diagnoses was not documented on study subjects. This information will be included on future prospective data collection and subsequent reports.

Despite these limitations, our study has certain specific strengths. Very little is known about adolescent opiate-dependent patients. Prior research has primarily focused on Rx opiate use among a general adolescent population. Our study uniquely focuses on a population of adolescents with a diagnosis of opiate dependence. In addition, to our knowledge, our study is the first to utilize a state-automated prescription reporting database for documentation of prescriptions filled by an opiate-dependent population. We cannot know for certain what role filled prescriptions for controlled medications played in our study population. These prescriptions could have been for legitimate medical indications, nonmedical use (abuse), or diversion. However the small subset of subjects in our study who filled multiple prescriptions is concerning. It is possible that for this subset of subjects prescriptions were abused or diverted. McCabe et al. found that among youth receiving a controlled medication approximately 13.8% had ever sold, traded, loaned, or given away their medications [9]. The prevalence of substance use and abuse was significantly higher among prescribed users of controlled medications who had diverted their medications compared to their peers. Further research is needed to better understand the nature of use of prescribed medications among opiate-dependent youth.

Prescription surveillance systems like OARRS can be effectively utilized to better understand patterns of prescriptions of controlled substances among a dependent population and to identify "high volume" patients and providers. We found that a subset of our subjects had filled multiple prescriptions for controlled substances. Similarly, previous researchers found that 3% of physicians accounted for 62% of the narcotics prescribed in one study [10]. Since 1993 federal legislation has supported the formation of state-based prescription drug monitoring programs (PDMPs). To date, 42 states have operational PDMPs, and 6 have enacted legislation to develop programs. Both medical providers and patients would benefit from early identification of nonmedical prescription drug use and intervention prior to the problem escalating. Physicians should screen all adolescents or young adults for nonmedical use whenever prescribing a controlled medication including obtaining a controlled prescription report in states where available. Next steps should include identification of characteristics associated with transitioning from proper use of controlled medications to abuse and ultimate dependence. PDMPs like OARRS could possibly be utilized in the future to identify points at which individuals transition from proper use to abuse.

5. Implications and Contributions

The nonmedical use of prescription opiates by adolescents and young adults has surpassed all illicit drugs except marijuana. The exact contribution of prescribed medications to the development of opiate dependence is not clear. Our findings provide some evidence that physician-provided prescriptions may be a source of abuse or diversion in a subset of opiate-dependent youth.

Abbreviations

MATA: Medication-assisted treatment for addiction
OARRS: The Ohio automated Rx reporting system
Rx: Prescription
PDMP: Prescription drug monitoring program.

Conflict of Interests

The authors declare they have no conflict of interests.

Authors' Contribution

Drs. S. C. Matson and A. E. Bonny had full access to all the data in the study and take responsibility for the integrity of the data and the accuracy of the data analysis; Dr. S. C. Matson, Ms. C. Bentley, and Ms. V. H. Dughman contributed to study concept and design; Ms. C. Bentley and Ms. V. H. Dughman contributed to acquisition of data; Dr. A. E. Bonny performed the statistical analyses; Drs. S. C. Matson and A. E. Bonny contributed to interpretation of data and drafting of the paper; all authors contributed to critical revision of the paper for important intellectual content.

Acknowledgments

The authors thank Sarah Higgins for her assistance with paper preparation. This paper was a poster presentation at the Annual Meeting of the American Society for Addiction Medicine, Washington, DC, USA, April 2011.

References

[1] Substance Abuse and Mental Health Services Administration, *Results From the 2010 National Survey on Drug Use and Health: Summary of National Findings*, NSDUH Series H-41, HHS Publication (SMA) 11-4658, Substance Abuse and Mental Health Services Administration, Rockville, Md, USA,

[2] E. A. Meier, J. P. Troost, and J. C. Anthony, "Extramedical use of prescription pain relievers by youth aged 12 to 21 years in the United States: national estimates by age and by year," *Archives of Pediatrics & Adolescent Medicine*, vol. 166, no. 9, pp. 803–807, 2012.

[3] L. Johnston, P. O'Malley, J. Bachman et al., *Monitoring the Future National Results on Adolescent Drug Use: Overview of Key Findings*, The University of Michigan, Institute for Social Research, Ann Arbor, Mich, USA.

[4] R. J. Fortuna, B. W. Robbins, E. Caiola, M. Joynt, and J. S. Halterman, "Prescribing of controlled medications to adolescents and young adults in the United States," *Pediatrics*, vol. 126, no. 6, pp. 1108–1116, 2010.

[5] S. E. McCabe, B. T. West, C. J. Teter, and C. J. Boyd, "Medical and nonmedical use of prescription opioids among high school seniors in the United States," *Archives of Pediatrics & Adolescent Medicine*, vol. 166, no. 9, pp. 797–802, 2012.

[6] S. E. McCabe, B. T. West, J. A. Cranford et al., "Medical misuse of controlled medications among adolescents," *Archives of Pediatrics and Adolescent Medicine*, vol. 165, no. 8, pp. 729–735, 2011.

[7] American Psychiatric Association, *Diagnostic and Statistical Manual of Mental Disorders*, American Psychiatric Publishing, Washington, DC, USA, 4th edition, 2000.

[8] S. E. McCabe, C. J. Boyd, and A. Young, "Medical and nonmedical use of prescription drugs among secondary school students," *Journal of Adolescent Health*, vol. 40, no. 1, pp. 76–83, 2007.

[9] S. E. McCabe, B. T. West, and C. J. Teter, "Characteristics associated with the diversion of controlled medications among

adolescents," *Drug and Alcohol Dependence*, vol. 118, pp. 452–458, 2011.

[10] A. Swedlow, J. Ireland, and G. Johnson, *PreScribing Patterns of Schedule II Opioids in California Worker's Compensation*, California Worker's Compensation Institute, Oakland, Calif, USA, 2011.

6

An Epidemiological Investigation of Male-Female Differences in Drinking and Drinking-Related Problems between US-Born and Foreign-Born Latino and Asian Americans

Hui G. Cheng,[1] and Orla McBride[2]

[1] *Shanghai Mental Health Center, Shanghai Jiao Tong University, 3210 Humin Road, Shanghai 201108, China*
[2] *Division of Population Health Sciences, Department of Psychology, Royal College of Surgeons in Ireland, 123 Street Stephen's Green, Dublin 2, Ireland*

Correspondence should be addressed to Hui G. Cheng; xchengyaojin@gmail.com

Academic Editor: Jennifer B. Unger

Background. It has been widely documented that males were more likely to drinking alcohol and have alcohol use disorders (AUD). The degrees of the male-female differences in drinking and AUD have varied across countries. The reasons behind these variations have not been fully understood. The current study compared the estimated male-female differences across US-born and foreign-born Latino and Asian Americans with respect to alcohol drinking behavior and AUD. *Method.* Data come from the National Latino and Asian American Study (NLAAS), a national household survey of adults with Latinos and Asian decent in the United States. Male-female differences were estimated for drinking behavior and AUD among drinkers for US-born and foreign-born individuals, respectively. Zero-inflated Poisson regressions were utilized to estimate male-female differences in the number of AUD clinical features once it occurs. *Results.* Larger male-female differences were found for foreign-born individuals as compared to US-born individuals, especially the occurrence of AUD among drinkers. Once AUD clinical feature occurs, there was no male-female difference for foreign-born individuals, while there was a males excess in the number of clinical features for US-born individuals. *Conclusion.* Results from this study supports the importance of sociocultural influence in drinking and AUD. Implications for prevention and intervention programs were discussed.

1. Introduction

Worldwide, it has been extensively documented that alcohol consumption and alcohol use disorders (AUD) are more common in males as compared to females [1–6]. The reason of this male-female difference is both biological and sociocultural. Biological factors include differences in average volume of body water where ethanol can be distributed, levels of enzymes and their activities to metabolize ethanol, neurotransmitters and receptors through which ethanol affects the brain, and others [7–10]. Sociocultural factors include different levels of stigma attached to female drinking, social expectation toward different gender roles, alcohol availability, and others [11–13]. That is, drinking has been used as a way to express masculinity among males. In contrast, the traditional role for female is family-oriented. Also, female drinking has been associated with higher vulnerability of sexual assault [14, 15]. Thus, female drinking is discouraged socially due to the fear that it may interfere with their responsibilities [15]. These factors interplay with each other leading to the observed male-female differences in drinking and the occurrence of AUD. Despite the consistent finding that males are more likely to experience drinking-related problems, wide variations in male-female differences have been found across cultures and populations and this variation in male-female differences across countries is considered to be too wide to be explained solely by biological differences [4–6, 15, 16]. Besides theoretical value, studies of male-female differences in drinking and AUD are also of public health importance. Some studies have recently documented a possible convergence in male and female drinking patterns in the US, which may in turn increase disease burden associated with alcohol drinking in females (e.g., [17]). Understanding the observed male-female differences may provide useful information for the design of future prevention.

Previous studies have shown that the male-female difference in AUD is considerably smaller in the United States as compared to Latin American and Asian countries, suggesting female drinking is tolerated more in the USA when compared to Latin American and Asian countries [11, 16, 18–22]. For example, a study using data from the National Latino and Asian American Study (NLAAS) found male-female ration in substance use disorders in foreign-born Latinos living in the US was at least 3 times higher compared to their US-born counterparts [6]. Furthermore, among foreign-born individuals drinking problem increases as the number of generations since immigration to the USA as well as the age of immigration decreases [6, 23]. Some research has hypothesized that this difference is due to acculturation process into a society where female drinking is more tolerated. Some studies found supporting evidence that acculturation is positively associated with heavy drinking in females [24, 25], while others found no such association [26, 27].

Reviewing previous literature, some exploration may aid further understanding of drinking and AUD. As suggested by previously studies, male-female difference may vary across various stages of alcohol involvement [28, 29]. Thus, comparing male-female difference between US-born and foreign-born individuals with respect to the transition from the earlier alcohol involvement to the occurrence of AUD may provide useful information. Alcohol use disorder includes socially maladaptive drinking (in line with DSM-IV alcohol abuse) and alcohol dependence, both of which involve multiple clinical features. Among AUD cases, the number of clinical features can vary widely. Studies have found that greater numbers of clinical features predict the persistence of AUD [30] and the occurrence of new clinical features [31]. In this context, it is of interest to probe if males are more likely to have more clinical features of AUD as compared to females after the occurrence of AUD. In this context, aims of the current study are (1) to estimate variations in male-female difference in terms of earlier alcohol involvement and the transition from alcohol drinking to the occurrence of AUD comparing US-born to foreign-born Latino and Asian Americans (LAA) (2) to assess if males are more likely to have a greater number of AUD clinical features once it occurs.

2. Method

2.1. Study Design and Sample Selection. Latinos and Asians are two of the fastest growing ethnic groups within the USA. The US census bureau projects that by 2050, each group will nearly triple in size (e.g., Latinos to 133 million, Asians to 34 million), accounting for more than one-third (37.9%) of the total US population jointly [32]. However, much is unknown about psychiatric disorders among the LAA population. Against this background, the NLAAS was conducted to assess the prevalence and correlates of psychiatric disorders

among LAA via standardized interviews and survey methodology [33]. The sampling procedure was designed to yield a nationally representative sample of household-dwelling LAA adults, aged 18 years and older. The sampling approach consisted of multistage nationwide probability sampling and supplemental sampling from high density geographical areas of LAA. High-density supplemental samples were added to the nationwide sampling to optimize the statistical efficiency. One eligible adult was randomly selected as main respondent from each identified household. In a subsample, one additional adult was selected as second respondent. The sampling procedure resulted in 4345 main respondents and 1234 second respondents. Of all 5579 identified individuals, 4649 individuals completed interview. Weighted response levels were 75.7% and 80.3% among main respondents and second respondents, respectively. Comprehensive details about the samples and calculation of response levels are available elsewhere [33]. The study protocol was reviewed and approved by the cognizant institutional review board for protection of human subjects in research. Data collection took place during May 2002 to December 2003.

3. Measures

The study utilized a version of the World Health Organization's (WHO) World Mental Health Composite International Diagnostic Interview (WMH-CIDI) [34]. The WMH-CIDI is a comprehensive fully structured diagnostic interview designed to be administered by trained lay interviewers for the assessment of mental disorders according to DSM-IV criteria. To minimize the number of interview refusals due to insufficiency with the English language, the CIDI was translated into three other languages: Spanish, Chinese, and Vietnamese. Respondents were interviewed in their own homes.

In this study, key response variables are lifetime history of AUD including DSM-IV alcohol abuse and alcohol dependence. The endorsement of any of the four clinical features of socially maladaptive drinking qualifies the individual of lifetime history of DSM-IV alcohol abuse. To ease discussion and presentation, they were labeled as "responsibility interference," "drink despite social problems", "hazardous use", and "legal problems." Lifetime DSM-IV alcohol dependence was defined as the occurrence of at least three of the seven clinical features of alcohol dependence during the same 12 months. Lifetime occurrence of clinical features of alcohol dependence is defined as the occurrence of at least one of the seven DSM-IV clinical features and "irresistible desire to drink." Opportunity to drink alcohol is defined as ever having opportunity to drink alcohol; more than minimum (MTM) drinking is defined as having at least 12 drinks in a given year; heavier drinking is defined as at least 5 drinks per day for males and 4 for females. This latter definition is consistent with the definition of "binge drinking" used by the US National Institute of Alcohol Abuse and Alcoholism (NIAAA) and the most commonly used definitions for "binge drinking" and "heavy episodic drinking" in previous studies [35].

Gender and place of birth were the main covariates in this analysis. Other covariates include age (in years), ethnicity (Latino or Asian), and number of parents born in the USA. All of these variables were based upon the respondent's self-report.

4. Analysis

During the first steps, we provided a description of the sample and lifetime estimates of AUD, as well as stratified estimates by male-female and place of birth. In subsequent steps, a series of logistic regressions were conducted to estimate the variation in male-female differences in alcohol involvement and the occurrence of AUD among drinkers. The male-female gap in drinking and AUD is estimated in the form of odds ratios (ORs). Statistical comparisons are made to investigate the variation of OR in US-born and foreign-born LAA by the inclusion of a product term. First, bivariate logistic regression was conducted to produce the unadjusted OR. Second, age, ethnicity, and number of parents born in the US, was introduced to the regression model. (The variable "number of grandparents born in the US" was initially included as well, but it is not associated with the outcomes. It was not included in the final models in order to obtain a parsimonious model.) In these steps, since the occurrence of outcomes, especially early alcohol involvement (e.g., opportunities to drink and trying alcohol when given the opportunity) was quite high, the odds ratio (OR) is not a good simulation for relative risk (RR). In order to be able to attach a more substantive meanings to estimates, we used the formula suggested by Zhang and Yu [36] to transform the OR into RR.

The final steps consisted of using the zero-inflated Poisson (ZIP) regressions to estimate male-female differences for foreign-born and US-born LAA with respect to both the occurrence of AUD and the increment in numbers of clinical features of AUD among drinkers. Due to the fact that a vast majority of individuals did not have any clinical feature of AUD (a count of zero) there was an "over-dispersion" of zeros in the outcome, the number of AUD clinical features. The ZIP model can account for this "inflation" of zeros [37]. The ZIP model assumes that there are two groups of individuals, one consists of those who never have a value greater than zero (the zero group), another consists of those who have a value greater than 0 (the nonzero group). This assumption is appropriate in this context because the majority of the LAA population never had any clinical feature of AUD due to characteristics such as light or moderate drinking. The ZIP model produces two sets of estimates: one set of estimates to associate the likelihood of being in the nonzero group (or the zero group), the other set to associate covariates with the increment of outcome given the nonzero group. The main covariate was gender. Other covariates included age, ethnicity, and number of parents born in the USA for adjustment.

The complex survey sampling strategy and selection probabilities were accounted for by applying proper sampling weights and post stratification adjustments. In this work,

the precision of estimates was expressed by 95% confidence intervals. Stata software was used for all analyses (version 9.2, Stata Corporation, 2009).

5. Results

5.1. The Sample Description. The sample included 1378 US-born LAA (924 Latinos and 454 Asians) and 3268 foreign-born LAA (1629 Latinos and 1659 Asians). With respect to alcohol use and related problems, males were more likely to drink and were more likely to have drinking-related problems than females in both US-born and foreign-born LAA (see Table 1).

US-born Individuals were more likely to drink when compared to foreign-born individuals (86.8% and 63.4% for US-born males and females, resp., 75.7% and 30.3% for foreign-born males and females, resp.). The same pattern was found for the lifetime occurrence of AUD.

Smaller male-female ratios were found for US-born LAA in the occurrence of AUD as compared to foreign-born LAA: the male-female ratio was above 20 (e.g., 8.3% and 0.4% for socially maladaptive drinking for males and females, resp.) for foreign-born LAA and approximately three in US-born LAA.

Table 2 presents estimated relative risks ratios (RRs) in relation to the transition from opportunity toward the occurrence of AUD for foreign-born and US-born LAA, respectively. For each outcome studied here, statistically significant variation in RR was found across foreign-born LAA and US born LAA ($P < 0.05$). Larger RR were found for the foreign-born LAA. Nonetheless, point estimates indicate that the male excessive risk is rather small in earlier alcohol involvement (i.e., the opportunity to drink alcohol and tried alcohol provided opportunities) in both groups. In contrast, as alcohol drinking progresses, much larger male-female gaps were found for foreign-born LAA (e.g., from 1.3 for alcohol opportunity to 8.7 for DSM-IV alcohol abuse among MTM drinkers), while moderately larger male-female gaps were found for US-born LAA (e.g., from 1.1 for alcohol opportunity to 2.0 for DSM-IV alcohol abuse among MTM drinkers). In foreign-born LAA, as one female drinker developed any socially maladaptive drinking, there were almost 10 male drinkers did so; in US-born LAA, this ratio was two. Similar pattern was found in the occurrence of alcohol dependence. Interestingly, the male excessive risk of heavy drinking, which is an indicator of problematic drinking, was much smaller, especially in foreign-born LAA. Variations across Latinos and Asians were tested, but the results were not statistically significant ($P > 0.05$).

As presented in Table 3, the male-female difference for foreign-born LAA lies mainly in the occurrence of clinical feature of AUD (adjusted OR = 9.5, 95% CI = 4.3, 21.0); once AUD clinical feature occurs, there was no male-female difference anymore with respect to the increment in the number of clinical features. In contrast, for US-born LAA, males were more likely to have any AUD clinical feature as compared to females (adjusted OR = 3.6, 95% CI = 2.5, 5.1). Among individuals who had ever experienced at least one

TABLE 1: Description of sociodemographic characteristics and drinking-related outcomes in males and females. Data from NLAAS, 2002-2003.

Demographics		The entire sample			US-born Males		US-born Females		Foreign-born Males		Foreign-born Females	
		n of cases	Mean[1]	se	n of cases	Mean[1]	n of cases	Mean[1]	n of cases	Mean[1]	n of cases	Mean[1]
Age (years)		4649	38.9	0.5	629	35.9	749	37.8	1494	39.0	1774	41.2
		n	%[1]	se	n	%[1]	n	%[1]	n	%[1]	n	%[1]
Race/Ancestry	Hispanic	2554	73.6	2.0	403	83.6	521	83.1	723	70.1	906	65.71
	Asian	2095	26.5		226	16.4	228	16.9	771	29.9	868	34.29
Born in the US	Yes	1378	36.6	2.0								
	No	3268	63.4									
Alcohol drinking and alcohol use disorders												
MTM drinking[2]		3730	61.2	1.2	540	86.8	484	63.4	1062	75.7	528	30.3
Past year drinking		1332	32.4	1.2	326	56.0	220	27.2	587	43.0	197	10.8
Ever DSM-IV alcohol abuse		299	8.7	0.9	130	23.8	61	8.7	97	8.2	11	0.4
Ever DSM-IV alcohol dependence		107	3.4	0.4	46	8.8	26	3.3	30	3.5	5	0.1
Ever dependence clinical feature		267	8.0	0.9	119	22.0	53	7.8	85	7.4	10	0.3

[1] Weighted percentage.
[2] MTM: more than minimum drinking.

TABLE 2: Male-female relative risks for transitions of alcohol drinking and AUD stratified by the place of birth. Data from NLAAS, 2002-2003.

		Foreign-born							US-born						
		wt%[1]	uRR	95% C.I.		aRR[2]	95% C.I.		wt%[1]	uRR	95% C.I.		aRR[2]	95% C.I.	
Opportunities	Female	76.7							94.0						
	Male	95.9	1.3	1.2	1.3	1.2	1.2	1.3	98.9	1.1	1.0	1.1	1.1	1.0	1.1
Tried alcohol given opportunity (n = 4098)	Female	84.5							92.3						
	Male	95.0	1.1	1.1	1.1	1.1	1.1	1.1	95.1	1.0	1.0	1.1	1.0	1.0	1.1
MTM drinking among those who tried (n = 3708)	Female	47.5							73.9						
	Male	83.4	1.8	1.7	1.8	1.8	1.7	1.8	92.4	1.3	1.2	1.3	1.3	1.2	1.3
Heavy drinking among MTM drinkers (n = 2617)	Female	18.2							39.1						
	Male	41.4	2.3	1.9	2.7	2.3	1.9	2.7	53.3	1.4	1.2	1.5	1.4	1.2	1.6
DSM-IV alcohol abuse among MTM drinkers	Female	1.3							14.3						
	Male	11.0	8.7	4.1	16.9	8.7	4.2	16.8	28.5	2.0	1.6	2.5	2.1	1.7	2.6
DSM-IV alcohol dependence among MTM drinkers	Female	0.4							5.2						
	Male	4.6	12.4	4.5	32.7	12.2	4.4	32.4	10.1	1.9	1.2	3.0	2.0	1.3	3.1
Any alcohol dependence clinical feature among MTM drinkers	Female	1.1							12.4						
	Male	9.8	8.8	4.0	18.2	8.8	4.1	18.0	25.3	2.1	1.6	2.6	2.2	1.7	2.7

[1] Weighted percentage.
[2] Estimates were adjusted for age, number of parents born in USA, and ethnicity.

clinical feature, males were more likely to experience a greater number of AUD clinical features overall.

6. Discussion

The main findings of this study maybe summarized succinctly. First, substantially larger male-female differences in drinking and AUD were found for foreign-born LAA compared to their US-born counterparts. Second, the male-female difference in foreign-born LAA occurs mainly in later stages that involve the occurrence of AUD. In contrast, the male-female difference is much more homogeneous across all stages of alcohol involvement among US-born LAA. Third, in foreign-born LAA, once AUD clinical feature occurs, there

TABLE 3: Estimates for male-female ratios from the zero-inflated poisson regression among drinkers. Data from NLAAS, 2002-2003.

	Foreign-born LAA		US-born LAA	
	Model 1[1]	Model 2[1]	Model 1[1]	Model 2[1]
OR to be in the nonzero group (95% CI)	9.4 (4.2, 21.0)	9.5 (4.3, 21.0)	2.4 (1.7, 3.4)	2.6 (1.9, 3.6)
P value	<0.001	<0.001	<0.001	<0.001
Coefficient for the increment in the count of clinical features (95% CI)	0.17 (−0.13, 0.46)	0.21 (−0.12, 0.53)	0.35 (0.02, 0.68)	0.39 (0.03, 0.70)
P value	0.26	0.22	0.04	0.03

[1] Model 1 adjusted for age and ethnicity; model 2 additionally adjusted for number of parents born in the USA.

was no male-female in the increment in number of clinical features; for US-born LAA, males were more likely to have a larger number of AUD clinical features once it occurs.

The current study found male-female ratios in foreign-born LAA were close to those from Latin and Asian countries [16, 18–21], while the male-female ratio in US-born LAA was almost the same as estimates for the US population [38]. These estimates were not due to differential distribution of age, ethnicity or "the number of parents born in the US." Given that the male-female differences were much similar at the early stages of alcohol involvement as compared to later stages (i.e., when maladaptive drinking occurred) across foreign- and US-born LAA, it is unlikely that the observed male-female differences in alcohol involvement is solely due to biological variations. Findings from this study correspond with previous knowledge and provide further evidence about male-female differences in drinking behavior highlighting the importance of social-environmental factors in alcohol drinking behavior and the occurrence of AUD [6, 11, 15, 16]. Indeed, the finding that males were more likely to have opportunity to drink alcohol is a direct piece of evidence about the social-environmental impact on alcohol involvement. Based on the United Nation Development Programme (UNDP)'s report, United State outranked most of the Latin American and Asian countries, especially those contributed large numbers of immigrants to the USA, in gender-related human development Indices, such as gender-related development index (GDI), and gender empowerment measure (GEM) [39]. The former is a gender inequality adjusted index to measure social and economic development of a country. The latter evaluates women's participation in politics and economics. As such, the convergence in social role expectation between males and females would have resulted in a convergence in alcohol drinking, which is traditionally viewed as a demonstration of masculine, including over-drinking. Another possibly important underlying mechanism is acculturation which may influence female drinking behavior more compared to males [24, 25].

This study provided some empirical evidence on the male-female differences for US-born and foreign-born LAAs in relation to stages of alcohol involvement and what happen after the occurrence of the first clinical feature of AUD. The results signal that the differential social expectation may

impact drinking behavior more in the later stages when maladaptive drinking pattern is manifested rather than early stages of alcohol involvement. It is interesting that the male-female difference in heavy drinking is not as large as that for AUD after MTM drinking has occurred. This suggests that occasional heavy episodic drinking in female may not be socially discouraged behavior as long as it does not evolve into a pattern of maladaptive drinking. However, heavy episodic drinking is associated with substantial disease burden through various routes [40]. The results call for attention to the importance of intervention of female heavy drinking. The distinct pattern in the increment of clinical features of AUD after the fist clinical feature has occurred across foreign-born and US-born LAA is novel. It is possible that for foreign-born LAA, female drinkers have to "cross a higher hurdle" to manifest a maladaptive drinking pattern (compared to US-born LAA) due to strong traditional social expectations toward females. Once the hurdle is crossed the impact of social expectation is not relevant to female drinkers anymore, and this results in the observed absence of male-female difference in the increment of AUD clinical features.

Several study limitations merit attention while interpreting findings. Of central concern is the cross-sectional nature of the study. Possible recall bias and survival bias cannot be ruled out [41]. Thus, the male-female difference in the transition of different alcohol involvement stages is best understood as the reported male-female difference in alcohol involvement stages among survivors. Nonetheless, there has been no evidence for a male-female associated differential reporting of drinking. All estimates were adjusted for age as well. With respect to the population under study, institutional people and adolescents were not included in this study. Thus, the results cannot be generalized to these populations. With respect to sample size, although this study has the largest sample size of LAA, there was limited number of AUD cases in the foreign-born female group ($n = 11$ as presented in Table 1). Thus, the estimates for the foreign-born LAA may not be precise. This also precluded the possibility to study acculturation variables (e.g., language efficiency) or the cross-ethnic variations in this study. Nonetheless, the robust variations in male-female ratios between foreign-born LAA and US-born LAA were not likely to be due to chance. With respect to reporting bias, it is possible that foreign-born females held higher level of self-stigma toward drinking and AUD as compared to US-born females [11, 12]. Unfortunately, to our knowledge, there has been no study about the degree and direction that self-stigmatization might influence reporting in a survey context. Regarding the assessment, although CIDI interviews were conducted using four languages, it is possible that some interviewees did not understand questions fully due to insufficient language ability given the multilinguistic nature of the LAA population. Last but not least, information about drinking levels before the occurrence of AUD cannot be obtained, although it holds great relevance in understanding the natural history of drinking problems. Future prospective studies with little attrition are needed to address this issue.

Counterbalancing strengths include that NLAAS is a nationally representative study. With statistical adjustments, such as sample weights and poststratification adjustment, the selection bias was minimized and thus results were generalizable to the LAA population as a whole. Based on findings like these, it is of interest to probe the role of acculturation in order to shed some light on the mechanism of the observed male-female differences among foreign-born LAAs. Also, studies on the male-female differences stratified by fine-grained grouping of ethnicity (e.g., different Asian and Latino ethnicities) may yield more relevant results for each subgroups of LAA.

References

[1] G. Rahav, R. Wilsnack, K. Bloomfield, G. Gmel, and S. Kuntsche, "The influence of societal level factors on men's and women's alcohol comsumption and alcohol problems," *Alcohol and Alcoholism*, vol. 41, no. 1, pp. i47–i55, 2006.

[2] A. D. Lopez, C. D. Mathers, M. Ezzati, D. T. Jamison, and C. J. Murray, "Global and regional burden of disease and risk factors, 2001: systematic analysis of population health data," *The Lancet*, vol. 367, no. 9524, pp. 1747–1757, 2006.

[3] M. Zilberman, H. Tavares, and N. El-Guebaly, "Gender similarities and differences: the prevalence and course of alcohol- and other substance-related disorders," *Journal of Addictive Diseases*, vol. 22, no. 4, pp. 61–74, 2003.

[4] W. A. Vega, G. Canino, Z. Cao, and M. Alegria, "Prevalence and correlates of dual diagnoses in U.S. Latinos," *Drug and Alcohol Dependence*, vol. 100, no. 1-2, pp. 32–38, 2009.

[5] M. Alegría, G. Canino, P. E. Shrout et al., "Prevalence of mental illness in immigrant and non-immigrant U.S. Latino groups," *American Journal of Psychiatry*, vol. 165, no. 3, pp. 359–369, 2008.

[6] G. Canino, W. A. Vega, W. M. Sribney, L. A. Warner, and M. Alegría, "Social relationships, social assimilation, and substance use disorders among adult Latinos in the U.S.," *Journal of Drug Issues*, vol. 38, no. 1, pp. 69–101, 2008.

[7] L. L. Devaud, F. O. Risinger, and D. Selvage, "Impact of the hormonal milieu on the neurobiology of alcohol dependence and withdrawal," *Journal of General Psychology*, vol. 133, no. 4, pp. 337–356, 2006.

[8] M. Ely, R. Hardy, N. T. Longford, and M. E. J. Wadsworth, "Gender differences in the relationship between alcohol consumption and drink problems are largely accounted for by body water," *Alcohol and Alcoholism*, vol. 34, no. 6, pp. 894–902, 1999.

[9] A. Yoshida, "Genetic polymorphisms of alcohol metabolizing enzymes related to alcohol sensitivity and alcoholic diseases," *Alcohol and Alcoholism*, vol. 29, no. 6, pp. 693–696, 1994.

[10] H. W. Goedde and D. P. Agarwal, "Polymorphism of aldehyde dehydrogenase and alcohol sensitivity," *Enzyme*, vol. 37, no. 1-2, pp. 29–44, 1987.

[11] K. Bloomfield, G. Gmel, R. Neve, and H. Mustonen, "Investigating gender convergence in alcohol consumption in Finland, Germany, The Netherlands, and Switzerland: a repeated survey analysis," *Substance Abuse*, vol. 22, no. 1, pp. 39–53, 2001.

[12] M. Holmila and K. Raitasalo, "Gender differences in drinking: why do they still exist?" *Addiction*, vol. 100, no. 12, pp. 1763–1769, 2005.

[13] S. Isidore and R. R. Obot, *Alcohol, Gender, and Drinking Problems. Perspectives from Low and Middle Income Countries*, World Health Organization, Genava, Switzerland, 2005.

[14] C. A. Christie-Mizell and R. L. Peralta, "The gender gap in alcohol consumption during late adolescence and young adulthood: gendered attitudes and adult roles," *Journal of Health and Social Behavior*, vol. 50, no. 4, pp. 410–426, 2009.

[15] R. W. Wilsnack, S. C. Wilsnack, A. F. Kristjanson, N. D. Vogeltanz-Holm, and G. Gmel, "Gender and alcohol consumption: patterns from the multinational GENACIS project," *Addiction*, vol. 104, no. 9, pp. 1487–1500, 2009.

[16] R. W. Wilsnack, N. D. Vogeltanz, S. C. Wilsnack et al., "Gender differences in alcohol consumption and adverse drinking consequences: cross-cultural patterns," *Addiction*, vol. 95, no. 2, pp. 251–265, 2000.

[17] K. M. Keyes, B. F. Grant, and D. S. Hasin, "Evidence for a closing gender gap in alcohol use, abuse, and dependence in the United States population," *Drug and Alcohol Dependence*, vol. 93, no. 1-2, pp. 21–29, 2008.

[18] I. S. Obot and R. Room, Eds., *Alcohol, Gender and Drinking Problems*, World Health Organization, Genava, Switzerland, 2005.

[19] N. Kawakami, H. Shimizu, T. Haratani, N. Iwata, and T. Kitamura, "Lifetime and 6-month prevalence of DSM-III-R psychiatric disorders in an urban community in Japan," *Psychiatry Research*, vol. 121, no. 3, pp. 293–301, 2004.

[20] M. E. Medina-Mora, G. Borges, C. Benjet, C. Lara, and P. Berglund, "Psychiatric disorders in Mexico: lifetime prevalence in a nationally representative sample," *British Journal of Psychiatry*, vol. 190, pp. 521–528, 2007.

[21] J. T. Park, B. G. Kim, and H. J. Jhun, "Alcohol consumption and the CAGE questionnaire in Korean adults: results from the second Korea National Health And Nutrition Examination Survey," *Journal of Korean Medical Science*, vol. 23, no. 2, pp. 199–206, 2008.

[22] K. Bloomfield et al., *Gender, Culture and Alcohol Problems: A Multi-National Study. Project Final Report*, Institute for Medical Informatics, Biometrics & Epidemiology, Charité Universitätsmedizin Berlin, Berlin, Germany, 2005.

[23] J. B. Peña, P. A. Wyman, C. H. Brown et al., "Immigration generation status and its association with suicide attempts, substance use, and depressive symptoms among Latino adolescents in the USA," *Prevention Science*, vol. 9, no. 4, pp. 299–310, 2008.

[24] R. Caetano, S. Ramisetty-Mikler, L. S. Wallisch, C. McGrath, and R. T. Spence, "Acculturation, drinking, and alcohol abuse and dependence among Hispanics in the Texas-Mexico border," *Alcoholism*, vol. 32, no. 2, pp. 314–321, 2008.

[25] P. A. Vaeth, R. Caetano, and L. A. Rodriguez, "The Hispanic Americans Baseline Alcohol Survey (HABLAS): the association between acculturation, birthplace and alcohol consumption across Hispanic national groups," *Addictive Behaviors*, vol. 37, no. 9, pp. 1029–1037, 2012.

[26] R. Caetano, P. A. C. Vaeth, and L. A. Rodriguez, "The Hispanic Americans baseline alcohol survey (HABLAS): acculturation, birthplace and alcohol-related social problems across Hispanic national groups," *Hispanic Journal of Behavioral Sciences*, vol. 34, no. 1, pp. 95–117, 2012.

[27] C. L. Ehlers, D. A. Gilder, J. R. Criado, and R. Caetano, "Acculturation stress, anxiety disorders, and alcohol dependence in a select population of young adult Mexican Americans," *Journal of Addiction Medicine*, vol. 3, no. 4, pp. 227–233, 2009.

[28] A. Kalaydjian, J. Swendsen, W. T. Chiu et al., "Sociodemographic predictors of transitions across stages of alcohol use, disorders, and remission in the National Comorbidity Survey Replication," *Comprehensive Psychiatry*, vol. 50, no. 4, pp. 299–306, 2009.

[29] S. Lee, W. J. Guo, A. Tsang et al., "Associations of cohort and socio-demographic correlates with transitions from alcohol use to disorders and remission in metropolitan China," *Addiction*, vol. 104, no. 8, pp. 1313–1323, 2009.

[30] R. Culverhouse, K. K. Bucholz, R. R. Crowe et al., "Long-term stability of alcohol and other substance dependence diagnoses and habitual smoking: an evaluation after 5 years," *Archives of General Psychiatry*, vol. 62, no. 7, pp. 753–760, 2005.

[31] M. A. Schuckit, T. L. Smith, and N. A. Landi, "The 5-year clinical course of high-functioning men with DSM-IV alcohol abuse or dependence," *American Journal of Psychiatry*, vol. 157, no. 12, pp. 2028–2035, 2000.

[32] United States Census Bureau, *U.S. Population Projections*, United States Census Bureau, 2008.

[33] S. G. Heeringa, J. Wagner, M. Torres, N. Duan, T. Adams, and P. Berglund, "Sample designs and sampling methods for the Collaborative Psychiatric Epidemiololgy Studies (CPES)," *International Journal of Methods in Psychiatric Research*, vol. 13, no. 4, pp. 221–240, 2004.

[34] R. C. Kessler and T. B. Ustün, "The world mental health (WMH) survey initiative version of the world health organization (WHO) composite international diagnostic interview (CIDI)," *International Journal of Methods in Psychiatric Research*, vol. 13, no. 2, pp. 93–121, 2004.

[35] NIAAA, "NIAAA council approves definition of binge drinking," *NIAAA Newsletter*, vol. 3, 2004, Bethesda: National Institute on Alcohol Abuse and Alcoholism.

[36] J. Zhang and K. F. Yu, "What's the relative risk? A method of correcting the odds ratio in cohort studies of common outcomes," *Journal of the American Medical Association*, vol. 280, no. 19, pp. 1690–1691, 1998.

[37] D. Lambert, "Zero-inflated poisson regression, with an application to defects in manufacturing," *Technometrics*, vol. 34, no. 1, pp. 1–14, 1992.

[38] B. F. Grant, D. A. Dawson, F. S. Stinson, S. P. Chou, M. C. Dufour, and R. P. Pickering, "The 12-month prevalence and trends in DSM-IV alcohol abuse and dependence: United States, 1991-1992 and 2001-2002," *Drug and Alcohol Dependence*, vol. 74, no. 3, pp. 223–234, 2004.

[39] United Nations Development Programme, *The Human Development Report*, Oxford University Press, New York, NY, USA, 2007.

[40] W. H. Organization, Ed., *WHO Global Status Report on Alcohol 2004*, World Health Organization. Department of Mental Health and Substance Abuse, Geneva, Switzerland, 2004.

[41] T. M. Caldwell, B. Rodgers, C. Power, C. Clark, and S. A. Stansfeld, "Drinking histories of self-identified lifetime abstainers and occasional drinkers: findings from the 1958 British Birth Cohort Study," *Alcohol and Alcoholism*, vol. 41, no. 6, pp. 650–654, 2006.

7

Initial Smoking Experiences and Current Smoking Behaviors and Perceptions among Current Smokers

Hugh Klein,[1,2] Claire E. Sterk,[2] and Kirk W. Elifson[2]

[1] Kensington Research Institute, 401 Schuyler Road, Silver Spring, Maryland, MD 20910, USA
[2] Rollins School of Public Health, Emory University, Atlanta, GA 30322, USA

Correspondence should be addressed to Hugh Klein; hughk@aol.com

Academic Editor: Jennifer B. Unger

Purpose. We examine early-onset cigarette smoking and how, if at all, it is related to subsequent smoking practices. *Methods*. From 2004 to 2007, face-to-face interviews were conducted with 485 adult cigarette smokers residing in the Atlanta metropolitan area. Data analysis involved a multivariate analysis to determine whether age of smoking onset was related to current smoking practices when the effects of gender, age, race, marital/relationship status, income, and educational attainment were taken into account. *Results*. The mean age for smoking onset was 14.8, and more than one-half of all smokers had their first cigarette between the ages of 12 and 16. Most people reported an interval of less than one month between their first and second time using tobacco. Earlier onset cigarette smoking was related to more cigarette use and worse tobacco-related health outcomes in adulthood. *Conclusions*. Early prevention and intervention are needed to avoid early-onset smoking behaviors. Intervening after initial experimentation but before patterned smoking practices are established will be challenging, as the interval between initial and subsequent use tends to be short.

1. Introduction

Research focusing on the age of initiation for various types of legal and illegal substances has shown that "average" Americans begin experimenting with substances, typically alcohol and/or tobacco, during their teenage years [1]. Increasingly, early-onset use appears to be occurring. By the time they are nine or ten years old, approximately 10% of the American children have begun drinking alcohol [2] and nearly one-third of all youths begin drinking prior to the age of thirteen [3]. By 10th grade (approximately aged 15 or 16), more than one-half (58.2%) of all American youths have used alcohol [1]; and by 12th grade (approximately aged 17 or 18), more than one-half (54.1%) of American adolescents have been drunk at least once [1]. Study findings have revealed that early-onset alcohol use oftentimes is associated with a greater likelihood of subsequent illegal drug use [4].

When it occurs, experimentation with illegal drugs typically begins, on average, a few years after initial alcohol consumption. Recent data suggest that 28.6% of 13 and 14 year olds, 40.6% of 15 and 16 year olds, and 49.9% of 17 and

18 year olds have used at least one illegal drug during their lifetime [1]. By far, the most commonly used of these drugs is marijuana. The median age of first marijuana use is 15.5 years [5]. Nearly two-thirds (62.6%) of all marijuana users first try the substance between the ages of 13 and 17, and the large majority of these persons (90.9%) report prior alcohol and/or tobacco use [5]. Early onset of marijuana use (defined here as experimentation prior to age 15) has been shown to be related to daily marijuana use as well as the use of heroin, cocaine, and other illegal drugs in adulthood [5, 6].

It is not uncommon for American youths to experiment with other types of drug use. While experimentation with cigarette smoking has declined sharply among young people since the 1990s [1], it remains the third ranked substance of experimentation among American adolescents, ranking only behind alcohol and marijuana. The average age of smoking initiation in the United States has been reported to be approximately 17 or 18 years [7]. In 2010, nearly one-half (42.2%) of all 12th graders reported having smoked a cigarette, with one-sixth (17.6%) reporting having tried some type of smokeless tobacco during their lifetime [1].

Approximately one-half of those who ever smoked reported having done so during the past month, and among them, approximately one-half smoked daily [1]. When all types of tobacco products are combined, more than one-quarter (26.0%) of all high school students are current users of tobacco [8].

Research on how age of initiation of cigarette smoking relates to subsequent smoking behaviors is sparse. In one study of early-onset cigarette smokers (defined as persons initiating use prior to age 12), about three-quarters of the young people (77.0%) became regular smokers by mid-adolescence [9]. Other researchers found that compared to people who began smoking at a later age, those who began smoking prior to age 16 were less than one-half as likely to quit smoking [10]. In their research on smoking initiation during the college years, Clarkin and colleagues [11] found that about one out of nine (11.7%) students had their first cigarette while in college years and 10.8% of college students began smoking regularly at some point during their college years. Having a positive experience (e.g., experiencing relaxation) when first smoking a cigarette has been associated with an increased risk of current smoking, daily smoking, nicotine dependence, and cue-induced cravings for a cigarette [12].

In this paper, using a community-based sample of adult current cigarette smokers, we examine (1) the age of onset of cigarette smoking, (2) people's recollections of their first smoking experiences, and (3) the potential link between age of onset and subsequent cigarette smoking behaviors. In doing so, we aim to add to the literature on smoking initiation and address important lessons that can be learned for prevention and intervention efforts.

2. Methods

2.1. Subjects and Design. The data presented in this paper are part of the Persistent Smokers Project (PSP) in Atlanta, Georgia. The community-based sample of 485 current smokers is distinct from those reported in many other studies, which have been based on younger, school-based research populations or those recruited at clinics or other institutional settings. Data were collected between September 2004 and July 2007. To be eligible, the participants had to be aged 18 years or older and reside in the Atlanta metropolitan area. Study participants had to have smoked at least 100 cigarettes during their lifetime (which is consistent with the National Health Interview Survey (NHIS) classification [13] as "ever smoked") and have smoked in the last week (which is consistent with the NHIS classification [13] as "current smoker").

Participant recruitment involved purposive sampling, including a combination of active and passive recruitment techniques. Using a short screening form, potential study participants were screened in the setting where they were recruited, such as near office buildings or other work locations, at restaurants, in social entertainment settings, in parks, and in other public settings. Passive recruitment involved posting flyers in local venues such as stores, restaurants, and community centers. Interested individuals, who called the project phone line listed on the flyers, initially were

screened over the phone using the same short form used in the active recruitment. Two-thirds of the respondents (n = 325) were brought into the study via active recruitment, with the remaining one-third being identified through passive recruitment (n = 160). We did not identify any significant difference in the sample characteristics or in the outcome variables based on the recruitment strategy.

Once a person was identified as eligible, the staff member described the study and time required to participate. The most common reason for ineligibility was having smoked an insufficient number of cigarettes to qualify, either during the person's lifetime or during the preceding week. The interviews took place at a mutually convenient location, such as one of the project offices, the respondent's home, a local restaurant or coffee shop, or community centers. Additional information was provided on the nature of the study, the time required, and the informed consent and other confidentiality procedures. The questionnaire contained items covering the respondent's social background characteristics, smoking behaviors, attitudes, and opinions, as well as items about alcohol and other drugs, a health inventory, and self and identity items. The average length of the interview was 90 minutes and respondents received $20 as compensation for their time and participation. Prior to implementation in the field, all study protocols were reviewed and approved by the institutional review board at Emory University and Georgia State University.

2.2. Measures Used. Three variables focused on initial smoking behaviors: Age of onset of cigarette smoking was a continuous measure assessed by respondents' answers to the question "How old were you when you smoked your first cigarette?" This question was asked separately from one in which respondents were asked when they had their first puff or two from a cigarette. Age of first cigarette purchase was measured similarly. The amount of time that elapsed between the first and the second time a person smoked was a seven-level ordinal measure, with the following response options: (1) "less than a day," (2) "one day," (3) "more than one day but less than a week," (4) "one week but less than one month," (5) "one month but less than three months," (6) "three months but less than twelve months," and (7) "one year or more." All of these measures (and all other measures of earlier-life smoking behaviors) were based on retrospective reports which, by their very nature, cannot be corroborated.

Initial smoking experiences were assessed using the following measures: source of first cigarette was a categorical measure asking respondents to indicate how they obtained their first cigarette: bought a cigarette on their own, got a cigarette from another person (e.g., parent, sibling, other relative, or friend), took/stole a cigarette from someone (e.g., parent, sibling, other relative, or friend), or some other way. Reality versus expectations regarding the first smoking experience was a categorical measure in which study participants selected one of the following response choices: more negative than expected, just as expected, or more positive than expected. Recollection of the first smoking experience included yes/no responses to items identified in our formative research on smoking initiation: coughing, feeling calm or relaxed, feeling dizzy, having more energy, feeling panicked, and so forth. Reasons for smoking again after the initial cigarette included yes/no responses to items such as: (a) I liked what it did for me, (b) I liked how it tasted, (c) I thought the next time would be better than the first time, (d) a friend offered it to me and I felt I could not decline, (e) it was cool to smoke, and (f) I wanted to be with friends, all of whom were smokers.

Current smoking behaviors were assessed with several measures. Number of cigarettes smoked was assessed based on the number of cigarettes smoked per week (continuous measure). This was computed from the number of days respondents reported having smoked during the preceding month, the average number of cigarettes smoked on a typical weekday, and the average number of cigarettes smoked over the course of a typical weekend. Smoking while ill was assessed from a question that asked "Do you smoke if you are so ill that you are in bed most of the day?" The response choices were "no" (coded as 0), "much less" (coded as 1), "somewhat less" (coded as 2), "the same as when I am not ill and need to stay in bed" (coded as 3), "a little more" (coded as 4), and "much more" (coded as 5). Needing a cigarette to function was derived from the question "How often do you feel that you need a cigarette to help you function?" Response choices were: "never" (coded as 0), "less than once a month" (coded as 1), "about once a month" (coded as 2), "a few times a month" (coded as 3), "about once a week" (coded as 4), "several times a week" (coded as 5), "daily" (coded as 6), and "every 2-3 hours or more often" (coded as 7). Taking a special trip to get cigarettes involved the question "How often do you make special trips to get cigarettes?" Chain smoking frequency was assessed by asking "How often do you chain-smoke, that is, smoke one cigarette right after another?" Smoking more than intended was derived from the question "How often do you smoke more cigarettes than you intend to smoke?" Response choices for these last three measures were "never" (coded as 0), "less than once a month" (coded as 1), "about once a month" (coded as 2), "a few times a month" (coded as 3), "about once a week" (coded as 4), "several times a week" (coded as 5), and "daily" (coded as 6).

Perceptions related to smoking were examined with several measures. Perceived benefits of smoking were measured using a scale consisting of twelve items that were adapted from the work of Myers and colleagues [14] and Copeland and colleagues [15]. All items were scored using a five-point Likert scale, with responses ranging from "strongly disagree" to "strongly agree." Items comprising the perceived benefits scale included: (a) "When I'm angry, smoking a cigarette calms me down"; (b) "Smoking calms me down when I feel nervous"; (c) "Smoking energizes me"; (d) "Cigarettes can really make me feel good"; (e) "When I am worrying about something, smoking a cigarette is helpful"; (f) "When I'm feeling happy, smoking helps keep that feeling"; (g) "I enjoy parties more when I am smoking"; (h) "I feel more at ease with other people if I have a cigarette"; (i) "(Smoking helps me) in social situations"; (j) "I am afraid that I will be unable to function if I stop smoking"; (k) "I do better work when I am allowed to smoke"; and (l) "I feel like I am part of a group when I'm around smokers." The scale was found to be reliable (Cronbach's alpha = 0.80). Perceived harms of cigarette smoking were based on four items from the *Smoking Consequences Questionnaire* [15]: (a) "Smoking is taking years off my life"; (b) "The more I smoke, the more I risk my health"; (c) "By smoking I risk heart disease and lung cancer"; and (d) "Smoking is hazardous to my health." The scale was found to be reliable (Cronbach's alpha = 0.82). Response categories ranged from "strongly disagree" (coded as 1) to "strongly agree" (coded as 5), with higher scores indicating more health concerns.

In the multivariate analyses, six demographic variables were included: gender (male versus female), age (continuous), race (white versus nonwhite), marital/relationship status ("involved" with someone versus not "involved"), educational attainment (college graduate versus less education), and monthly income (continuous).

2.3. Statistical Analysis. For the first part of the analysis (focusing on the onset of smoking behaviors), descriptive statistics are presented. In the second part of the analysis (examining the relationship between age of smoking onset and subsequent smoking behaviors), bivariate analyses were conducted. Correlation coefficients (Pearson's r) were computed to examine the relationship between initial smoking characteristics (age of smoking first cigarette, age of first purchasing cigarettes, and lapse time between first and subsequent cigarette smoking) and current smoking practices (number of cigarettes smoked, chain smoking, smoking while bed-ridden due to illness, smoking more than intended, making trips to procure cigarettes, needing cigarettes in order to function, perceived benefits of smoking, and perceived harms of smoking). In the final part of the analysis, multivariate analyses were undertaken to determine whether the age-of-onset measures were important contributors to the measures (a) number of cigarettes smoked and (b) smoking while sick in bed, when the effects of gender, age, race, marital/relationship status, income, and educational attainment were taken into account. These analyses were conducted via multiple regression, adding the age-of-onset measures alongside the demographic control variables. Throughout this paper, results are reported as statistically significant whenever $P < .05$.

3. Results

3.1. Sample Characteristics. Slightly more than one-half (56.8%) of the study participants were male ($n = 275$). Participants ranged in age from 18 to 70, with a mean age of 36.4 (median = 34, SD = 12.3). Most of the respondents were either Caucasian (54.6%) or African American (39.0%) ($n = 265$ and 189, resp.). Most respondents (83.5%) were heterosexual ($n = 405$). Overall, this was a fairly well-educated research sample, with only 25.2% of the people having completed no more than a high school education ($n = 122$). Of those who had attended college ($n = 363$), nearly one-half (34.2% of the total sample) were college graduates or people with postgraduate education ($n = 166$). About one-half of the study participants were employed on a full-time basis at the time of their interview (55.1%); about one-third (32.9%) were employed on a part-time basis; and most of the remaining people (12.0%) were unemployed (n = 266, 159, and 58, resp.). On balance, this was a relatively low-income sample, with annual median income being approximately $21,500 (mean = $30,475, SD = $28,183, and range = $0 to $216,000). Compared to national data reported by the Centers for Disease Control and Prevention, the study sample included more women and was better educated. Otherwise, the sample reflected the characteristics of smokers nationally [16].

3.2. Age of Smoking Onset.

The mean age at which people first reported smoking was 14.8 (median = 14, SD = 4.6). More than one-half (56.5%) of the study participants said that they smoked their first cigarette between the ages of 12 and 16, and the large majority (81.4%) reported having tried cigarettes before they were of legal age to smoke.

Study participants reported purchasing their first cigarette approximately two years after they smoked their first cigarette (mean age = 17.0, median = 16, SD = 3.9). More than one-half of the study participants (59.6%) said that they bought a cigarette for the first time between the ages of 15 and 18. Overall, slightly more than three-fifths of the study participants (61.9%) indicated that they were underage when they bought their first cigarette.

After trying their first cigarette, approximately one-half of the study participants (53.2%) reported having smoked their next cigarette within one week. These persons were relatively evenly divided amongst those who said that the interval between their first and second cigarettes was less than one day (15.5%), approximately one day (16.8%), and more than one day but less than one week (20.9%). Another 18.0% of the study participants reported smoking their second cigarette within one month of their first one. Comparatively few people reported a first-to-second cigarette interval of one to three months (6.8%), three months to one year (6.8%), or a year or more (15.1%).

3.3. Initial Smoking Experiences.

Approximately one-half (51.6%) of the study participants said that they received their first cigarette from a friend. Another one-quarter (25.8%) said that they secretly took or stole their first cigarette from someone (e.g., a parent, another relative, or a friend). Much less commonly reported for the first cigarette has having purchased it on one's own (5.6%) or having gotten it from a sibling (4.5%), a relative other than a sibling or a parent (3.9%), or a parent (2.1%).

When asked to think back about their first time smoking a cigarette, approximately one-half (50.7%) of the study participants said that the experience was more negative than they had expected. Nearly one-third (30.2%) said that the experience was about what they thought it would be like, and the remainder (19.1%) said that it was more positive than expected. The most common negative experience remembered about their first time smoking was becoming dizzy (66.9%). Many study participants (53.7%) recalled that they disliked the taste of their first cigarette, while

almost as many (52.1%) mentioned that it made them cough extensively. Conversely, approximately three-quarters of the study participants (77.9%) said that their first cigarette made them feel calm and relaxed.

When asked about the reasons for continuing to smoke after their initial cigarette, dominant explanations were the study participants felt that it was "cool" to smoke (57.5%) and they wanted to be with friends of theirs, who happened to be smokers (49.9%). Approximately one-quarter of the study participants (27.4%) said that they continued to smoke because they liked what cigarettes/smoking did for them. Peer pressure, in the form of being offered a cigarette from a friend whose offer they felt they could not refuse, explained continued use for 16.3% of the study participants. A comparable proportion of the people interviewed (16.1%) said that they decided to continue smoking after their initial experience because they thought that their subsequent experiences with cigarettes would be better than their first. Citing a liking for the taste of cigarettes as the reason for continued use occurred among 12.6% of the study participants.

3.4. Initial Smoking Experiences and Subsequent Smoking Behaviors and Perceptions.

Table 1 presents Pearson's r correlation coefficients for the relationships between the three main age-of-onset measures (age of first cigarette smoked, age of first cigarette purchased, and lapse time between first and next cigarettes) and current smoking behaviors and smoking perceptions (e.g., number of cigarettes smoked, chain smoking, needing a cigarette in order to function, and perceived harms/benefits of smoking). The younger people were when they first smoked a cigarette, the more cigarettes they currently smoked (P < .05). Similarly, the younger they were when they first purchased a cigarette, the more they currently smoked (P < .001). Moreover, the shorter the interval between people's first and second cigarette smoking experiences, the greater their current tobacco use was likely to be (P < .10).

Likewise, as Table 1 shows, the younger people were the first time they smoked, the more likely they were to smoke during adulthood when they were so ill that they could not get out of bed (P < .001). Similarly, the younger they were when they first purchased a cigarette, the more likely they were to smoke as adults when they were bed-ridden due to illness (P < .001). The shorter the interval between people's first and second time ever using cigarettes, the more likely they were, as adults, to smoke when they were too sick to get out of bed (P < .001).

Similar results are shown for needing a cigarette in order to function properly. The younger study participants were when they first smoked a cigarette, the more often they currently reported needing a cigarette to function properly (P < .05). A younger age of first purchased cigarettes was associated with a greater current need to smoke a cigarette in order to function properly (P < .001). Additionally, the shorter the period between the person's first and second time smoking cigarettes, the more likely the person was to report needing to smoke in order to function properly (P < .05).

In contrast, initial smoking experiences were not found to be related to the frequency with which people made

TABLE 1: Age of onset of tobacco use and subsequent smoking behaviors.

	Age of first cigarette use	Age of first cigarette purchase	Interval between 1st and 2nd cigarette
Number of cigarettes smoked per week	.14**	.19***	.08†
Smoking when so ill that the person is unable to get out of bed	.16***	.21***	.16***
Needing a cigarette in order to function	.11*	.16***	.09*
Making special trips to purchase cigarettes	.03	.07	.06
Chain smoking	.03	.06	.01
Smoking more cigarettes than intended	.03	.03	.04
Perceived benefits derived from continuing to smoke	.10*	.16***	.09*
Perceived harms resulting from continuing to smoke	.05	.02	.06

†$P < .10$, *$P < .05$, **$P < .01$, and ***$P < .001$.

special trips to purchase cigarettes, chain smoking, smoking more cigarettes than intended, or with perceived negative health consequences resulting from smoking. As Table 1 shows, however, in terms of the perceived benefits of cigarette smoking, a younger age of cigarette smoking initiation and a younger age of first cigarette purchase were associated with perceiving more benefits from smoking in adulthood ($P < .05$ and $P < .001$, resp.). Additionally, the longer the interval between the person's first-ever and second-ever cigarettes, the more benefits of smoking the person perceived himself/herself to derive ($P < .05$).

Table 2 presents the results of the multivariate analyses, which were undertaken to determine whether the age of onset measures that were statistically significant (as shown in Table 1) were robust enough to remain statistically significant when the effects of key demographic variables such as gender, age, race, marital/relationship status, educational attainment, and income were taken into account. Standardized regression coefficients (i.e., beta values) are provided so that relative effects sizes can be compared. In each instance, the initial smoking experiences measures (age of first cigarette smoked, age of first purchasing a cigarette, and time lapse between first and second cigarettes smoked) were found to be significant even when the demographic control variables were included in the analyses. The results for two of the main outcome measures are presented in Table 2; dependent variables not included in this table (e.g., chain smoking, perceived benefits resulting from continuing to smoke, smoking more than intended, etc.) were omitted in the interest of conserving space, but comparable findings were obtained for those measures as well.

In this table, the dependent variables presented are the number of cigarettes smoked and smoking when one is so ill that one is bed-ridden. Both the age of first smoking and the age of first purchasing a cigarette were found to be statistically significant predictors despite the inclusion of two highly significant demographic control variables, namely, being Caucasian and being older, as well as the inclusion of gender, educational attainment, income, and marital status. The R-squared data indicate that more variance was accounted for with regard to the number of cigarettes smoked per week than smoking when ill and bed-ridden.

4. Discussion

Our findings show that the current smokers in our study typically smoked their first cigarette during adolescence, specifically in mid-adolescence. The mean age at which the study participants smoked their first cigarette was just shy of 15 years of age, with approximately one-half of all persons having initiated smoking behaviors between the ages of 12 and 16 years. This is a few years younger than the 17-18 years old age range reported by Fernander and colleagues [7] and Johnston and colleagues [1], but it is relatively close to the mean age of onset reported by Zabor and colleagues [17]. It is quite possible that people whose cigarette smoking ended with or shortly after initial experimentation, or people whose early-life smoking experiences did not turn into years-long smoking "habits," began smoking at later ages than those who took part in the present study. The present study, in contrast, was characterized by persistent smokers who, on average, began their smoking careers at a young age.

Our findings pertaining to the interval between first tobacco use and subsequent smoking behaviors showed that, ordinarily, only a short period of time elapsed between smoking initiation or experimentation and the continuation of tobacco use practices. Nearly three-quarters (71.2%) of the people in this study reported having "progressed" from their first tobacco use incident to their second one in less than one month's time. This brief interval will make it very difficult for smoking prevention and intervention programs to have an impact, because they will have very little time to identify youths who are using cigarettes for the first time and then do something to intervene in their behaviors so as to prevent subsequent use. Parental vigilance and involvement in their children's (especially their teenage children's) lives, and acute awareness on the part of teachers and other school officials who have daily contact with youths, are likely to be the principal avenues by which early intervention can occur once smoking behaviors have been initiated. Previously published studies support this contention [18–22]. Educating parents and teachers about how to identify the signs that a young person is experimenting with tobacco and then providing them with strategies that they can use to broach the subject of smoking in an effective

TABLE 2: Multivariate analysis for selected age-of-onset measures and adult smoking behaviors.

	No. of cigarettes smoked per week	No. of cigarettes smoked per week	Smoking when bed-ridden due to illness	Smoking when bed-ridden due to illness
Age of smoking first cigarette	−.12**	—	−.17***	—
Age of purchasing first cigarette	—	−.19***	—	−.22***
Gender (male)	.03	.03	−.06	−.07
Race (Caucasian)	.26***	.26***	.05	.05
Educational attainment (college graduate)	−.07	−.07	−.04	−.04
Income	.05	.05	.01	.02
Marital status ("involved")	−.04	−.04	.02	.02
Age	.21***	.22***	.06	.08
R-squared	**.112**	**.131**	**.037**	**.056**

**P < .01, and ***P < .001.

way with the youth(s) in question are essential if initial experiences with tobacco are to be prevented from turning into longer-term smoking behaviors. Supporting this type of approach, some studies have shown school-based smoking prevention/education/intervention programs to be effective at reducing tobacco use rates among children and adolescents [18, 23, 24].

The present study also revealed that the initial smoking experiences of about one-half of the study participants were more negative than they expected. Consistent with other published reports [17, 25], most of the people taking part in this study said that their first time smoking caused them to feel dizzy, made them cough, and/or left them with a bad taste. Despite these negative experiences and sensations, they chose to smoke again anyway. Other researchers have found, as the present study did, that even negative initial experiences with smoking are related to subsequent smoking behaviors later in life [26]. Also of relevance here is the fact that many studies have found that large proportions of the people who eventually went on to become regular smokers experienced a variety of negative effects from their initial tobacco use, such as nausea, dizziness, and coughing (among others) [17, 26, 27]. More research is needed to understand the myriad factors that lead people whose initial smoking experiences are negative to continue to experiment with smoking and subsequently to become regular smokers. Peer pressure-related explanations alone do not explain this occurrence, because only about one-sixth of the study participants, thinking in retrospect, said that this was an important reason why they continued to smoke after their initial experiences using tobacco. The study findings show that peer influences or peer pressure to smoke was less powerful than what has been claimed in other researches, a finding that has been reported by others as well [28, 29]. Indeed, it may be that it is not so much peer pressure *per se* that leads young people to experiment with smoking as it is peer norms that are tolerant of smoking that eases adolescents and young adults into the process of normalizing their opinions regarding smoking practices, which in turn leads some of them to be less resistant to experiment with tobacco. Media messages that normalize or glamorize smoking may contribute to this process as well

[28, 30, 31]. Likewise, parents who serve as in advertent role models for smoking behaviors or who provide weak or mixed messages with regard to adolescent smoking practices also play a role in fostering smoking-positive norms or belief structures for some youths, thereby increasing their odds of experimenting with tobacco [32–34].

In our study, there were two primary reasons cited by study participants as to why they elected to smoke again after their initial experiences with cigarettes: perceiving smoking to be "cool" and wanting to spend time with friends who were smokers. These reasons are consistent with those reported by other researchers (e.g., [25, 35, 36]), who have mentioned such factors as enjoying "the buzz" created by smoking, smoking to cope with stress, considering smokers to look "cool" or to appear to be grown-up, enjoying the taste of cigarettes, feeling more "perked up" or alert after smoking, and enjoying the social/friendship aspects of smoking behaviors (among others) as being the main reasons cited by people in their studies for their initial use of cigarettes. Relating to the present study, youth-focused antismoking campaigns need to work to counteract messages about the "coolness" of smoking, and they need to provide realistic but scare-tactic-free messages about the "down side" to smoking. This latter point is particularly important because research has shown that health promotion efforts to reduce smoking among young people are less effective if they are too harsh with regard to their efforts to induce fear and/or disgust in their target audience [37]. That research demonstrated that the inclusion of some fear components or some disgust-inducing messages can be effective, but that using too much of this type of content is counterproductive. Developing fun, engaging, eye-catching, attention-keeping multimedia campaigns (e.g., online informational websites, and video games) that address smoking in a way that is age-appropriate and engaging for youths are likely to be effective ways of helping to curtail youth smoking. An example of one such program that has been shown to be effective [38] is the Adolescent Smoking Cessation Escaping Nicotine and Tobacco (ASCENT) Program, originally created by researchers at Danya International. Another example of a promising multifaceted, multimedia approach to preventing smoking among youths has been named ASPIRE (A Smoking Prevention Interactive Experience). It, too, has been shown to be effective [39]. Results from a mobile phone-based multimedia program to foster smoking cessation among youths have also demonstrated efficacy [40]. More innovative programs like these, which utilize multimedia platforms and take into account the need to be creative in the various ways they try to engage young persons in the smoking prevention/cessation process, are needed.

Finally, we wish to discuss our findings pertaining to the age of onset of smoking behaviors and subsequent tobacco use practices. The strong tendency in this study was for earlier onset of smoking to be related to worse tobacco-related outcomes in adulthood. This is consistent with findings reported in the substance abuse literature generally (cited earlier) and in the tobacco literature specifically [9, 10, 12]). This finding highlights the importance of heading off early experimentation with cigarettes and to find ways to delay such experimentation to the greatest extent possible. Researchers and smoking prevention experts need to learn more about the factors that place people at risk for early-onset smoking. This is a topic about which little has been written (exceptions include the work of [9, 41]) and it is an area that would be fruitful for future researchers to explore. By learning more about who it is who is likely to experiment with smoking at an earlier age, we can increase the odds of reaching at-risk individuals and delaying (if not altogether preventing) their experimentation with cigarettes. Our findings suggest that, the longer this process can be delayed, the greater the likelihood is that better longer-term outcomes can be achieved.

Before concluding, we would like to acknowledge four potential limitations of this research. First, the data collected as part of this study of adult persistent smokers were all based on uncorroborated self-reports. Therefore, the extent to which respondents underreported or overreported their involvement in various smoking-related behaviors is unknown. In all likelihood, the self-reported data can be trusted, as numerous authors have noted that persons in their smoking studies have provided reasonably accurate information about their tobacco-using behaviors [42–44].

A second possible limitation pertains to recall bias. Respondents were asked to report about their beliefs, attitudes, and behaviors during the past 30 days or the past year, depending upon the measure in question. These time frames were chosen specifically: (1) to incorporate a large enough amount of time in the risk behavior questions' time frames so as to facilitate meaningful variability from person to person, and (2) to minimize recall bias. The exact extent to which recall bias affected the data cannot be assessed although other researchers collecting various types of smoking-related data have reported that recall bias is sufficiently minimal that its impact upon study findings is likely to be small [45]. This includes recall of earlier-life experiences pertaining to smoking onset [45].

On this same subject, recall bias may also affect the data in terms of the amount of time that elapsed between people's initial smoking behaviors and the present. For example, on average, when people were responding to questions about their first time smoking, they were reporting on events that occurred slightly more than 20 years ago (mean = 21.6, SD = 12.6, and median = 20.2). As another example, when providing information about the first time that they purchased a cigarette, respondents were reporting on events that took place slightly less than 20 years ago (mean = 19.4, SD = 12.4, median = 17.5). Although initial usage of cigarettes is the kind of behavior that people oftentimes are able to remember fairly clearly [46], there is no way for us to know or assess specifically how accurate their recall is of these earlier-life events. Thus, the extent to which this aspect of recall bias affects the data used in this study is unknown. Other authors have addressed this issue in their own studies of smoking behaviors, however, and they have indicated that recall bias regarding earlier-life smoking behaviors appears to be minimal [45, 47].

A third possible limitation of these data comes from the sampling strategy used. All interviews were conducted in the Atlanta, Georgia metropolitan area. There may very well be local or regional influences or subcultural differences between these persons and those residing elsewhere that could affect the generalizability of the data.

A fourth possible limitation of these data comes in the form of potential cohort effects and the influence that this potential source of bias could have on the findings. Specifically of concern here is the influence that changing social attitudes towards smoking, along with the concomitant changes in social policies regarding smokers and smoking in public places, might have on the younger smokers (who grew up and began smoking in a relatively antitobacco culture) versus the older smokers (many of whom grew up and began smoking in a relatively prosmoking culture). To examine this possible source of bias in the data, we conducted additional ad hoc analyses of our data, dividing the sample into two groups: those aged 18–39 and those aged 40 and older. The multivariate analyses shown in Table 2 were then undertaken separately for the two age cohorts, to determine whether or not there was evidence of this type of bias in our data. Although of course the specific coefficients obtained in the multivariate analyses did change when we examined the data for cohort effects, the actual, substantive findings pertaining to the first smoking and first cigarette purchase experiences did not change. Thus, we did not find statistical evidence of cohort effects influencing our findings, which lends credibility to the data and the findings as they currently are presented in the paper and helps to quell concerns about the impact of cohort effects on this study's main findings.

Acknowledgments

This research was supported by a grant from the National Institutes of Health, and the National Institute on Drug Abuse (Grant no. R01 DA015707, Principal Investigator: Claire Sterk).

References

[1] L. D. Johnston, P. O.'Malley, J. G. Bachman, and J. E. Schulenberg, *Monitoring the Future National Results on Adolescent*

Drug Use: Overview of Key Findings, 2010, Institute for Social Research, Ann Arbor, Miss, USA, 2011.

[2] J. E. Donovan, S. L. Leech, R. A. Zucker et al., "Really underage drinkers: alcohol use among elementary students," *Alcoholism*, vol. 28, no. 2, pp. 341–349, 2004.

[3] J. A. Grunbaum, L. Kann, S. Kinchen et al., "Youth risk behavior surveillance–United States, 2003," *Surveillance Summaries*, vol. 53, no. 2, pp. 1–96, 2004.

[4] J. W. LaBrie, A. Rodrigues, J. Schiffman, and S. Tawalbeh, "Early alcohol initiation increases risk related to drinking among college students," *Journal of Child and Adolescent Substance Abuse*, vol. 17, no. 2, pp. 125–141, 2008.

[5] Substance Abuse Mental Health Services Administration (SAMHSA), "Initiation of marijuana use: trends, patterns, and implications," 2008, http://www.oas.samhsa.gov/MJinitiation/highlights.htm.

[6] P. L. Ellickson, E. J. D'Amico, R. L. Collins, and D. J. Klein, "Marijuana use and later problems: when frequency of recent use explains age of initiation effects (and when it does not)," *Substance Use and Misuse*, vol. 40, no. 3, pp. 343–359, 2005.

[7] A. Fernander, M. K. Rayens, M. Zhang, and S. Adkins, "Are age of smoking initiation and purchasing patterns associated with menthol smoking?" *Addiction*, vol. 105, pp. 39–45, 2010.

[8] D. K. Eaton, L. Kann, S. Kinchen et al., "Youth risk behavior surveillance: United States, 2009," *Morbidity and Mortality Weekly Report*, vol. 59, no. 5, pp. 1–142, 2010.

[9] W. A. Vega and A. G. Gil, "Revisiting drug progression: long-range effects of early tobacco use," *Addiction*, vol. 100, no. 9, pp. 1358–1369, 2005.

[10] S. A. Khuder, H. H. Dayal, and A. B. Mutgi, "Age at smoking onset and its effect on smoking cessation," *Addictive Behaviors*, vol. 24, no. 5, pp. 673–677, 1999.

[11] P. F. Clarkin, L. A. Tiech, and A. S. Glicksman, "Socioeconomic correlates of current and regular smoking among college students in Rhode Island," *Journal of American College Health*, vol. 57, no. 2, pp. 183–190, 2008.

[12] W. W. Sanouri Ursprung, J. A. Savageau, and J. R. Difranza, "What is the significance of experiencing relaxation in response to the first use of nicotine," *Addiction Research and Theory*, vol. 19, no. 1, pp. 14–21, 2011.

[13] Centers for Disease Control and Prevention, "NHIS-Adult tobacco use information: smoking status recodes," 2009, http://www.cdc.gov/nchs/nhis/tobacco/tobacco_recodes.htm.

[14] M. G. Myers, D. M. McCarthy, L. MacPherson, and S. A. Brown, "Constructing a short form of the smoking consequences questionnaire with adolescents and young adults," *Psychological Assessment*, vol. 15, no. 2, pp. 163–172, 2003.

[15] A. L. Copeland, T. H. Brandon, and E. P. Quinn, "The smoking consequences questionnaire-adult: measurement of smoking outcome expectancies of experienced smokers," *Psychological Assessment*, vol. 7, no. 4, pp. 484–494, 1995.

[16] Centers for Disease Control and Prevention, "A for program early release of selected estimates from the National Health Interview Survey," 2009, http://www.cdc.gov/nchs/data/nhis/earlyrelease/ER_Booklet.htm.

[17] E. C. Zabor, Y. Li, L. M. Thornton et al., "Initial reactions to tobacco use and risk of future regular use," *Nicotine and Tobacco Research*, vol. 15, pp. 509–517, 2013.

[18] D. S. DeGarmo, J. M. Eddy, J. B. Reid, and R. A. Fetrow, "Evaluating mediators of the impact of the Linking the Interests of Families and Teachers (LIFT) multimodal preventive intervention on substance use initiation and growth across adolescence," *Prevention Science*, vol. 10, no. 3, pp. 208–220, 2009.

[19] N. Jairath, K. Mitchell, and B. Filleon, "Childhood smoking: the research, clinical and theoretical imperative for nursing action," *International Nursing Review*, vol. 50, no. 4, pp. 203–214, 2003.

[20] M. J. Karcher and L. Finn, "How connectedness contributes to experimental smoking among rural youth: developmental and ecological analyses," *Journal of Primary Prevention*, vol. 26, no. 1, pp. 25–36, 2005.

[21] E. M. Mahabee-Gittens, Y. Xiao, J. S. Gordon, and J. C. Khoury, "The dynamic role of parental influences in preventing adolescent smoking initiation," *Addictive Behaviors*, vol. 38, pp. 1905–1911, 2013.

[22] S. M. Suldo, S. Mihalas, H. Powell, and R. French, "Ecological predictors of substance use in middle school students," *School Psychology Quarterly*, vol. 23, no. 3, pp. 373–388, 2008.

[23] G. J. Botvin, K. W. Griffin, E. Paul, and A. P. Macaulay, "Preventing tobacco and alcohol use among elementary school students through life skills training," *Journal of Child and Adolescent Substance Abuse*, vol. 12, no. 4, pp. 1–17, 2003.

[24] A. Richardson, J.-P. He, L. Curry, and K. Merikangas, "Cigarette smoking and mood disorders in U.S. adolescents: sex-specific associations with symptoms, diagnoses, impairment and health services use," *Journal of Psychosomatic Research*, vol. 72, no. 4, pp. 269–275, 2012.

[25] R. Finkenauer, C. S. Pomerleau, S. M. Snedecor, and O. F. Pomerleau, "Race differences in factors relating to smoking initiation," *Addictive Behaviors*, vol. 34, no. 12, pp. 1056–1059, 2009.

[26] C. F. Ríos-Bedoya, C. S. Pomerleau, R. J. Neuman, and O. F. Pomerleau, "Using MIMIC models to examine the relationship between current smoking and early smoking experiences," *Nicotine and Tobacco Research*, vol. 11, no. 9, pp. 1035–1041, 2009.

[27] J. R. DiFranza, J. A. Savageau, K. Fletcher et al., "Recollections and repercussions of the first inhaled cigarette," *Addictive Behaviors*, vol. 29, no. 2, pp. 261–272, 2004.

[28] V. L. P. Clark, D. L. Miller, J. W. Creswell et al., "In conversation: high school students talk to students about tobacco use and prevention strategies," *Qualitative Health Research*, vol. 12, no. 9, pp. 1264–1283, 2002.

[29] M.-H. Go, H. D. Green, D. P. Kennedy, M. Pollard, and J. S. Tucker, "Peer influence and selection effects on adolescent smoking," *Drug and Alcohol Dependence*, vol. 109, no. 1–3, pp. 239–242, 2010.

[30] W. G. Shadel, S. C. Martino, A. Haviland, C. Setodji, and B. A. Primack, "Smoking motives in movies are important for understanding adolescent smoking: a preliminary investigation," *Nicotine and Tobacco Research*, vol. 12, no. 8, pp. 850–854, 2010.

[31] S. E. Tanski, M. Stoolmiller, S. D. Cin, K. Worth, J. Gibson, and J. D. Sargent, "Movie character smoking and adolescent smoking: who matters more, good guys or bad guys?" *Pediatrics*, vol. 124, no. 1, pp. 135–143, 2009.

[32] D. F. Herbert and K. M. Schiaffino, "Adolescents' smoking behavior and attitudes: the influence of mothers' smoking communication, behavior and attitudes," *Journal of Applied Developmental Psychology*, vol. 28, no. 2, pp. 103–114, 2007.

[33] C. K. Holub, J. I. Candelaria, and R. Laniado-Laborin, "Prevention strategies for parents on adolescent smoking: a gap between what they know and what they practice," in *New Developments*

in Parent-Child Relations, D. M. Devore, Ed., pp. 147–162, Nova Science Publishers, Hauppauge, NY, USA, 2006.

[34] A. V. Wilkinson, S. Shete, and A. V. Prokhorov, "The moderating role of parental smoking on their children's attitudes toward smoking among a predominantly minority sample: a cross-sectional analysis," *Substance Abuse*, vol. 3, article 18, 2008.

[35] S. S. Brady, A. V. Song, and B. L. Halpern-Felsher, "Adolescents report both positive and negative consequences of experimentation with cigarette use," *Preventive Medicine*, vol. 46, no. 6, pp. 585–590, 2008.

[36] D. Freeman, M. Brucks, and M. Wallendorf, "Young children's understandings of cigarette smoking," *Addiction*, vol. 100, no. 10, pp. 1537–1545, 2005.

[37] G. Leshner, P. Bolls, and E. Thomas, "Scare "em or disgust" em: the effects of graphic health promotion messages," *Health Communication*, vol. 24, no. 5, pp. 447–458, 2009.

[38] J. Hoffman, S. Nemes, J. Weil, S. Zack, K. Munly, and L. Hess, "Evaluation of the ASCENT smoking cessation program for adolescents," *Journal of Smoking Cessation*, vol. 3, pp. 2–8, 2008.

[39] A. V. Prokhorov, S. H. Kelder, R. Shegog et al., "Impact of A Smoking Prevention Interactive Experience (ASPIRE), an interactive, multimedia smoking prevention and cessation curriculum for culturally diverse high school students," *Nicotine and Tobacco Research*, vol. 10, no. 9, pp. 1477–1485, 2008.

[40] R. Whittaker, R. Maddison, H. McRobbie et al., "A multimedia mobile phone-based youth smoking cessation intervention: findings from content development and piloting studies," *Journal of Medical Internet Research*, vol. 10, no. 5, article e49, 2008.

[41] E. Z. Hanna, H.-Y. Yi, M. C. Dufour, and C. C. Whitmore, "The relationship of early-onset regular smoking to alcohol use, depression, illicit drug use, and other risky behaviors during early adolescence: results from the youth supplement to the Third National Health and Nutrition Examination Survey," *Journal of Substance Abuse*, vol. 13, no. 3, pp. 265–282, 2001.

[42] T. P. Johnson and J. A. Mott, "The reliability of self-reported age of onset of tobacco, alcohol and illicit drug use," *Addiction*, vol. 96, no. 8, pp. 1187–1198, 2001.

[43] J. D. Klein, R. K. Thomas, and E. J. Sutter, "Self-reported smoking in online surveys: prevalence estimate validity and item format effects," *Medical Care*, vol. 45, no. 7, pp. 691–695, 2007.

[44] C. A. Stanton, G. Papandonatos, E. E. Lloyd-Richardson, and R. Niaura, "Consistency of self-reported smoking over a 6-year interval from adolescence to young adulthood," *Addiction*, vol. 102, no. 11, pp. 1831–1839, 2007.

[45] O. F. Pomerleau, C. S. Pomerleau, A. M. Mehringer, S. M. Snedecor, and O. G. Cameron, "Validation of retrospective reports of early experiences with smoking," *Addictive Behaviors*, vol. 30, no. 3, pp. 607–611, 2005.

[46] N. Bradburn, S. Sudman, and B. Wansink, *Asking Questions: The Definitive Guide To Questionnaire Design-For Market Research, Political Polls, and Social and Health Questionnaires*, Jossey-Bass, New York, NY, USA, 2004.

[47] K. A. Perkins, C. Lerman, S. Coddington, and J. L. Karelitz, "Association of retrospective early smoking experiences with prospective sensitivity to nicotine via nasal spray in nonsmokers," *Nicotine and Tobacco Research*, vol. 10, no. 8, pp. 1335–1345, 2008.

8

A Preliminary Study of Functional Brain Activation among Marijuana Users during Performance of a Virtual Water Maze Task

Jennifer Tropp Sneider,[1,2,3] Staci A. Gruber,[2,3,4] Jadwiga Rogowska,[3] Marisa M. Silveri,[1,2,3] and Deborah A. Yurgelun-Todd[3,5]

[1] Neurodevelopmental Laboratory on Addictions and Mental Health, McLean Hospital, 115 Mill Street, Mail Stop 204, Belmont, MA 02478-1064, USA
[2] McLean Imaging Center, McLean Hospital, Boston, MA, USA
[3] Department of Psychiatry, Harvard Medical School, Belmont, MA, USA
[4] Cognitive and Clinical Neuroimaging Core, McLean Hospital, Belmont, MA, USA
[5] The Brain Institute, University of Utah Medical School, Salt Lake City, UT, USA

Correspondence should be addressed to Jennifer Tropp Sneider; jtsneider@mclean.harvard.edu

Academic Editor: Jennifer B. Unger

Numerous studies have reported neurocognitive impairments associated with chronic marijuana use. Given that the hippocampus contains a high density of cannabinoid receptors, hippocampal-mediated cognitive functions, including visuospatial memory, may have increased vulnerability to chronic marijuana use. Thus, the current study examined brain activation during the performance of a virtual analogue of the classic Morris water maze task in 10 chronic marijuana (MJ) users compared to 18 nonusing (NU) comparison subjects. Imaging data were acquired using blood oxygen level-dependent (BOLD) functional MRI at 3.0 Tesla during retrieval (hidden platform) and motor control (visible platform) conditions. While task performance on learning trials was similar between groups, MJ users demonstrated a deficit in memory retrieval. For BOLD fMRI data, NU subjects exhibited greater activation in the right parahippocampal gyrus and cingulate gyrus compared to the MJ group for the Retrieval-Motor Control contrast (NU > MJ). These findings suggest that hypoactivation in MJ users may be due to differences in the efficient utilization of neuronal resources during the retrieval of memory. Given the paucity of data on visuospatial memory function in MJ users, these findings may help elucidate the neurobiological effects of marijuana on brain activation during memory retrieval.

1. Introduction

Research on marijuana (MJ) use continues to be a major area of investigation, since MJ remains the most widely used illicit drug in several countries, including the United States [1]. Daily, long-term, and frequent MJ use can have serious adverse effects on mental and physical health and can affect work performance, family, and school functioning [2]. In 2009, epidemiological data (Treatment Episode Data Set) indicated that MJ was associated with 740,800 substance abuse treatment admissions, with daily use being reported in 23% of treatment entries [2]. Nearly half (46.3%) of daily MJ admissions occurred in individuals between ages 26 and 40 years old and 34.2% between ages 18 and 25 years old [2]. In addition, there has been a rise in the prevalence of MJ use among youth, with 36.4% and 22.6% of high school seniors reporting past year and past 30 days use, respectively. Given that rapid brain maturation occurs from adolescence into the early twenties [3, 4], a time when MJ use is often initiated and tends to increase, identifying neurobiological vulnerabilities associated with MJ use is critical.

Short-term effects of MJ have been reported across a number cognitive domains (for review [5, 6]), including deficits in memory [7], attention and mental flexibility [8], response inhibition [9], decision making [10, 11], emotional processing [12], and impulsivity [13]. However, to date there have been limited studies examining the effects of MJ on spatial memory processing. While chronic MJ users have been shown to exhibit deficits on tests of visual recognition, delayed visual recall, and prospective memory [14], a meta-analytic study failed to find substantial long-term neurocognitive deficits, except in the domains of learning and forgetting [15]. To this end, significant structural and functional changes have been reported in young MJ users in brain regions implicated in learning and memory [16–19].

The hippocampus may be notably vulnerable to the effects of MJ, given the high density of cannabinoid receptors in this area [20]. Findings from animal studies have provided evidence supporting cannabinoid-induced impairments on hippocampal-mediated memory tasks [21–27]. For instance, activation of cannaninoid-1 (CB_1) receptors in mice in the hippocampal region inhibited long-term potentiation (LTP), which is a neurobiological model for learning and memory [28]. Administration of delta-9-tetrahydrocannabinol (Δ^9-THC) impaired spatial memory in mice tested on the Morris water maze task (WMT), while the CB_1 receptor antagonist SR141716A reversed the impairment [26]. Similar Morris water maze impairments were reported in mice after injection of Δ^9-THC or inhalation of marijuana smoke [24]. These findings provide evidence of cannabinoid-induced impairments on hippocampus-dependent spatial learning tasks, likely due to interference in learning acquisition and retrieval processing.

The hippocampus is necessary for processing spatial layout and configural representation of an environment [29–35], as rodents with hippocampal lesions demonstrate spatial memory deficits, evidenced as an inability to find a hidden platform in the Morris WMT [30, 36, 37]. In addition to compelling animal literature indicating that MJ exposure impacts hippocampal function [23, 25, 38], humans with medial temporal lobe damage, including the hippocampus and associated areas, exhibit impaired declarative memory, such that patients have an inability to describe time, place, and meaning of events [39]. Patients with unilateral hippocampal resections demonstrate impaired spatial navigation during performance of a virtual Morris WMT [40]. Studies employing functional magnetic resonance imaging (fMRI) techniques provide evidence for altered brain activation patterns in memory-related processing regions associated with heavy MJ use. Long-term, heavy MJ users exhibit greater widespread blood oxygen level-dependent (BOLD) activation compared to NU during a spatial working memory task after short-term drug withdrawal [41]. In a study using a visuospatial 2-back working memory fMRI task, MJ users and NU exhibited similar task performance; however, MJ users demonstrated greater activation in the inferior and middle frontal gyri, areas associated with visuospatial working memory, and increased activation in the right superior temporal gyrus, an area not typically recruited for visuospatial working memory [42]. The parahippocampal area also plays an important role in spatial memory, namely, allocentric memory processing, especially during viewing of complex scenes with objects

and landmarks (e.g., [43–45]). An increased response in the parahippocampal gyrus has been reported for objects at relevant locations (i.e., at decision making points) during an object-location memory task [46], suggesting that neural activation in the parahippocampus is associated with the navigational relevance of an object's location.

The frontal cortex, specifically, the dorsolateral prefrontal cortex, has been implicated in spatial working memory tasks [47, 48]. While MJ effects on spatial working memory have been the subject of several investigations, the objective of the present study was to investigate MJ-related effects on spatial memory (learning and retrieval) to examine differences in neural activation during the performance of a virtual analogue of the Morris water maze task. Based on the work by Jager and colleagues [49], it was hypothesized that MJ users would demonstrate hypoactivity in the hippocampal/parahippocampal region relative to NU participants. Further, exploratory analysis of the cingulate gyrus was performed, given that this region is activated during WMT performance [50], but also frontal-related alterations associated with MJ use have been previously reported [42, 51, 52].

2. Methods

2.1. Participants. The study sample consisted of ten chronic marijuana (MJ) users (8 males) and eighteen nonusing (NU) comparison subjects (11 males). Participants were recruited through local advertisement and screened by telephone interview to ensure they met criteria for inclusion in the study. All aspects of the clinical research protocol were reviewed and approved by the Institutional Review Board of McLean Hospital (Belmont, MA, USA). After a complete description of the study, participants provided written informed consent. All participants received monetary compensation ($100) for study completion. Participant demographics are presented in Table 1.

To qualify for study entry, MJ smokers had to have smoked MJ a minimum of 2500 times, used MJ at least five of the last seven days prior to the study visit, test positive for urinary cannabinoids, and meet DSM-IV criteria for MJ abuse on the day of scanning. MJ users were asked to refrain from smoking for 12 hours immediately preceding the study visit and were told a urine sample would be collected at the initiation of the study visit, in order to improve compliance. The NU participants reported fewer than 5 lifetime episodes of MJ use and did not use any other illicit substances. Exclusion criteria for all subjects included history of head injury, loss of consciousness, history of organic mental disorder, seizure disorder or central nervous system disease, and contraindications to MR scanning (e.g., pacemaker, aneurysm clips, metallic implants, pregnancy, or claustrophobia). MJ users reported consuming 4.4 ± 4.3 alcoholic beverages per week, while NU participants reported consuming 1.8 ± 2.5 alcoholic beverages per week ($F(1, 26) = 4.2$, $P = .05$). Four MJ users reported recent nicotine use (ranging from 1 pack per day; 1 pack every 2 weeks; 1 pack per month; occasional/social use). NU adults did not report any use of nicotine.

TABLE 1: Demographic and marijuana use data.

	MJ ($n = 10$)	NU ($n = 18$)
Age (years)	20.3 ± 3.6	22.8 ± 5.0
	(Age range: 18–30)	(Age range: 18–33)
Education (years)	13.4 ± 1.5	15.5 ± 2.4
Ethnicity (Caucasian/non-Caucasian)[a]	9/0	11/7
SES[b]	43.4 ± 10.6	49.1 ± 12.2
Age of MJ onset	15.6 ± 1.2	—
Smokes per week	10.7 ± 5.5	—
Grams per week[c]	4.8 ± 4.9	—
Duration of use (yrs)	4.0 ± 2.4	—
ASI (MJ use out of 30 days)	25.5 ± 4.0	—
MWC	2.0 ± 2.1	—
THC (ng/mL)	193.5 ± 219.2	—

Data represent mean ± standard deviation. MJ: marijuana; NU: nonusers; SES: Socioeconomic status; ASI: Addiction Severity Index; MWC: Marijuana Withdrawal Check List. [a]One missing data point for MJ user. Non-Caucasian classification consisted of Asian, African American, and others. [b]One missing data point for NU. [c]Two missing data points for grams per week.

The Barratt Simplified Measure of Social Status (BSMSS) was used to measure socioeconomic status (SES) [53]. Clinical interviews were conducted using the Structured Clinical Interview for DSM-IV (SCID; [54]). All participants were free of Axis 1 diagnosis, except the MJ group, who were required to meet criteria for MJ abuse. Participants completed the Positive and Negative Affect Scale (PANAS; [55]), a 20-item scale measuring positive and negative affects, and the Hamilton Anxiety Scale (HAM-A; [56]), a 14-item scale measuring anxiety level. The Addiction Severity Index (ASI) was used to evaluate substance abuse using a 5-point scale (0 = not at all; 4 = extremely) for questions regarding seven areas in their life that include medical condition, employment, drug use, alcohol use, illegal activity, family/social relations, and psychiatric function [57]. The Marijuana Withdrawal Checklist (MWC), a 12-item scale, was used to assess withdrawal symptom during the early stages of abstinence is a 12-item scale used [58]. Clinical data are presented in Table 1.

All participants provided a urine sample to be tested for amphetamines, barbiturates, benzodiazepines, cocaine, opiates, phencyclidine, and tetrahydrocannabinol (THC) (Triage Drugs of Abuse Panel: Immediate Response Diagnostics, Biosite, San Diego, CA, USA). A positive result for THC confirmed recent MJ use in the MJ group, while a negative result was required for the NU group. Standard laboratory urinalysis assessed an aliquot of the urine sample, which included gas chromatography-mass spectroscopy in order to quantify the level of 11-nor-9-carboxy-delta 9-tetrahydrocannabinol (THC-COOH) and creatinine (Quest Diagnostics, Cambridge, MA, USA). To allow for differences in urinary concentration among the participants, levels of THC-COOH were normalized to urinary creatinine levels.

A measure of general intellectual ability (IQ) was derived using two of the four subtests (vocabulary and matrix reasoning) from the Wechsler Abbreviated Scale of Intelligence (WASI, [59]). Visuospatial ability and spatial perception were assessed using the Mental Rotation Task [60] and the Santa Barbara Sense-of-Direction Scale (SBSOD) [61]. The Mental Rotation Task is a four-minute paper-pencil test in which participants match a target item to two of four rotated versions. One point is given for a correct response, with a maximum score of 24. The SBSOD is a 15-item self-report measure of environmental spatial ability. The questionnaire consists of several statements about spatial and navigational abilities, preferences, and experiences. Subjects circle a number to indicate their level of agreement with each statement using a seven-point scale ranging from "1: strongly agree" to "7: strongly disagree".

A PC-compatible laptop was used for testing and operating the virtual water maze program (NeuroInvestigations, Inc., Lethbridge, Canada). The virtual environment was comprised of a circular pool located in the center of a square room, with four large abstract pictures positioned on the walls, which served as landmarks (Figure 1(a)). Subjects viewed the virtual environment from a first-person perspective and navigated through the environment using an MR-compatible joystick that allowed right, left, and forward, but not backward, movements. Participants began each trial facing the wall of the pool, from each of four starting positions: north, south, east, and west. The platform was always located in the northeast (NE) quadrant for all trials for all participants.

Prior to the start of the experiment (nonscanning and scanning conditions), participants completed a training phase outside of the MR suite, which consisted of two trials with the platform visible in the NE quadrant, in order to familiarize them with the task and the use of the joystick. The virtual environment used for training had landmarks that were unique from those in the virtual environment presented during nonscanning and during fMRI. The experimental phase consisted of three conditions: Learning (Hidden Trials—conducted outside the magnet/nonscanning); Retrieval (Hidden Trials—conducted in the magnet); Motor Control (Visible Trials—conducted in the magnet). During the Learning condition, each participant completed 4 blocks of hidden platform trials (4 trials per block, each trial beginning from a different location), in which the platform was hidden under the surface of the water and the participants were instructed to navigate to the platform as quickly as possible. The platform was always located in the same position. Once the participant successfully navigated to the area where the platform was located, a message on the computer displayed "Platform found." If the platform was not located within 60 sec, the platform became visible and the following message was displayed on the screen: "The platform is visible, swim to it." The next trial began 1 sec after the previous trial ended (1 sec intertrial interval (ITI)). After completion of the Learning trials, the Probe trial began, in which the platform was removed from the virtual environment unbeknownst to participants. The probe trial ended after participants navigated around the environment for 30 sec.

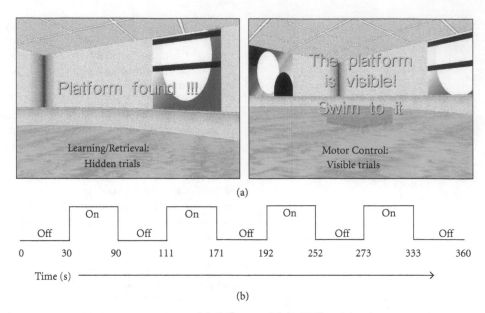

(a)

(b)

FIGURE 1: (a) Screen captures of the water maze task during the Learning and Retrieval conditions (hidden trials) (left) and the Motor Control condition (visible trials) (right). (b) BOLD fMRI scanning sequence used during Retrieval and Motor Control conditions.

The Retrieval Condition was similar to the Learning condition and participants were instructed to navigate to the hidden platform as quickly as they could. The platform was always located in the same location as during the learning condition. During the Motor Control condition, each participant completed 2 blocks of visible platform trials (4 trials per block, each trial beginning from a different location). The platform was visibly above the surface of the water and participants were instructed to navigate to the platform as quickly as possible, without paying attention to environmental landmarks. The location of the platform was the same as in the hidden condition, thereby minimizing the potential for encoding novel information during navigation in the environment. The scanning sequence lasted for 360 sec and consisted of alternating "on" (4 active "on" periods) and "off" periods (5 rest "off" periods). During the "on" periods participants navigated through the virtual environment and completed as many trials as possible within each of the four 60 sec "on" periods. Therefore, the number of completed trials varied between participants. During "off" periods, participants viewed a black screen that displayed the message "please wait for instructions" (Figure 1(b)).

Dependent measures for Learning, Retrieval, and Motor Control conditions on the WMT included path length, navigation latency, and first movement latency. Path length (relative to pool diameter) was measured as the distance to reach the platform. Navigation latency was measured as the total time (sec) to complete the task minus the total elapsed time (sec) prior to the first movement. Latency to first movement was measured as the time (sec) before the participant initiated navigation in the pool. Path length (distance to the platform), navigation latency, and latency to first movement measures were averaged across trials per block for the Learning, Retrieval, and Motor Control conditions. For the Probe trial, dependent measures included

percent of total distance traversed within the correct platform quadrant (NE), reflecting as an index of spatial learning, and heading error towards the platform, calculated as the angular deviation from a straight path to the center of the platform from the starting position. Heading error was measured at the first occurrence that participant distance was greater than 25% of the pool diameter from the starting position. The number of trials completed during the Retrieval and Motor Control conditions was also recorded.

Two independent raters blind to participant diagnosis rated navigation strategies used by participants during the Probe trial. The strategy chosen to solve the water maze could affect behavioral performance [62]. Participant navigation strategies were rated as a direct strategy, where participants navigated directly to the platform location, or a nondirect strategy, where participants navigated in a circuitous or random route that was not in the direction of the platform quadrant (NE) (Figure 2). Interrater reliability for strategy coding was $r = .53$, $P = .004$ (Pearson's r correlation coefficient, two-tailed).

2.2. Functional MRI Acquisition. Functional MRI scanning was performed on a 3T Siemens Trio whole-body MR scanner (Siemens Healthcare, Erlangen, Germany), using a birdcage quadrature RF head coil for acquisition of echo planar imaging (EPI) blood oxygen level-dependent (BOLD) fMRI. Sagittal scout images were first acquired for alignment and localization using a fast spin echo sequence (FSE) with the following parameters: repetition time (TR) = 3 msec, echo time (TE) = 40 msec, field of view (FOV) = 20 cm, matrix size = 64 × 64, slice thickness = 7 mm (1 mm gap), and flip angle = 90°. Images were acquired from the whole brain using the following parameters: 100 images per slice using a single-shot, gradient pulse-echo sequence, slice thickness = 5 mm, 0 mm skip, flip angle = 90°, TE = 30 msec, and

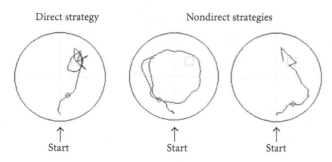

FIGURE 2: Sample strategies used by participants during the WMT Probe trial. For the direct strategy (left), participants navigated directly to the platform, and for the nondirect strategy (right), participants navigated in a circuitous or random route that was not in the direction of the platform quadrant.

TR = 3000 msec. For each participant, matched T1 and T2 EPI image sets were also obtained: T1-matrix size = 256×256, TR = 5760 msec; TE = 80 msec, number of shots = 4, flip = 90°; T2-matrix size = 256 × 256, TR = 6680 msec, TE = 75 msec, number of shots = 4, flip = 90°; 64×64 image matrix, 3 mm × 3 mm in plane resolution. In order to maximize the amplitude of the task-induced signal intensity changes, a gradient echo pulse sequence was utilized. The virtual water maze environment was projected via an LCD video projector (Resonance Technology Inc., Northridge, CA, USA) onto a translucent screen located at the rear of the bore, visible to subjects using a mirror mounted on the head coil.

2.3. Functional MRI Analyses. SPM5 (Wellcome Department of Imaging Neuroscience, University College, London, UK) was run in Matlab (MathWorks, Natick, MA, USA) for analysis of functional MRI data. To correct for motion in BOLD fMRI data, an intrarun realignment algorithm was utilized, which uses the first image as a reference. An exclusionary criterion of 2 mm of head motion in any direction was used. An EPI template in Montreal Neurological Institute (MNI) stereotactic space was employed to normalize the realigned images, which were resampled into 2 mm cubic voxels. To spatially smooth the normalized images, an isotropic Gaussian filter (full width half maximum [FWHM] = 10 mm) was then applied [63]. In SPM5, high-pass temporal filtering, with a cut-off of 128 sec was applied, and serial autocorrelations were modeled using an AR(1) model. Global scaling was not utilized. Using the framework of the general linear model, statistical analysis for individual subjects was performed [64, 65] using a box-car reference function convolved with the hemodynamic response function.

The motor control condition of the water maze paradigm was used as a control condition since there was no learning or memory component (i.e., subjects simply navigate to the visible platform). Age was entered as a covariate into the analysis. To identify brain areas activated during hidden conditions, predetermined condition effects were calculated at each voxel by the fixed model and a single image of mean activation for Retrieval-Motor Control was created for each

subject. The group data were then analyzed using a random-effects model on a second level to account for interindividual variance. Comparisons between groups (NU > MJ; MJ > NU) were performed using a two-sample t-test with a priori threshold of $P < .005$, uncorrected, with a minimum extent threshold (k) set at 20 contiguous voxels. Anatomic regions (hippocampus, parahippocampal gyrus, and cingulate gyrus) for the region of interest analyses were automatically defined using the Automated Anatomical Labeling atlas [66] in SPM5 using a threshold of $P < .05$ and $k = 20$. Thresholds were based on previously published methods used in BOLD fMRI studies of MJ users [12, 41, 50, 67].

2.4. Statistical Analysis. One-way analyses of variance (ANOVAs) were used to compare MJ users and NU on demographic, clinical measures, cognitive measures, and behavioral measures. SPSS 18.0 (SPSS, Chicago, IL) was used for all statistical analyses (α = .05). Two-way (Group × Block) repeated measures analyses of variance (ANOVAs) were conducted for path length, navigation latency, first movement latency on WMT Learning trials. One-way ANOVAs were conducted for all other WMT performance measures. Chi-square nonparametric analyses were conducted to compare navigation strategies, that is, direct strategy versus the nondirect strategy, between groups. Significant group differences were observed for age ($F(1, 27) = 5.0$, $P = .03$) and education ($F(1, 27) = 5.10$, $P = .03$), and, therefore, fMRI analyses included age as a covariate.

3. Results

3.1. Demographic Variables. As illustrated in Table 1, data for the MJ group confirm near daily MJ use, as indicated by ASI scores of MJ use in the last 30 days, smoking episodes per week, total grams of MJ used per week and average urinary cannabinoid levels (ng/mg). MJ users also reported very low scores (out of a total 36) on the MWC, suggesting no significant withdrawal symptoms were present on study day.

3.2. Clinical and Cognitive Measures. No significant differences were observed between the groups for IQ, as measured by WASI, or for mood, as measured by the HAM-A, or on PANAS (positive or negative affect subscales) (Table 2). Further, no significant performance differences were detected between the MJ and NU groups on the Mental Rotation Test Total Score, or on the SBSOD Total Score (Table 2).

3.3. Virtual Water Maze Behavioral Performance

3.3.1. Pre-fMRI Hidden Platform Trials: Learning. There was a significant effect of Block ($F(3, 78) = 5.1$, $P < .005$), with both groups displaying shorter path lengths to reach the hidden platform by the fourth block (Figure 3). For navigation latency, there also was a significant main effect of Block ($F(3, 78) = 3.8$, $P < .05$), again with both

TABLE 2: Clinical and cognitive measures.

	MJ ($n = 10$)	NU ($n = 18$)	F	P
PANAS				
Positive affect	30.9 ± 6.6	33.9 ± 7.5	1.1	0.29
Negative affect	12.2 ± 3.2	11.7 ± 2.4	0.2	0.66
HAM-A	2.7 ± 2.3	1.5 ± 1.7	2.5	0.12
Mental rotation total score	16.6 ± 4.6	14.7 ± 4.9	1.0	0.33
SBSOD total score[a]	4.8 ± 0.7	4.6 ± 1.0	0.2	0.68
WASI IQ	121.3 ± 8.3	120.2 ± 8.9	0.1	0.74

Data represent mean ± standard deviation. MJ: marijuana; NU: nonusers. PANAS: positive and negative affect scale; HAM-A: Hamilton Anxiety Scale; SBSOD: Santa Barbara Sense-of-Direction Scale; WASI: Wechsler Abbreviated Scale of Intelligence. [a]MJ = 8; NU = 14.

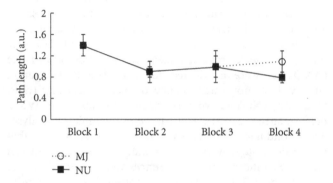

FIGURE 3: Average path lengths on WMT hidden trials during the Learning condition in MJ (open circles) and NU (closed squares) groups across trial blocks.

groups displaying shorter navigation latencies to successfully complete the trial with increasing number of completed trials (Block 1: 16.0 ± 9.2; Block 2: 11.0 ± 6.9; Block 3: 12.9 ± 13.2; Block 4: 9.8 ± 6.4). There was a significant main effect of Block ($F(3, 78) = 17.1, P < .001$) for latency to first movement, with both groups displaying shorter latencies to initiate movement by the fourth block (Block 1: 5.6.0 ± 1.8; Block 2: 4.1 ± 1.8; Block 3: 4.1 ± 1.7; Block 4: 3.8 ± 1.9). No interactions Block × Group interactions reached statistical significance for any of these measures.

3.3.2. Pre-fMRI Probe Trial: Retention. The Group effect for Retention trended towards significance, with MJ users displaying a lower percentage of total navigation distance within the NE (correct) platform quadrant on the Probe trial relative to NU (41.6% ± 15.6 versus 50.7% ± 10.6, resp.; include F value, $P = .08$). Heading error did not differ significantly between MJ and NU groups (27.9 degrees° ± 28.6 and 20.6° ± 21.5, resp.).

3.3.3. fMRI Hidden Platform Trials: Retrieval. The number of hidden platform trials completed during fMRI did not differ between groups, with MJ users completing 10.3 ± 3.6 and NU completing 11.4 ± 2.7 hidden platform trials during fMRI BOLD acquisition. Despite a lack of difference in the number of trials completed, there was a significant group

effect for latency to first movement. MJ users demonstrated shorter latencies to first movement (3.2 sec ± 1.2) relative to NU (4.6 ± 1.6) ($F(1, 26) = 5.9, P < .05$) and longer path lengths to reach the hidden platform (MJ: 1.7 ± 1.5 versus NU: 0.8 ± 0.4; $F(1, 26) = 4.8, P < .05$). There were no significant group differences for navigation latency (MJ users: 15.1 ± 12.9; NU: 9.9 ± 5.5).

3.3.4. fMRI Visible Platform Trials: Motor Control. The number of visible platform trials completed also did not differ between groups, with MJ users completing 15.7 ± 1.3 and NU completing 15.0 ± 1.4 visible platform trials during fMRI BOLD acquisition. There were no significant group differences observed for path length (MJ users: 0.5 ± 0.1; NU: 0.4 ± 0.01), navigation latency (MJ users: 3.9 ± 0.5; NU: 3.9 ± 0.7), or latency to first movement (MJ users: 3.3 ± 1.4; NU: 4.4 ± 1.7).

3.3.5. fMRI Navigation Strategies. There was a significant preference observed for the use of a direct versus a nondirect strategy during the Probe Trial in the NU group, with 78% ($n = 14$) employing a direct search strategy and 22% ($n = 4$) employing a nondirect strategy ($\chi^2(1, 18) = 5.6, P < .05$). A strategy preference was not observed in the MJ group, 50% ($n = 5$) utilized a direct strategy and 50% ($n = 5$) utilized a nondirect strategy.

3.3.6. fMRI BOLD Activation. Whole-Brain Analysis: Retrieval-Motor Control Condition. NU, relative to MJ group, demonstrated greater BOLD activation in the bilateral inferior frontal pars triangularis and bilateral inferior frontal pars opercularis, left superior frontal gyrus, left superior frontal pars orbitalis, bilateral middle frontal gyrus, right pallidum, and right putamen for the Retrieval-Motor Control contrast (Table 3). However, the MJ group relative to NU did not show greater BOLD activation in any region (Table 3).

Region of Interest Analysis: Retrieval-Motor Control Condition. NU, relative to MJ group, displayed significantly greater BOLD activation in the right parahippocampal gyrus (cluster size (k) = 26, $x = 24, y = -4, z = -28$, P uncorrected = 0.018) for the Retrieval-Motor Control contrast (Figure 4(a)). However, no significant group differences in BOLD activation were detected in the hippocampus. In addition, MJ users demonstrated no regions of greater BOLD activation relative to the NU group in either the parahippocampal gyrus or hippocampus. For the exploratory analysis of the cingulate gyrus, the NU group relative to the MJ group also demonstrated greater bilateral anterior cingulate gyrus and bilateral midcingulate gyrus activation (Figure 4(b)), however, MJ users showed no greater activation in this area relative to the NU group (Table 4).

4. Discussion

This pilot study compared current, chronic MJ users and NU during performance of a virtual water maze task of spatial learning and memory. While task performance on learning

TABLE 3: Foci of maximally activated brain regions—Retrieval-Motor Control.

Whole brain Region	BA	MNI coordinates			Cluster size (k)	T-max	Voxel P uncorrected	Cohen's d
		x	y	z				
NU > MJ								
L inferior frontal pars triangularis	45	−46	20	12	44	4.46	<.001	1.78
L inferior frontal pars opercularis								
L superior frontal pars orbitalis	47	−26	46	−2	36	3.78	<.001	1.51
L superior frontal gyrus								
L middle frontal gyrus	46	−42	40	28	201	3.67	.001	1.47
L inferior frontal pars triangularis								
R pallidum	48	18	6	−4	25	3.42	.001	1.37
R putamen								
R inferior frontal pars triangularis								
R inferior frontal pars orbitalis	47	40	42	0	25	3.24	.002	1.30
R middle frontal gyrus								
MJ > NU		—	—	—		—	n.s.	

L: left hemisphere; R: right hemisphere. BA: Brodmann area. $P < .005$ (uncorrected).

TABLE 4: Region of interest analysis of bold activation—Retrieval-Motor Control.

Region	MNI coordinates			Cluster size (k)	T-max	Voxel P uncorrected	Cohen's d
	x	y	z				
NU > MJ							
Hippocampus	—	—	—		—	n.s.	
R. parahippocampal gyrus	24	−4	−28	26	2.20	.018	0.88
Anterior cingulate gyrus	10	38	−4	316	3.11	.002	1.24
Midcingulate gyrus	12	−12	40	563	2.97	.003	1.19
MJ > NU							
Hippocampus	—	—	—		—	n.s.	
Parahippocampal gyrus	—	—	—		—	n.s.	
Cingulate gyrus	—	—	—		—	n.s.	

L: left hemisphere; R: right hemisphere. $P < .05$ (uncorrected).

trials was similar between groups, there was a trend for MJ users to display a lower percentage of total navigation distance within the correct quadrant during the probe trial relative to NU, suggesting a subtle difference in memory retention. During performance on hidden trials during fMRI, although the number of completed trials did not differ between groups, MJ users exhibited significantly longer path lengths and shorter latencies to first movement, which also indicates a deficit in memory retrieval. Performance on visible trials did not differ between groups, however, suggesting that groups had comparable motor abilities. Visuospatial perception (i.e., mental rotation) and environmental spatial ability (i.e., Santa Barbara Sense of Direction Scale) also did not differ between groups, which is consistent with a previous investigation that failed to find differences in orientation skills in MJ users [68]. Importantly, this first pilot fMRI investigation of water maze performance in current MJ users revealed that in addition to some behavioral performance differences during memory retrieval, brain activation patterns differed significantly during task performance, with

MJ users demonstrating less BOLD activation in the right parahippocampus and the cingulate gyrus relative to NU.

The parahippocampal area is necessary for the processing associations between landmark objects and the environment (landmark-based memory), or contextual memory [69]. In the current study, the NU group demonstrated greater recruitment of the parahippocampus during the retrieval of the hidden platform location, which was located between two relevant landmarks (e.g., abstract paintings) within the environment, which provides consistent support for this brain region being involved in spatial navigation in healthy adults [50]. Although there are no existing data on MJ effects on BOLD activation during a spatial memory task, alterations in hippocampal activation in MJ users relative to nonusers have been reported for nonspatial, associative memory tasks. Jager and colleagues [49] reported that despite normal memory performance, abstinent MJ users displayed hypoactivity in the hippocampal/parahippocampal area compared to NU during the learning phase of a pictorial memory pairing task [49]. In contrast, hyperactivation of

Parahippocampal gyrus
NU > MJ users

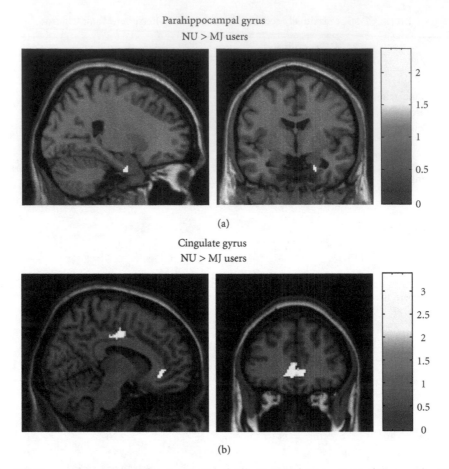

(a)

Cingulate gyrus
NU > MJ users

(b)

FIGURE 4: Representative SPM images depicting significant activation for the Retrieval-Motor Control contrast for NU > MJ contrast. (a) NU displayed greater activation in the right parahippocampal gyrus relative to the MJ group. (b) NU displayed greater activation in the bilateral anterior cingulate gyrus and bilateral midcingulate gyrus relative to the MJ group. For the MJ > NU contrast, the MJ group showed no regions of greater BOLD activation relative to NU group. All images are in neurological orientation, that is, left = left and right = right; the color bar at the right reflects the suprathreshold value of the SPM (t) statistic for the analysis.

the hippocampal/parahippocampal area was reported during the learning phase in a face-name matching task in MJ users compared to nonusers [51]. Similarly, hyperactivation in the left parahippocampal gyrus was observed during the encoding of face-profession pairs in high-frequency versus low-frequency MJ users [70]. Overall, these data suggest evidence for hippocampal/parahippocampal activation differences associated with MJ use during the performance of memory tasks, although memory for objects versus memory for faces may underlie the MJ-related differences in the direction of BOLD activation effects (hypoactivation versus hyperactivation) across these previously published studies.

In the present study, exploratory analysis of the cingulate gyrus revealed greater activation of the anterior cingulate and the midcingulate gyrus during memory retrieval in the NU group compared to the MJ group. The anterior cingulate cortex is an executive region that plays a critical role in modulation of attention, with reciprocal connections with the amygdala, providing support for its role in arousal and motivation [71]. These preliminary data suggest that NU may differentially activate this frontal region to meet the attentional demands posed by this task, which subsequently

leads to a greater utilization of attentional resources during memory retrieval as compared to MJ users. These findings are consistent with previous studies, in which frontal hypoactivation was observed in MJ users relative to nonusers [51]. Nestor and colleagues [51] demonstrated hypoactivation in the frontal gyrus in MJ users relative to nonusers during the learning phase in a face-name association task. The majority of remaining available data on brain activation differences associated with MJ use are based on investigations of spatial working memory, which employs a different neural circuitry that is more frontally mediated, compared to more traditional memory tasks that involve the medial temporal lobe. Nonetheless, adolescents with recent MJ use exhibit greater activation of the medial and left superior prefrontal cortex and bilateral anterior insula, despite similar task performance, and as compared to an abstinent group and nonusers during the performance of a 2-back spatial working memory task [52]. In addition, young adult MJ users were reported to demonstrate greater activation in the inferior and middle frontal gyri, as well as the right superior temporal gyrus, an area not typically recruited for visual spatial working memory during the performance of a visuospatial 2-back working memory task [42]. Long-term heavy MJ users also exhibit increased activation in the prefrontal cortex and anterior cingulate, as well as the basal ganglia, compared to non-users, during performance of a spatial working memory task [41]. Taken together, these data suggest that MJ users exhibit altered neural functioning during spatially-related cognitive challenges, with deficits being observed in both frontal and temporal cortices and suggesting evidence for compensatory and adaptive functioning to overcome inefficient activation of the neural network associated.

Brain activation changes associated with MJ use appear to be task specific, with some studies demonstrating hyper-activation, suggestive of increased recruitment, and other studies demonstrating hypoactivation, suggestive of inefficient neural networking [42, 51, 52]. Overall, studies that have reported hyperactivation of brain areas suggest functional compensation and possible neural recruitment of additional brain areas [5]. Alterations in brain activation (e.g., hypoactivation) can also be affected by differences in cerebral blood volume (CBV) and cerebral blood flow (CBF) [72]. Studies using dynamic susceptibility contrast magnetic resonance imaging (DSC MRI) have provided important insight into the effects of marijuana on cerebral hemodynamics, demonstrating that while CBV levels begin to normalize with continued abstinence from marijuana in frontal areas, temporal and cerebellar brain regions show slower CBV decreases [73, 74]. These findings have important implications for understanding the effects of changes in the microvasculature blood volume and/or blood flow that can affect fMRI BOLD signal in chronic marijuana users and nonusers [73, 74].

At least in the current study, the strategy chosen to solve the water maze could have affected behavioral performance [62]. A significantly greater percentage of NU than MJ users employed a direct navigation strategy, which relies on spatial cues and is the most efficient means to reach the platform quadrant. Indeed, only half of the MJ users used a direct approach to complete the task, which may have contributed to the trend for worse performance on the Probe trial and greater path lengths during retrieval. It is plausible that choosing a less efficient strategy to solve the water maze could have likewise contributed to differences in BOLD activation during spatial navigation. These preliminary findings should therefore be replicated in a larger sample of MJ and NU subjects, which would permit the ability to examine strategy choice in relationship to BOLD activation during spatial memory task performance.

There are a number of strengths and weakness associated with this pilot study. A strength of this study is that it is the first investigation of hippocampal brain activation during the performance of a virtual analogue of the well-established Morris water maze task in MJ users, who were well characterized, clinically diagnosed with marijuana abuse, and who did not meet criteria for any other substance abuse disorders. Furthermore, self-report of marijuana use was confirmed by urine drug toxicology screen and results from the SCID and the MWC suggest that in this sample of chronic, heavy MJ smokers, they were not experiencing significant withdrawal symptoms at the time of assessment. In terms of

limitations, only a modest number of subjects were examined in this pilot study, which limits generalizability and precludes the ability to examine sex differences within the groups. Performance measures of spatial ability typically have large variability and, therefore, the current investigation should be replicated using a larger sample of subjects. However, despite the modest sample size, significant BOLD activation differences in the parahippocampal and cingulate region were detected. Although differences in age may have been a potential confound, fMRI analyses were corrected for age and differences remained significant between groups. The MJ group also endorsed more alcohol and tobacco use than the NU comparison group, albeit at modest, nonclinical levels. Nonetheless, effects on BOLD activation cannot be ruled out, particularly since nicotinic alpha-7 acetylcholine receptors are highly distributed in the hippocampus [75] and alcohol use has been reported to block the induction of long-term potentiation in hippocampal rat slices [76]. Although subjects from the current study were well characterized with regard to their clinical, demographic and MJ-use status, formal personality testing was not completed with instruments designed to specifically assess Axis II pathology, which may impact neurocognitive performance. It is of note, however, that the majority of these subjects (80%) were enrolled in a separate, multiweek study, which repeatedly assessed clinical state through clinical scales and interviews, and none appeared to meet criteria or demonstrate any symptoms of a personality disorder [67, 77]. In terms of fMRI data processing, the Automated Anatomical Labeling (AAL) atlas was used to define region of interest (ROIs). It is difficult to localize activation in small areas such as the hippocampus, since areas such as the parahippocampal cortex, fusiform gyrus, and lingual gyrus surround this area. Thus, the atlas map chosen for analysis could have contributed to varied results across studies.

The length of the period of abstinence from marijuana use has been shown to impact performance on memory tasks and brain function [78]. Even though, the MWC suggests that the MJ users are not experiencing significant withdrawal symptoms, it cannot be discounted that the observed group differences could still reflect residual effects of MJ use and may account for the disparate findings amongst studies. While the MJ users in the Jager et al. study [49] were abstinent for at least 7 days prior to testing, participants in the current pilot study abstained for only a minimum of 12 hours. Regardless, both studies demonstrated hypoactivation of the hippocampus and parahippocampal gyrus in MJ users relative to nonusers during a learning and memory task. In order to examine the potential adverse effects of MJ use on neural activity beyond a week of abstinence, a logical next step to this work would be to examine subjects who have undergone a longer period of abstinence to explore whether functional changes in BOLD signal between MJ users and NU result from potential washout effects associated with drug abstinence.

In summary, data from this pilot study demonstrate significant differences in BOLD activation in MJ users compared to a NU comparison group during memory retrieval on a spatial navigation task. These data suggest that MJ users utilize neuronal resources in a manner that differs from NU, as suggested by the observed hypoactivation of the/parahippocampal area during navigation, but perhaps also from frontal hypoactivation due to the attentional demands of the task. Further research is warranted to determine the potential mechanism of action by which MJ use may affect brain activation during memory retrieval. Nevertheless, the current findings demonstrate that MJ use exerts a significant effect on neural activity, which is relevant to public health concerns associated with understanding the long-term consequences of chronic marijuana use on brain function in young adults. Indeed, altered brain function in the absence of gross behavioral performance differences may be an early indicator of future long-term consequences associated with continued use, particularly given that relatively short history of MJ use in the current study sample. Early alterations in neuronal function may potentially be related to the later manifestation of MJ-related cognitive impairments, as well as an increased risk for psychiatric conditions [79], which underscores the need for additional investigations focusing on the neurobiological consequences of MJ use.

Acknowledgments

This work was supported by NIDA Grant no. R03 DA022482 (J. T. Sneider). The authors wish to thank Dr. Derek Hamilton for his technical assistance with the virtual water maze task. In addition, the authors thank Dr. William D. S. Killgore for programming the virtual water maze for use with fMRI as well as his helpful feedback.

References

[1] National Institute on Drug Abuse, *NIDA InfoFacts*, U.S. Department of Health and Human Services, Bethesda, MD, USA, 2009.

[2] TEDS, *Substance Abuse and Mental Health Services Administration (Center for Behavioral Health Statistics and Quality), the TEDS Report*, Marijuana Admissions Reporting Daily Use at Treatment Entry, Rockville, Md, USA, 2012.

[3] C. M. Bennett and A. A. Baird, "Anatomical changes in the emerging adult brain: a voxel-based morphometry study," *Human Brain Mapping*, vol. 27, no. 9, pp. 766–777, 2006.

[4] E. V. Sullivan, A. Pfefferbaum, T. Rohlfing, F. C. Baker, M. L. Padilla, and I. M. Colrain, "Developmental change in regional brain structure over 7 months in early adolescence: comparison of approaches for longitudinal atlas-based parcellation," *NeuroImage*, vol. 57, no. 1, pp. 214–224, 2011.

[5] R. Martin-Santos, A. B. Fagundo, J. A. Crippa et al., "Neuroimaging in cannabis use: a systematic review of the literature," *Psychological Medicine*, vol. 40, no. 3, pp. 383–398, 2010.

[6] R. J. van Holst and T. Schilt, "Drug-related decrease in neuropsychological functions of abstinent drug users," *Current Drug Abuse Reviews*, vol. 4, no. 1, pp. 42–56, 2011.

[7] R. A. Battisti, S. Roodenrys, S. J. Johnstone, C. Respondek, D. F. Hermens, and N. Solowij, "Chronic use of cannabis and poor neural efficiency in verbal memory ability," *Psychopharmacology*, vol. 209, no. 4, pp. 319–330, 2010.

[8] H. G. Pope and D. Yurgelun-Todd, "The residual cognitive effects of heavy marijuana use in college students," *Journal of the American Medical Association*, vol. 275, no. 7, pp. 521–527, 1996.

[9] S. A. Gruber and D. A. Yurgelun-Todd, "Neuroimaging of marijuana smokers during inhibitory processing: a pilot investigation," *Cognitive Brain Research*, vol. 23, no. 1, pp. 107–118, 2005.

[10] K. I. Bolla, D. A. Eldreth, J. A. Matochik, and J. L. Cadet, "Neural substrates of faulty decision-making in abstinent marijuana users," *NeuroImage*, vol. 26, no. 2, pp. 480–492, 2005.

[11] C. T. Whitlow, A. Liguori, L. Brooke Livengood et al., "Long-term heavy marijuana users make costly decisions on a gambling task," *Drug and Alcohol Dependence*, vol. 76, no. 1, pp. 107–111, 2004.

[12] S. A. Gruber, J. Rogowska, and D. A. Yurgelun-Todd, "Altered affective response in marijuana smokers: an FMRI study," *Drug and Alcohol Dependence*, vol. 105, no. 1-2, pp. 139–153, 2009.

[13] S. A. Gruber, M. M. Silveri, M. K. Dahlgren, and D. Yurgelun-Todd, "Why so impulsive? White matter alterations are associated with impulsivity in chronic marijuana smokers," *Experimental and Clinical Psychopharmacology*, vol. 19, no. 3, pp. 231–242, 2011.

[14] S. McHale and N. Hunt, "Executive function deficits in short-term abstinent cannabis users," *Human Psychopharmacology*, vol. 23, no. 5, pp. 409–415, 2008.

[15] I. Grant, R. Gonzalez, C. L. Carey, L. Natarajan, and T. Wolfson, "Non-acute (residual) neurocognitive effects of cannabis use: a meta-analytic study," *Journal of the International Neuropsychological Society*, vol. 9, no. 5, pp. 679–689, 2003.

[16] M. Ashtari, B. Avants, L. Cyckowski et al., "Medial temporal structures and memory functions in adolescents with heavy cannabis use," *Journal of Psychiatric Research*, vol. 45, no. 8, pp. 1055–1066, 2011.

[17] L. K. Jacobsen, K. R. Pugh, R. T. Constable, M. Westerveld, and W. E. Mencl, "Functional correlates of verbal memory deficits emerging during nicotine withdrawal in abstinent adolescent cannabis users," *Biological Psychiatry*, vol. 61, no. 1, pp. 31–40, 2007.

[18] J. Jacobus, S. Bava, M. Cohen-Zion, O. Mahmood, and S. F. Tapert, "Functional consequences of marijuana use in adolescents," *Pharmacology Biochemistry and Behavior*, vol. 92, no. 4, pp. 559–565, 2009.

[19] K. L. Medina, A. D. Schweinsburg, M. Cohen-Zion, B. J. Nagel, and S. F. Tapert, "Effects of alcohol and combined marijuana and alcohol use during adolescence on hippocampal volume and asymmetry," *Neurotoxicology and Teratology*, vol. 29, no. 1, pp. 141–152, 2007.

[20] M. Herkenham, A. B. Lynn, and M. D. Little, "Cannabinoid receptor localization in brain," *Proceedings of the National Academy of Sciences of the United States of America*, vol. 87, no. 5, pp. 1932–1936, 1990.

[21] R. E. Hampson and S. A. Deadwyler, "Role of cannabinoid receptors in memory storage," *Neurobiology of Disease*, vol. 5, no. 6, part B, pp. 474–482, 1998.

[22] R. E. Hampson and S. A. Deadwyler, "Cannabinoids, hippocampal function and memory," *Life Sciences*, vol. 65, no. 6-7, pp. 715–723, 1999.

[23] L. Iversen, "Cannabis and the brain," *Brain*, vol. 126, part 6, pp. 1252–1270, 2003.

[24] F. Niyuhire, S. A. Varvel, B. R. Martin, and A. H. Lichtman, "Exposure to marijuana smoke impairs memory retrieval in mice," *Journal of Pharmacology and Experimental Therapeutics*, vol. 322, no. 3, pp. 1067–1075, 2007.

[25] J. M. Sullivan, "Cellular and molecular mechanisms underlying learning and memory impairments produced by cannabinoids," *Learning and Memory*, vol. 7, no. 3, pp. 132–139, 2000.

[26] S. A. Varvel, R. J. Hamm, B. R. Martin, and A. H. Lichtman, "Differential effects of Δ9-THC on spatial reference and working memory in mice," *Psychopharmacology*, vol. 157, no. 2, pp. 142–150, 2001.

[27] L. E. Wise, A. J. Thorpe, and A. H. Lichtman, "Hippocampal CB(1) receptors mediate the memory impairing effects of Δ9 - tetrahydrocannabinol," *Neuropsychopharmacology*, vol. 34, no. 9, pp. 2072–2080, 2009.

[28] D. L. Misner and J. M. Sullivan, "Mechanism of cannabinoid effects on long-term potentiation and depression in hippocampal CA1 neurons," *Journal of Neuroscience*, vol. 19, no. 16, pp. 6795–6805, 1999.

[29] N. Burgess, "Spatial cognition and the brain," *Annals of the New York Academy of Sciences*, vol. 1124, pp. 77–97, 2008.

[30] L. E. Jarrard, "On the role of the hippocampus in learning and memory in the rat," *Behavioral and Neural Biology*, vol. 60, no. 1, pp. 9–26, 1993.

[31] E. A. Maguire, "Hippocampal and parietal involvement in human topographical memory: evidence from functional neuroimaging," in *The Hippocampal and Parietal Foundations of Spatial Cognition*, N. Burgess, K. J. Jeffery, and J. O'keefe, Eds., pp. 404–415, Oxford University Press, Oxford, UK, 1999.

[32] E. A. Maguire, D. G. Gadian, I. S. Johnsrude et al., "Navigation-related structural change in the hippocampi of taxi drivers," *Proceedings of the National Academy of Sciences of the United States of America*, vol. 97, no. 8, pp. 4398–4403, 2000.

[33] J. O'Keefe and L. Nadel, *The Hippocampus as a Cognitive Map*, Oxford University Press, Oxford, UK, 1978.

[34] R. J. Sutherland, R. J. McDonald, and C. R. Hill, "Damage to the hippocampal formation in rats selectively impairs the ability to learn cue relationships," *Behavioral and Neural Biology*, vol. 52, no. 3, pp. 331–356, 1989.

[35] J. Tropp Sneider, J. J. Chrobak, M. C. Quirk, J. A. Oler, and E. J. Markus, "Differential behavioral state-dependence in the burst properties of CA3 and CA1 neurons," *Neuroscience*, vol. 141, no. 4, pp. 1665–1677, 2006.

[36] R. G. M. Morris, P. Garrud, J. N. P. Rawlins, and J. O'Keefe, "Place navigation impaired in rats with hippocampal lesions," *Nature*, vol. 297, no. 5868, pp. 681–683, 1982.

[37] D. S. Olton, J. A. Walker, and F. H. Gage, "Hippocampal connections and spatial discrimination," *Brain Research*, vol. 139, no. 2, pp. 295–308, 1978.

[38] N. Solowij and R. Battisti, "The chronic effects of cannabis on memory in humans: a review," *Current drug abuse reviews*, vol. 1, no. 1, pp. 81–98, 2008.

[39] N. J. Cohen and H. Eichenbaum, *Memory, Amnesia, and the Hippocampal System*, The MIT Press, Cambridge, UK, 1993.

[40] R. S. Astur, L. B. Taylor, A. N. Mamelak, L. Philpott, and R. J. Sutherland, "Humans with hippocampus damage display severe spatial memory impairments in a virtual Morris water task," *Behavioural Brain Research*, vol. 132, no. 1, pp. 77–84, 2002.

[41] G. Kanayama, J. Rogowska, H. G. Pope, S. A. Gruber, and D. A. Yurgelun-Todd, "Spatial working memory in heavy cannabis users: a functional magnetic resonance imaging study," *Psychopharmacology*, vol. 176, no. 3-4, pp. 239–247, 2004.

[42] A. M. Smith, C. A. Longo, P. A. Fried, M. J. Hogan, and I. Cameron, "Effects of marijuana on visuospatial working memory: an fMRI Study in young adults," *Psychopharmacology*, vol. 210, no. 3, pp. 429–438, 2010.

[43] N. Burgess, E. A. Maguire, and J. O'Keefe, "The human hippocampus and spatial and episodic memory," *Neuron*, vol. 35, no. 4, pp. 625–641, 2002.

[44] G. Janzen and C. G. Weststeijn, "Neural representation of object location and route direction: an event-related fMRI study," *Brain Research*, vol. 1165, no. 1, pp. 116–125, 2007.

[45] E. A. Maguire, N. Burgess, J. G. Donnett, R. S. J. Frackowiak, C. D. Frith, and J. O'Keefe, "Knowing where and getting there: a human navigation network," *Science*, vol. 280, no. 5365, pp. 921–924, 1998.

[46] G. Janzen and M. Van Turennout, "Selective neural representation of objects rellevant for navigation," *Nature Neuroscience*, vol. 7, no. 6, pp. 673–677, 2004.

[47] A. D. Schweinsburg, B. C. Schweinsburg, E. H. Cheung, G. G. Brown, S. A. Brown, and S. F. Tapert, "fMRI response to spatial working memory in adolescents with comorbid marijuana and alcohol use disorders," *Drug and Alcohol Dependence*, vol. 79, no. 2, pp. 201–210, 2005.

[48] T. D. Wager and E. E. Smith, "Neuroimaging studies of working memory: a meta-analysis," *Cognitive, Affective and Behavioral Neuroscience*, vol. 3, no. 4, pp. 255–274, 2003.

[49] G. Jager, H. Van Hell Hendrika, M. L. De Win Maartje et al., "Effects of frequent cannabis use on hippocampal activity during an associative memory task," *European Neuropsychopharmacology*, vol. 17, no. 4, pp. 289–297, 2007.

[50] J. T. Sneider, S. Sava, J. Rogowska et al., "A preliminary study of sex differences in brain activation during a spatial navigation task in healthy adults," *Perceptual and Motor Skills*, vol. 113, no. 2, pp. 461–480, 2011.

[51] L. Nestor, G. Roberts, H. Garavan, and R. Hester, "Deficits in learning and memory: parahippocampal hyperactivity and frontocortical hypoactivity in cannabis users," *NeuroImage*, vol. 40, no. 3, pp. 1328–1339, 2008.

[52] A. D. Schweinsburg, B. C. Schweinsburg, K. L. Medina, T. McQueeny, S. A. Brown, and S. F. Tapert, "The influence of recency of use on fMRI response during spatial working memory in adolescent marijuana users," *Journal of Psychoactive Drugs*, vol. 42, no. 3, pp. 401–412, 2010.

[53] W. Barratt, *Barratt Simplified Measure of Social Status (BSMSS)*, Indiana State University, 2006.

[54] M. B. First, J. B. . Williams, and R. L. Spitzer, *Structured Clinical Interview for DSM-IV Axis I Disorders, (Clinical Version)*, American Psychiatric Press, Washington, DC, USA, 1997.

[55] D. Watson, L. A. Clark, and A. Tellegen, "Development and validation of brief measures of positive and negative affect: the PANAS scales," *Journal of Personality and Social Psychology*, vol. 54, no. 6, pp. 1063–1070, 1988.

[56] M. Hamilton, "The assessment of anxiety states by rating," *The British Journal of Medical Psychology*, vol. 32, no. 1, pp. 50–55, 1959.

[57] A. T. McLellan et al., *Guide To the Addiction Severity Index: Background, Administration, and Field Testing Results, in Treatment Research Report*, National Institute on Drug Abuse, Rockville, Md, USA, 1985.

[58] A. J. Budney, B. A. Moore, R. G. Vandrey, and J. R. Hughes, "The time course and significance of cannabis withdrawal," *Journal of Abnormal Psychology*, vol. 112, no. 3, pp. 393–402, 2003.

[59] D. Wechsler, *Wechsler Abbreviated Scale of Intelligence Manual*, The Psychological Corporation, Hartcourt Brace and Company, San Antonio, Tex, USA, 1999.

[60] S. G. Vandenberg and A. R. Kuse, "Mental rotations, a group test of three-dimensional spatial visualization," *Perceptual and Motor Skills*, vol. 47, no. 2, pp. 599–604, 1978.

[61] M. Hegarty, A. E. Richardson, D. R. Montello, K. Lovelace, and I. Subbiah, "Development of a self-report measure of environmental spatial ability," *Intelligence*, vol. 30, no. 5, pp. 425–447, 2002.

[62] R. S. Astur, J. Tropp, S. Sava, R. T. Constable, and E. J. Markus, "Sex differences and correlations in a virtual Morris water task, a virtual radial arm maze, and mental rotation," *Behavioural Brain Research*, vol. 151, no. 1-2, pp. 103–115, 2004.

[63] K. J. Fristen, K. J. Worsley, R. S. J. Frackowiak, J. C. Mazziotta, and A. C. Evans, "Assessing the significance of focal activations using their spatial extent," *Human Brain Mapping*, vol. 1, pp. 214–220, 1994.

[64] K. J. Friston, C. D. Frith, R. S. J. Frackowiak, and R. Turner, "Characterizing dynamic brain responses with fMRI: a multivariate approach," *NeuroImage*, vol. 2, no. 2 I, pp. 166–172, 1995.

[65] K. J. Friston, C. D. Frith, R. Turner, and R. S. J. Frackowiak, "Characterizing evoked hemodynamics with fMRI," *NeuroImage*, vol. 2, no. I, pp. 157–165, 1995.

[66] N. Tzourio-Mazoyer, B. Landeau, D. Papathanassiou et al., "Automated anatomical labeling of activations in SPM using a macroscopic anatomical parcellation of the MNI MRI single-subject brain," *NeuroImage*, vol. 15, no. 1, pp. 273–289, 2002.

[67] S. A. Gruber, M. K. Dahlgren, K. A. Sagar et al., "Age of onset of marijuana use impacts inhibitory processing," *Neuroscience Letters*, vol. 511, no. 2, pp. 89–94, 2012.

[68] L. Palermo, B. Filippo, I. Giuseppe et al., "Assessing topographical orientation skills in cannabis users," *The Scientific World Journal*, vol. 2012, Article ID 137071, 7 pages, 2012.

[69] G. Rauchs, P. Orban, E. Balteau et al., "Partially segregated neural networks for spatial and contextual memory in virtual navigation," *Hippocampus*, vol. 18, no. 5, pp. 503–518, 2008.

[70] B. Becker, D. Wagner, E. Gouzoulis-Mayfrank, E. Spuentrup, and J. Daumann, "Altered parahippocampal functioning in cannabis users is related to the frequency of use," *Psychopharmacology*, vol. 209, no. 4, pp. 361–374, 2010.

[71] B. A. Vogt, D. M. Finch, and C. R. Olson, "Functional heterogeneity in cingulate cortex: the anterior executive and posterior evaluative regions," *Cerebral Cortex*, vol. 2, no. 6, pp. 435–443, 1992.

[72] P. C. M. Van Zijl, S. M. Eleff, J. A. Ulatowski et al., "Quantitative assessment of blood flow, blood volume and blood oxygenation effects in functional magnetic resonance imaging," *Nature Medicine*, vol. 4, no. 2, pp. 159–167, 1998.

[73] J. T. Sneider, H. G. Pope, M. M. Silveri, N. S. Simpson, S. A. Gruber, and D. A. Yurgelun-Todd, "Altered regional blood volume in chronic cannabis smokers," *Experimental and Clinical Psychopharmacology*, vol. 14, no. 4, pp. 422–428, 2006.

[74] J. T. Sneider, H. G. Pope, M. M. Silveri, N. S. Simpson, S. A. Gruber, and D. A. Yurgelun-Todd, "Differences in regional blood volume during a 28-day period of abstinence in chronic cannabis smokers," *European Neuropsychopharmacology*, vol. 18, no. 8, pp. 612–619, 2008.

[75] T. L. Wallace and R. H. P. Porter, "Targeting the nicotinic alpha7 acetylcholine receptor to enhance cognition in disease," *Biochemical Pharmacology*, vol. 82, no. 8, pp. 891–903, 2011.

[76] H. S. Swartzwelder, W. A. Wilson, and M. I. Tayyeb, "Age-dependent inhibition of long-term potentiation by ethanol in immature versus mature hippocampus," *Alcoholism, Clinical and Experimental Research*, vol. 19, no. 6, pp. 1480–1485, 1995.

[77] S. A. Gruber, K. A. Sagar, and M. K. Dahlgren, "Age of onset of marijuana use and executive function," *Psychology of Addictive Behaviors*, vol. 26, no. 3, pp. 496–506, 2012.

[78] R. Gonzalez, "Acute and non-acute effects of cannabis on brain functioning and neuropsychological performance," *Neuropsychology Review*, vol. 17, no. 3, pp. 347–361, 2007.

[79] J. A. McLaren, E. Silins, D. Hutchinson, R. P. Mattick, and W. Hall, "Assessing evidence for a causal link between cannabis and psychosis: a review of cohort studies," *International Journal of Drug Policy*, vol. 21, no. 1, pp. 10–19, 2010.

9

Understanding Nonprescription and Prescription Drug Misuse in Late Adolescence/Young Adulthood

Sasha A. Fleary,[1] Robert W. Heffer,[1] and E. Lisako J. McKyer[2]

[1] Department of Psychology, Texas A&M University, MS 4235, College Station, TX 77843, USA
[2] Department of Health and Kinesiology, Texas A&M University, Dulie Bell, College Station, TX 77843, USA

Correspondence should be addressed to Sasha A. Fleary; sfleary@tamu.edu

Academic Editor: Jennifer B. Unger

This study explored the extent to which nonprescription and prescription drugs misuse among adolescents/young adults are related to their perception that it is safer than illicit drugs, ease of access, and lower societal stigma. Adolescents/young adults ($N = 465$; $M_{age} = 18.57$, SD = 0.86) completed an online survey about their nonprescription and prescription drug misuse, other substance use, and correlates of use. Perceived risk, societal stigma, and access to nonprescription and prescription drugs were predictive of misuse. Results support program planners working towards targeting perceived risk and societal stigma in reducing misuse and the need to restrict and monitor access to nonprescription and prescription drugs for adolescents/young adults.

1. Introduction

Prescription drugs are becoming the drugs of choice for adolescents and young adults with a reported increase in misuse of 212% from 1992 to 2003 [1]. The Substance Abuse and Mental Health Services Administration [2] and Johnston et al. [3] have reported that the misuse or nonmedical use of prescription drugs has a greater prevalence rate than illicit drugs use with the exception of marijuana use, with the highest prevalence rates being reported among adolescents and young adults. The increased incidence and prevalence of nonprescription and prescription drug misuse among young people led to the Office of National Drug Control Policy's [4] prescription drug abuse prevention campaign to target parents of adolescents in 2008.

Friedman [5] and Manchikanti [6] argued that continued prescription drug misuse among adolescents may be attributed to adolescents' perception that this type of drug use is safer than illicit drugs, the ease of access to these drugs, and lower societal stigma about misuse compared to illicit drugs use. These three variables are directly related to peer influence and are consistent with Kandel's [7] adolescent socialization theory, particularly imitation and social reinforcement. Kandel [7] described peer influence, rather than parent

influence, as being the most important influence to adolescents' immediate lifestyle, hence peers being more relevant in understanding adolescents' health risk behaviors. Regarding Kandel's [7] theory, imitation involves adolescents modeling their behaviors and attitudes based on others' behaviors and social reinforcement involves adolescents internalizing and displaying behaviors and attitudes approved by others. Both are applicable to adolescents' perception of prescription drug use being safer than illicit drugs and lower stigma about misuse, since these perceptions are based on attitudes displayed by others in conjunction with adolescents' own beliefs. The theory also applies to ease of access to drugs, such that if parents and peers are engaging in prescription drug use, drugs may be more easily accessible to adolescents. Also noteworthy is the developmental level of adolescents/young adults, and according to E. H. Erikson and J. M. Erikson [8] peers are key counterplayers during this stage of life. Adolescents/young adults are forming their identity which may be based on in-group or out-group values. If adolescents'/young adults' group values involve prescription drug use, then there will be norms for use and ease of access to drugs. Understanding the roles of adolescents' perception that this type of drug use is safer than illicit drugs, the ease of access to these drugs, and lower societal stigma about misuse compared to illicit drugs use may provide additional targetable areas for intervention. Hence, the purpose of this study is to explore the extent to which these variables are predictive of adolescents'/young adults' prescription drug misuse.

In the health risk behaviors and substance abuse literature, abuse has been shown to be related to perceived risk (PR) such that as PR of substance use increases, use decreases [9–12]. PR of nonprescription and prescription drugs have not been extensively explored with most studies addressing PR of nonprescription and prescription drug misuse in relation to illicit drugs.

Arria et al. [13] conducted a longitudinal study on perceived harmfulness of stimulants and analgesics in college students and found that 25.2% and 27.8% of students attributed a descriptor of "great risk" to the occasional nonmedical use of stimulant and analgesics misuse, respectively. Additionally, prescription stimulants and analgesics were viewed as less risky than cocaine but more risky than marijuana and binge drinking. The Partnership for a Drug Free America [14] (PDFA) reported that 40% of adolescents viewed prescription medication to be safer than illegal drugs. Additionally, adolescents did not believe that prescription pain relievers were addictive and believed that it was okay to use prescription drugs without a prescription once in a while [14]. Prescription drugs may be perceived as being safer than illicit drugs because they can be legitimately prescribed by doctors and are Food and Drug Administration approved [5, 6]. Manchikanti [6] also reported that the increase in social acceptability of medicating ailments may also be responsible for misperceptions of prescription drug misuse safety. Based on these findings, we hypothesize that PR of prescription drugs will be significantly lower than illicit drugs and that the belief that prescription drugs misuse is safer than illicit drug use will be positively related to nonprescription and prescription drug misuse. Additionally, we hypothesize that PR of misuse will be negatively predictive of misuse.

Another variable mentioned by Friedman [5] as being responsible for the increased prevalence in prescription drug misuse is lower societal stigma about misuse. Like PR, the role of parent and peer approval has been extensively studied in the substance abuse literature but few studies have focused on its relations with nonprescription and prescription drug misuse. Ford [15] found that adolescents who had parents and peers with pro-substance abuse attitudes were more likely to report engaging in prescription drug misuse. Additionally, the PDFA [14] highlighted that 21% of adolescents reported that their parents won't care if they caught them engaging in prescription pain reliever misuse. Researchers also found that adolescents whose friends engage in substance use were more likely to engage in prescription drugs misuse [15–18]. According to the PDFA [14], 33% of adolescents reported that there was less shame attached to using prescription pain relievers than illicit drugs. These findings reiterate imitation and social reinforcement as described in Kandel's [7] adolescent socialization theory and the influence of in-groups and out-groups. We hypothesize that perceived societal stigma (PSS) in the form of peer and parent disapproval and

perceived peer misuse would be related to nonprescription and prescription drug misuse. We also hypothesize that, similar to PR, participants will perceive peers to be more approving of prescription drug misuse than illicit drug use.

Ease of access to nonprescription and prescription drugs has been suggested as responsible for the increased prevalence of misuse; however, similar to PR and PSS, few researchers have studied the extent to which this is true. Weyandt et al. [19] found that half the sample they examined reported that prescription stimulants were easily accessible on campus with 21.2% and 9.8% reporting being offered stimulants or purchasing stimulants from other students, respectively. However, they did not explore the extent to which easy accessibility was predictive of misuse. Poulin [20] found that students who reported medical use of stimulants reported giving, selling, and being forced to give their medication to others. Giving and selling prescribed medication to others were positively related to increase in nonmedical stimulant use, thus providing evidence for the role of ease of access in stimulant misuse. Manchikanti [6] identified several modes of access to prescription drugs including internet pharmacies, drug theft, sharing among family and friends, doctor shopping, and improper prescribing. The PDFA [14] also provided evidence for the role of easy access to drugs in the increase in misuse prevalence. According to the PDFA [14], adolescents reported having easy access to prescription drugs via parents' medicine cabinets (62%), others' prescriptions (50%), and from the internet (32%). This provides further evidence for the role of imitation and social reinforcement in prescription drug misuse. Therefore, we hypothesize that ease of access to nonprescription and prescription drugs will be predictive of nonprescription and prescription drug misuse.

Based on Kandel's [7] adolescent socialization theory and the proposals by Friedman [5] and Manchikanti [6] about the role of PR, PSS, and ease of access in the increased prevalence of nonprescription and prescription drug misuse, we hypothesize that these variables will be predictive of misuse. Specifically, PR and PSS will be negatively related to misuse and ease of access will be positively related to misuse.

2. Method

2.1. Participants. The sample was taken from a public college in the Southwestern US. The sample consisted of 465 college students between the ages of 18 and 24 years ($M = 18.57$, SD = 0.86). The majority of the participants (90.5%) were between 18 and 19 years. Participants were predominantly Caucasian (74%), female (60%), and freshmen (73%). Sixteen percent of participants ($N = 73$) reported some prescription drug misuse and 15% ($N = 71$) reported some nonprescription drug misuse. Note that cough and cold syrup and pills misuse (9%, $N = 42$) were not included in the frequency calculations because the question about cough and cold syrup and pills did not distinguish between prescription and nonprescription drugs. Twenty-six percent of participants ($N = 119$) reported some nonprescription and/or prescription drug misuse.

TABLE 1: Descriptive statistics for the sample.

	Users N (%)	Age of first use in years M (SD)	Perceived risk M (SD)	Perceived societal stigma, parent M (SD)	Perceived societal stigma, peer M (SD)
Prescription drugs					
Prescription pain	50 (10.7)	17.32 (1.48)	5.30 (1.71)	4.38 (.90)	3.93 (1.09)
Prescription sedatives and tranquilizers	22 (4.7)	17.23 (1.66)	5.84 (1.43)	4.71 (.60)	4.23 (.90)
Prescription stimulants	41 (8.8)	18.05 (2.30)	5.06 (1.83)	4.51 (.85)	3.98 (1.09)
Nonprescription drugs					
Nonprescription pain	61 (13.1)	15.18 (2.84)	3.60 (2.00)	2.43 (1.21)	3.19 (1.33)
Nonprescription sleeping pills	22 (4.7)	17.09 (1.60)	4.82 (1.74)	3.95 (1.12)	3.77 (1.11)
No distinction					
Cough/cold syrup	42 (9)	15.33 (3.18)	3.99 (2.00)	2.70 (1.31)	3.42 (1.31)
Illicit drugs					
Marijuana	134 (29.9)	17.78 (1.67)	5.07 (1.90)	4.87 (.48)	3.49 (1.37)
Crack or cocaine	10 (2.1)	17.80 (1.55)	6.76 (.71)	4.97 (.30)	4.73 (.58)

2.2. Measures. Misuses of nonprescription and prescription drugs were defined as use of medications to get high. PR was measured by perceived personal risk, which is the extent to which the participant felt they would be at risk of getting sick or hurt if they engaged in nonprescription, prescription, and illicit drug use. PR was measured on a 7-point evaluation scale ranging from *No risk at all (1)* to *Very much at risk (7)*. PSS was participants' self-report on their perceptions about how friends and parents felt about them engaging in nonprescription, prescription, and illicit drug use (i.e., parent and peer disapproval). Parent and peer approval was measured on a 5-point Likert scale ranging from *Strongly Approve (1)* to *Strongly Disapprove (5)*. PSS variables also included participants' perceptions of friends' nonprescription and prescription drug misuse. Friends misuse was participants' assessment of the percentage of friends who engaged in misuse in 10% increments (e.g., 0%, 1%–10%, 11%–20%). To measure accessibility of nonprescription and prescription drugs, participants answered questions on whether their friends brought medications to school for recreational use (access in school) and what nonprescription and prescription drugs were kept in the home. Participants were also asked about their perceptions about the safety of nonprescription and prescription drug misuse in relation to illicit drugs use.

Nonprescription and prescription drugs misuse and illicit drug use were measures of lifetime use on a 5-point frequency scale ranging from *Never (1)* to *More than 40 times (5)*. For nonprescription and prescription drugs, the question stem was "*Have you ever used the following medications recreationally?*" and for illicit drugs the question stem was "*Have you ever engaged in the following activity?*" Prescription drug misuse was measured for the following classifications of medications; prescription pain (e.g., Vicodin, Codeine, OxyContin, Percocet), prescription stimulants (Adderall, Dexedrine, Ritalin), and prescription sedatives and tranquilizers (Mebaral, Quaaludes, Xanax, Valium

(benzodiazepines), Nembutal, Fluoxetine). Nonprescription drug misuse was measured for nonprescription pain relievers (e.g., Tylenol, Motrin, Advil, Aleve, Ibuprofen, Aspirin) and nonprescription sleeping pills. Misuse was also measured for cough and cold syrup and pills; however, no distinction was made between prescription and nonprescription. Illicit drugs included marijuana, methamphetamines, crack or cocaine, and inhalants. Participants also completed a demographic questionnaire.

2.3. Procedures. This study was approved by the Institutional Review Board at the university. Data were collected as part of the "Media influences on health risk behaviors and prescription drug use in young adults" project. Data were collected using a survey developed by the authors specifically for this project; however, portions of the survey (e.g., PR and PSS) were modified from Omori and Ingersoll [21]. College students were recruited from the introduction to psychology course to participate in the study. Participants completed an online survey at a computer lab where workstations were separated by desk partitions. The survey was administered via surveymonkey.com and took approximately 35–50 minutes to complete. Participants received two research credits upon completion of the survey. To ensure participant privacy, respondent identification numbers were assigned.

2.4. Statistical Analyses. Descriptive statistics were computed (see Table 1). To test for differences in PR and perception of societal stigma for nonprescription and prescription drug misuse versus illicit drug use, paired sample t-tests were computed. Pearson correlations were computed to explore the relationship between participants PR and PSS for nonprescription and prescription drug misuse and that of illicit drug use. Nonprescription and prescription drug misuse was dichotomized into nonusers (participants who responded

Never to the questions) and users (participants who reported any misuse). Binary logistic regressions were calculated to differentiate PR, PSS, and access to nonprescription and prescription drugs on self-reported nonusers and misusers. Demographic variables including age, gender, and ethnicity were controlled for in the first step of the regression analyses.

3. Results

Results of correlations and paired sample *t*-tests are presented in Table 2. PR of nonprescription and prescription drugs misuse was positively correlated with PR of marijuana and crack or cocaine at the $P \leq 0.001$. Similarly, peer approval for nonprescription and prescription drug misuse was positively correlated with peer approval for marijuana and crack or cocaine use at the $P \leq 0.001$. Parent approval for prescription pain, prescription sedatives and tranquilizers, prescription stimulants, and nonprescription sleeping pills was positively correlated with marijuana and crack or cocaine use at the $P < 0.05$ to $P \leq 0.001$ range. Parent approval for nonprescription pain was significantly positively correlated with approval for marijuana use and uncorrelated with approval for crack or cocaine use. Parent approval for cough/cold syrup was uncorrelated with approval for marijuana use and crack or cocaine use.

PR of all nonprescription and prescription drugs examined were lower than the PR of crack or cocaine confirming the hypothesis that PR of prescription drugs is lower than that of illicit drugs. Participants also perceived risk from marijuana use to be higher than that from nonprescription pain, cough/cold syrup, and nonprescription sleeping pills misuse. Participants perceived risk from the misuse of prescription pain and prescription sedatives and tranquilizers to be higher than that of marijuana use.

Regarding PSS, participants reported parent disapproval of all nonprescription and prescription drugs misuse as significantly lower than parent disapproval of marijuana and crack or cocaine use. Participants reported that their peer disapproval of nonprescription and prescription drugs misuse was significantly lower than that of crack or cocaine. These results confirm that participants perceived peers and parents to be more approving of nonprescription and prescription drug misuse. Participants' PSS of all the nonprescription and prescription drugs measured with the exception of cough/cold syrups and pills and nonprescription pain medication was higher than that of marijuana use. Participants' perceived peers to be less disapproving of nonprescription pain misuse than marijuana use.

Results of binary logistic regression analyses predicting nonprescription and prescription drug misuse are presented in Table 3. Regarding prescription pain drugs misuse, Caucasians were more likely to be misusers than African-Americans/Black and Hispanics, while PR and peer disapproval were negatively associated with use. Access to prescription medications at home was positively associated with misuse. For prescription sedatives and tranquilizers, African-Americans/Blacks were less likely to be misuses than Caucasians, and parent disapproval and peer use were

positively associated with misuse. PR was negatively related to misuse of sedatives and tranquilizers. Age was positively related to misuse of stimulants while peer disapproval and perceived risk were negatively related to misuse. Regarding nonprescription pain medication, peer use was positively related to misuse. No other predictor variables were related to nonprescription pain medication. Access to nonprescription sleeping pills in the home was positively related to misuse. No other predictor variables were related to nonprescription sleep drugs misuse. For cough/cold syrup and pills, peer disapproval and peer use was negatively and positively related to misuse, respectively. Note that the odds ratio and confidence intervals could not be calculated for Asians for any of the prescription drugs, for Hispanics for nonprescription sleep, and for ethnicity and access in home for cold/cough syrup and pills due to extremely large standard errors.

4. Discussion

As discussed in Friedman [5] and Manchikanti [6], we proposed that PR, perception of illicit drugs being safer than street drugs, PSS, and access to nonprescription and prescription drug misuse would be significantly related to misuse. Our results provide some evidence that these variables provide a plausible explanation for increased prescription drug misuse among adolescents/young adults.

Both PR and PSS of nonprescription and prescription drugs misuse and illicit drug use were positively correlated, suggesting that adolescents/young adults recognize that nonprescription and prescription drugs misuse are risky. These findings also provide evidence for the high correlation of illicit drug use and nonprescription and prescription medication misuse [16, 18, 22]. Specifically, PR for one substance may influence PR for the other substance and subsequent decisions to engage in use of both substances. Additionally, adolescents/young adults may belong to in-groups and out-groups that are consistent in how they perceive substance abuse, for example, a group that disapproves of illicit drug use may also disapprove of prescription drug misuse. These results also provide evidence for social reinforcement and imitation of attitudes proposed in the adolescent socialization theory [7].

PR and PSS of nonprescription and prescription drugs being lower than crack or cocaine but not marijuana highlight an important trend that is somewhat consistent with Arria et al. [13] and should be explored further. Specifically, the potential of a substitution effect whereby adolescents/young adults perceive misuse of nonprescription and prescription drugs as a middle ground between too little and too much risk, as well as the formation of a new sub-culture should be explored. These findings also suggest a need to reevaluate and reconfigure programs targeting marijuana prevention with programs emphasizing PR and stigma (possibly via harsher penalties for use). In addition to reevaluating marijuana programs, more should also be done to increase awareness of the risks associated with nonprescription and prescription drug misuse. The Office of National Drug Control Policy's

TABLE 2: Significant correlations and mean differences of perceived risk and perceived societal stigma (peer disapproval) of non-prescription and prescription drug misuse with illicit drug use.

	Perceived risk[a]				Perceived societal stigma, peer[a]				Perceived societal stigma, parent[a]			
	Marijuana		Crack or cocaine		Marijuana		Crack or cocaine		Marijuana		Crack or cocaine	
	r	MD	r	MD	r	MD	r	MD	r	MD	r	MD
Prescription drugs												
Pain	.32	.22*	.30	-1.46	.45	.44	.35	-.80	.14**	-.43	.20	-.59
Sedatives and tranquilizers	.37	.77	.38	-.92	.44	.74	.43	-.50	.30	-.10**	.41	-.25
Stimulants	.46	-.01 (ns)	.27	-1.69	.50	.48	.34	-.76	.34	-.30	.31	-.45
Nonprescription Drugs												
Pain	.25	-1.47	.21	-3.15	.34	-.30	.17	-1.54	.12*	-2.38	.07 (ns)	-2.53
Sleeping pills	.31	-.25*	.24	-1.93	.41	.27	.32	-.97	.18	-.86	.18	-1.01
No distinction												
Cough/cold syrup and pills	.49	-1.09	.23	-2.77	.36	-.08 (ns)	.23	-1.31	.08 (ns)	-2.11	.05 (ns)	-2.26

MD: mean difference; ns: nonsignificant.
[a]$P \leq 0.001$ unless were indicated, * $P < 0.05$, ** $P < 0.01$.

TABLE 3: Results of binary logistic regression analyses predicting misuse from risk perception, societal stigma, and access.

	Prescription			Nonprescription		No Distinction
	Pain OR (95% CI)	Sedatives and Tranquilizers OR (95% CI)	Stimulants OR (95% CI)	Pain OR (95% CI)	Sleep OR (95% CI)	Cough/Cold OR (95% CI)
Step 1 {ΔR^2}	(.06)	(.10)	(.08)	(.02)	(.03)	(.04)
Age	1.06 (.75, 1.49)	1.20 (.76, 1.88)	1.73** (1.27, 2.36)	1.03 (.75, 1.41)	.85 (.47, 1.54)	1.21 (.89, 1.66)
Gender	.68 (.37, 1.25)	.59 (.24, 1.44)	.94 (.48, 1.84)	.61 (.35, 1.06)	1.65 (.63, 4.34)	.54 (.28, 1.04)
Ethnicity[a]						
Black	.20** (.07, .56)	.16** (.04, .63)	.50 (.13, 1.88)	2.54 (.33, 19.71)	.75 (.09, 6.02)	.00[b]
Asian	.00[b]	.00[b]	.00[b]	.95 (.05, 16.50)	.74 (.04, 12.95)	.00[b]
Hispanic	.19 (.03, 1.10)	.22 (.02, 2.37)	.18 (.02, 2.114)	3.63 (.37, 36.83)	.00[b]	.00[b]
Other	.30 (.09, 1.03)	.67 (.15, 2.96)	.32 (.06, 1.66)	2.67 (.31, 23.19)	1.02 (.11, 9.92)	.00[b]
Step 2 {ΔR^2}	(.28)	(.31)	(.31)	(.30)	(.29)	(.27)
Age	1.00 (.66, 1.51)	.90 (.45, 1.80)	2.18*** (1.48, 3.21)	.94 (.65, 1.35)	.77 (.42, 1.40)	1.28 (.89, 1.83)
Gender	.96 (.47, 1.99)	.49 (.15, 1.54)	1.23 (.55, 2.72)	.67 (.35, 1.26)	1.64 (.56, 4.80)	.52 (.25, 1.10)
Ethnicity[a]						
Black	.23* (.07, .76)	.09** (.02, .54)	.66 (.13, 3.41)	2.52 (.29, 21.93)	.38 (.04, 4.11)	.00[b]
Asian	.00[b]	.00[b]	.00[b]	.65 (.03, 13.66)	1.53 (.06, 40.06)	.00[b]
Hispanic	.09* (.01, .72)	.18 (.01, 3.15)	.21 (.01, 3.41)	3.35 (.28, 40.55)	.00[b]	.00[b]
Other	.29 (.07, 1.22)	.48 (.08, 3.07)	.85 (.12, 6.00)	.62 (.25, 1.51)	1.21 (.09, 17.02)	.00[b]
PR	.78* (.64, .96)	.63** (.46, .87)	.71** (.56, .91)	.84 (.67, 1.04)	.91 (.69, 1.20)	1.00 (.79, 1.27)
PSSD	1.42 (.42, 4.89)	.28 (.07, 1.14)	.62 (.19, 2.02)	.62 (.25, 1.51)	.56 (.14, 2.28)	.65 (.23, 1.81)
PSS:						
Parent	.92 (.63, 1.34)	21.03* (1.9, 229.7)	.77 (.52, 1.15)	1.08 (.77, 1.51)	.81 (.49, 1.34)	.93 (.64, 1.35)
Peer	.52*** (.36, .75)	.84 (.47, 1.50)	.56** (.36, .87)	.70 (.48, 1.02)	.69 (.39, 1.19)	.52** (.34, .79)
Peer use	1.12 (.97, 1.32)	1.50** (1.16, 1.94)	1.15 (.98, 1.35)	1.24*** (1.12, 1.36)	1.14 (.89, 1.46)	1.19** (1.06, 1.33)
Access						
School	2.09* (1.01, 4.35)	1.87 (.60, 5.76)	1.54 (.65, 3.63)	1.26 (.64, 2.47)	1.03 (.36, 2.90)	1.55 (.73, 3.30)
Home	1.69 (.84, 3.42)	3.57 (.75, 16.90)	1.14 (.36, 3.57)	.10 (.01, 1.27)	16.5 (3.4, 79.1)***	.00[b]

PR: perceived risk; PSS: perceived societal stigma; PSSD: prescription safer than street drug; ΔR^2: change in Nagelkerke R^2 at each step; [a] White/Caucasian is the comparison group; [b] odds ratio cannot be computed due to extremely large standard error.
* $P < 0.05$, ** $P < 0.01$, *** $P \leq 0.001$.

[4] media campaign targeted parents; however, the findings of this study suggest that adolescents/young adults may benefit from additional campaigns targeting them (adolescents/young adults) and their peers that highlight the risks associated with nonprescription and prescription drug misuse. Addressing misuse in this way may be very effective since it will reduce the amount of unhealthy or inappropriate social reinforcement and imitation of undesirable attitudes regarding prescription drug misuse currently displayed by adolescents/young adults.

The inconsistency in PR and PSS of nonprescription and prescription drugs when compared to marijuana may also explain why pain medication misuse is second only to marijuana use [23]. The only drugs perceived as being less risky than marijuana were nonprescription pain, nonprescription sleep, and cough and cold medications suggesting that adolescents'/young adults' perception of nonprescription and prescription drugs differ probably due to access or level of control imposed by the Food and Drug Administration. Also noteworthy is the nonsignificant relationship between parent disapproval for cough/cold syrup and pills and marijuana and crack or cocaine. Possible explanations for these nonsignificant relationships include parents not viewing these drugs as risky and worthy of discussion with adolescents, parents not recognizing that these drugs are subject to misuse, adolescents mistaking access for approval, or both parents and adolescent not connecting the relationship between misuse of cough/cold medications and illicit drugs. Future research should explore nonprescription drugs, including cough and cold medication, independently. Though nonprescription drugs are less risky than prescription drugs, it is imperative that programs and campaigns incorporate the dangers associated with the improper use of nonprescription drugs, particularly among adolescents and young adults, instead of focusing solely on prescription drugs.

To predict misuse, demographic variables were first controlled for. Given the restricted age range of our sample, it was interesting that there was a significant age difference for prescription stimulant misusers. We propose that since stimulants are known "study drugs", older participants may be engaging in more stimulant misuse due to demands of classes. Surprisingly, particularly for pain medication, gender was not a significant predictor of misuse. Several researchers have found that women tend to misuse pain medications more often than men [24, 25]. One possible reason for our nonsignificant results is our definition of misuse. In most studies, misuse is broadly defined as non-prescribed use [24], but because our definition was limited to recreational use we may have screened out the young women who misuse these medications for pain relief rather than getting high.

Consistent with Friedman [5], Manchikanti [6], and Ford [15], PSS was the strongest predictor of all nonprescription and prescription drug misuse with the exception of nonprescription sleeping pills. This reiterates the need for prevention programs to target adolescents/young adults; adolescents/young adults influence each other's decision to engage in use therefore increasing the PR and reducing acceptance of nonprescription and prescription drug misuse

in some adolescents and young adults may have a ripple effect. Of particular note is the significantly positive relationship between parent disapproval, peer use, and sedatives and tranquilizers misuse. These findings highlight that though parents may be important and instrumental in limiting access and exposure to medications, their disapproval may have the reverse effect on adolescents/young adults. It also further explains the role of peer groups and peer norms in misuse and further confirms Kandel [7] findings about the role of peers in immediate lifestyle choices adolescents/young adults make.

PR was only a significant predictor of prescription pain, prescription sedatives and tranquilizers, and prescription stimulants, suggesting that other variables may also be contributing to adolescents and young adults' decision to engage in misuse. PR may still be important but may be interacting with other variables in the decision-making process. Future studies should explore other correlates of misuse and how they interact with PR to influence misuse. Future studies should also replicate these findings using a smaller misuser to nonuser ratio. Noteworthy is the failure of the variable, prescription drug not being safer than illicit drug, to predict misuse. This suggests that PR in general may be more important than risk in relation to other substances for predicting misuse.

Regarding access to medication, medicine kept in the home was only significantly related with misuse of nonprescription sleeping pills. Separate regression analyses were conducted including access to medicine cabinets in the home and this was not significantly correlated to misuse for any classification of drug. We hypothesize therefore that medicine kept in the home being a significant predictor of misuse may be due to a combination of access and acceptability of use for medical reasons as suggested by Manchikanti [6] and consistent with social reinforcement and imitation [7]. Access in school was only predictive of prescription pain, and the authors suspect that these medications were probably the most accessible medications taken to school. Future studies should be more thorough in their definition in school.

5. Limitations and Future Directions

As mentioned before, this study was restricted to recreational users of nonprescription and prescription medication, these misusers do not encompass all non-medical use therefore generalizations about misuse are limited. Additionally, the findings of this study should be viewed as exploratory due to the restrictedness and non-representativeness of the sample. This study should be replicated using a multilocation community sample. Because of the higher misuser to nonuser ratio, statistical power to detect significant correlates of misuse may have been insufficient; therefore, future studies should replicate these analyses with lower misuse to nonuser ratios. A broader definition of PSS may also be warranted in future studies. Other future directions include using the results from this study as a basis for developing a peer-focused prevention intervention and a prescription drug misuse awareness intervention.

6. Conclusions

To conclude, adolescents'/young adults' PR and PSS of nonprescription and prescription drugs misuse differ from their perception of illicit drug use, particularly for crack or cocaine. Their perceptions are important because they are correlated with misuse and program planners should work towards targeting these perceptions to prevent and decrease misuse. Additionally, access to medications also influences misuse and this suggests that to prevent and decrease use, stronger measures should be taken to restrict access to OTC and prescription drugs.

References

[1] National Center on Addiction and Substance Abuse at Columbia University, *Under the Counter: The Diversion and Abuse of Controlled Prescription Drugs in the U.S.*, CASA, Columbia University, New York, NY, USA, 2005.

[2] Substance Abuse Mental Health Services Administration, *Results from the 2005 National Survey on Drug Use and Health: National Findings*, Office of Applied Studies, Washington, DC, USA, 2006.

[3] L. D. Johnston, P. M. O'Malley, J. G. Bachman, and J. E. Schulenberg, *Monitoring the Future National Results on Adolescent Drug Use: Overview of Key Findings, 2005*, National Institute on Drug Abuse, Bethesda, Md, USA, 2006.

[4] Office of National Drug Control Policy, *The ONDCP Launches Initiative to Combat Teen Prescription Drug Abuse*, White House Office of National Drug Control Policy, Rockville, Md, USA, 2008.

[5] R. A. Friedman, "The changing face of teenage drug abuse—the trend toward prescription drugs," *The New England Journal of Medicine*, vol. 354, no. 14, pp. 1448–1450, 2006.

[6] L. Manchikanti, "Prescription drug abuse: what is being done to address this new drug epidemic? Testimony before the subcommittee on criminal justice, drug policy and human resources," *Pain Physician*, vol. 9, no. 4, pp. 287–321, 2006.

[7] D. B. Kandel, "Drug and drinking behavior among youth," *Annual Review of Sociology*, vol. 6, pp. 235–285, 1980.

[8] E. H. Erikson and J. M. Erikson, *The Life Cycle Completed*, Extended ed, W. W. Norton, New York, NY, USA, 1997.

[9] J. G. Bachman, L. D. Johnston, and P. M. O'Malley, "Explaining recent increases in students' marijuana use: impacts of perceived risks and disapproval, 1976 through 1996," *American Journal of Public Health*, vol. 88, no. 6, pp. 887–892, 1998.

[10] S. A. Fleary, R. W. Heffer, E. L. J. McKyer, and D. A. Newman, "Using the bioecological model to predict risk perception of marijuana use and reported marijuana use in adolescence," *Addictive Behaviors*, vol. 35, no. 8, pp. 795–798, 2010.

[11] K. S. Leung, A. B. Abdallah, J. Copeland, and L. B. Cottler, "Modifiable risk factors of ecstasy use: risk perception, current dependence, perceived control, and depression," *Addictive Behaviors*, vol. 35, no. 3, pp. 201–208, 2010.

[12] G. E. Ryb, P. C. Dischinger, J. A. Kufera, and K. M. Read, "Risk perception and impulsivity: association with risky behaviors and substance abuse disorders," *Accident Analysis and Prevention*, vol. 38, no. 3, pp. 567–573, 2006.

[13] A. M. Arria, K. M. Caldeira, K. B. Vincent, K. E. O'Grady, and E. D. Wish, "Perceived harmfulness predicts nonmedical use of prescription drugs among college students: interactions

with sensation-seeking," *Prevention Science*, vol. 9, no. 3, pp. 191–201, 2008.

[14] Partnership for a Drug-Free America, *The Partnership Attitude Tracking Study*, Partnership for a Drug-Free America, New York, NY, USA, 2006.

[15] J. A. Ford, "Social learning theory and nonmedical prescription drug use among adolescents," *Sociological Spectrum*, vol. 28, no. 3, pp. 299–316, 2008.

[16] A. Kokkevi, A. Fotiou, A. Arapaki, and C. Richardson, "Prevalence, patterns, and correlates of tranquilizer and sedative use among European adolescents," *Journal of Adolescent Health*, vol. 43, no. 6, pp. 584–592, 2008.

[17] S. E. McCabe, C. J. Teter, C. J. Boyd, J. R. Knight, and H. Wechsler, "Nonmedical use of prescription opioids among U.S. college students: prevalence and correlates from a national survey," *Addictive Behaviors*, vol. 30, no. 4, pp. 789–805, 2005.

[18] H.-E. Sung, L. Richter, R. Vaughan, P. B. Johnson, and B. Thom, "Nonmedical use of prescription opioids among teenagers in the United States: trends and correlates," *Journal of Adolescent Health*, vol. 37, no. 1, pp. 44–51, 2005.

[19] L. L. Weyandt, G. Janusis, K. G. Wilson et al., "Nonmedical prescription stimulant use among a sample of college students: relationship with psychological variables," *Journal of Attention Disorders*, vol. 13, no. 3, pp. 284–296, 2009.

[20] C. Poulin, "Medical and nonmedical stimulant use among adolescents: from sanctioned to unsanctioned use," *Canadian Medical Association Journal*, vol. 165, no. 8, pp. 1039–1044, 2001.

[21] M. Omori and G. M. Ingersoll, "Health-endangering behaviours among Japanese college students: a test of psychosocial model of risk-taking behaviours," *Journal of Adolescence*, vol. 28, no. 1, pp. 17–33, 2005.

[22] J. A. Ford and M. C. Arrastia, "Pill-poppers and dopers: a comparison of non-medical prescription drug use and illicit/street drug use among college students," *Addictive Behaviors*, vol. 33, no. 7, pp. 934–941, 2008.

[23] W. M. Compton and N. D. Volkow, "Abuse of prescription drugs and the risk of addiction," *Drug and Alcohol Dependence*, vol. 83, supplement 1, pp. S4–S7, 2006.

[24] C. J. Boyd, S. Esteban McCabe, and C. J. Teter, "Medical and nonmedical use of prescription pain medication by youth in a Detroit-area public school district," *Drug and Alcohol Dependence*, vol. 81, no. 1, pp. 34–45, 2006.

[25] L. Simoni-Wastila, "The use of abusable prescription drugs: the role of gender," *Journal of Women's Health and Gender B*, vol. 9, no. 3, pp. 289–297, 2000.

10

The Interactive Effects of Affect Lability, Negative Urgency, and Sensation Seeking on Young Adult Problematic Drinking

Kenny Karyadi, Ayca Coskunpinar, Allyson L. Dir, and Melissa A. Cyders

Indiana University-Purdue University, Indianapolis, IN, USA

Correspondence should be addressed to Kenny Karyadi; kkaryadi@iupui.edu

Academic Editor: Michael Joseph Zvolensky

Prior studies have suggested that affect lability might reduce the risk for problematic drinking among sensation seekers by compensating for their deficiencies in emotional reactivity and among individuals high on negative urgency by disrupting stable negative emotions. Due to the high prevalence of college drinking, this study examined whether affect lability interacted with sensation seeking and negative urgency to influence college student problematic drinking. 414 college drinkers (mean age: 20, 77% female, and 74% Caucasian) from a US Midwestern University completed self-administered questionnaires online. Consistent with our hypotheses, our results indicated that the effects of sensation seeking and negative urgency on problematic drinking weakened at higher levels of affect lability. These findings emphasize the importance of considering specific emotional contexts in understanding how negative urgency and sensation seeking create risk for problematic drinking among college students. These findings might also help us better understand how to reduce problematic drinking among sensation seekers and individuals high on negative urgency.

1. Introduction

Young adult college students in the United States are at a heightened risk for alcohol use problems due to their hazardous patterns of alcohol use [1–4]. Particularly, among 14000 students from 119 universities, 31% endorsed criteria for alcohol abuse and 6% endorsed criteria for alcohol dependence [5]. However, few college students seek treatment for alcohol use problems [1, 5], suggesting a need to identify risk factors for problematic drinking among these students. The National Institute on Alcohol Abuse and Alcoholism (NIAAA) has stated that these young adults have personality traits and psychological vulnerabilities that place them at increased risk for problems with alcohol [6]. The present study examined three traits that have been associated with problematic drinking: negative urgency (tendency to behave impulsively in face of strong negative emotions), sensation seeking (tendency to pursue stimulation through impulsive behaviors), and affect lability (rapidly changing affective states) [7, 8].

Sensation seekers are thought to use alcohol to attain stimulation [9], whereas individuals who are high on negative urgency might use alcohol to alleviate negative emotions

[10], and affectively labile individuals might use alcohol to regulate affective fluctuations [7]. Even though these characteristics indicate different pathways for alcohol use, all three traits have been associated with problematic drinking. However, there are inconsistencies: although sensation seeking has been associated with problematic alcohol use cross-sectionally [11, 12] and prospectively [13], other studies have failed to find this association either cross-sectionally [10] or prospectively [14]. Similarly, negative urgency has been associated with problematic drinking [9, 15, 16], but some research has failed to find the negative urgency-problematic drinking association cross-sectionally [17, 18] and prospectively [14]. Finally, affectively labile individuals have also been shown to engage in problematic drinking [7, 19–21], but the affect lability-problematic drinking association is not always consistent [20, 22].

Taken together, these findings indicate that the effects of sensation seeking, negative urgency, and affect lability on problematic drinking are inconsistent. One potential explanation for these inconsistencies is the presence of an interactive effect. Indeed, prior findings indicated that affect lability interacted with broader impulsivity traits to influence problematic drinking [7, 23], supporting the possibility that

TABLE 1: Measures information.

Measures	Male		Female		Total		t-test
	M	SD	M	SD	M	SD	P
Sensation seeking	3.04	0.56	2.77	0.60	2.83	0.60	<0.0001
Negative urgency	2.35	0.57	2.41	0.62	2.39	0.61	0.44
Anxiety-depression	1.73	0.82	2.07	0.84	1.99	0.84	0.001
Depression-elation	2.07	0.69	2.17	0.69	2.15	0.69	0.25
Anger	1.73	0.76	1.88	0.81	1.84	0.80	0.10
Hazardous drinking	7.85	2.94	6.34	2.09	6.69	2.39	<0.0001
Alcohol problems	5.86	2.33	5.27	1.67	5.41	1.86	0.007

Note: Independent samples t-test were conducted to examine whether scale scores differ between men and women.

affect lability might also interact with more specific forms of impulsivity. However, those findings indicated that high levels of affect lability strengthened the effects of impulsivity traits on problematic drinking. In contrast, the present study proposed that higher levels of affect lability will attenuate the effects of sensation seeking and negative urgency on problematic alcohol use. Specifically, we proposed that affect lability would compensate for emotional reactivity deficiencies among sensation seekers and would disrupt stable negative emotions among individuals high on negative urgency, both of which would reduce the risk for problematic drinking.

It has been theorized that sensation seekers have deficiencies in emotional reactivity [24]. Indeed, prior studies indicated that sensation seekers are less reactive to aversive stimuli [25] and threatening images [26]. Sensation seekers might engage in risky behaviors, such as alcohol use [10], in order to achieve stimulation and to compensate for these deficiencies in emotional reactivity [24, 27]. At the same time, affect lability has been shown to be present in some sensation seekers [24] and has been characterized as enhanced emotional reactivity [28]. High levels of affect lability might compensate for deficiencies in emotional reactivity among sensation seekers. If this is the case, affectively labile sensation seekers may be less likely to use alcohol as a means of compensation. We hypothesized that high levels of affect lability would weaken the effect of sensation seeking on problematic drinking.

Individuals who are high on negative urgency have been thought to be emotionally dysregulated. The experience of negative emotions might cause these individuals to focus on their immediate emotional needs [29, 30] and to engage in risky behaviors, such as alcohol use, in order to address those emotional needs [10]. Furthermore, prior findings indicated that risky behaviors among individuals high on urgency are driven by strong and stable emotional states [31, 32], suggesting that problematic alcohol use among individuals high on negative urgency might also be driven by strong and stable negative emotions. In contrast, affect lability is characterized by fluctuations in affective states [7]. The presence of affect lability among individuals high on negative urgency might undermine the strong and stable negative emotions needed to drive alcohol use. We hypothesized that high levels of affect lability would weaken the effect of negative urgency on problematic drinking.

2. Materials and Methods

2.1. Participants and Procedure. Study data were obtained from undergraduate students (n = 785) enrolled in lower level psychology courses at a US Midwestern University. The final study sample was restricted to ages 18–25, in order to focus on young adults, as recommended by NIAAA [33]. Furthermore, the final study sample was also restricted to those who consumed alcohol on at least a monthly basis (n = 414), in order to ensure that observed effects were not confounded by abstention. About 77% of the final sample was female and 23% was male. The mean age of the sample was 20.11 years old (SD = 1.79). The sample was comprised of about 74% European American, 9% African American, 5% Hispanic American, and 3% Asian American—with the remaining 9% comprising other races. The original and final samples did not significantly differ on race or sex. The study was approved by the university's Institutional Review Board. Participants completed the study in one session using a web-based questionnaire and were awarded course credit for participation.

2.2. Measures (See Table 1)

2.2.1. Hazardous Alcohol Use and Alcohol-Related Problems. We decided to use two subscales of the Alcohol Use Disorder Identification Test rather than the full scale [34]. This is because the subscales allow us to measure specific constructs underlying problematic alcohol use, including alcohol-related problems and hazardous patterns of drinking, whereas the full scale assesses the risk for alcohol use disorders. Additionally, as suggested by Coskunpinar and colleagues [35], disaggregating alcohol outcomes will lead to more robust prediction by impulsivity-related traits. All items were rated on a 5-point Likert scale, with higher ratings indicating higher levels of alcohol involvement. The hazardous alcohol use subscale consists of 2 items (α = .83) and was calculated as a sum, with higher summed values indicating greater levels of hazardous alcohol use. This subscale assesses frequency of heavy drinking and typical quantity of drinking. Alcohol-related problems consist of 4 items (α = .67), with higher summed values indicating greater levels of alcohol-related problems. This subscale assesses whether participants have ever felt guilty after drinking, had blackouts

TABLE 2: Correlations among predictors and outcomes.

Variables	1	2	3	4	5	6	7
(1) HAU	1	.61**	.26**	.21**	.001	.02	.06
(2) ARP		1	.13**	.28**	.13**	.16**	.16**
(3) SS			1	.08	−.09	.07	.04
(4) NUR				1	.45**	.40**	.51**
(5) ADL					1	.68**	.69**
(6) DEL						1	.63**
(7) AL							1

Note: *indicates $P < 0.05$, **indicates $P < 0.01$. HAU: hazardous alcohol use, ARP: alcohol-related problems, SS: sensation seeking, NUR: negative urgency, ADL: anxiety-depression lability, DEL: depression-elation lability, and AL: anger lability.

and other alcohol-related injuries, and have had others expressed concerns about their drinking.

2.2.2. Sensation Seeking and Negative Urgency.

Sensation seeking and negative urgency were assessed using subscales of the UPPS-P Impulsive Behavior Scale—which is a 59-item inventory designed to measure personality pathways to impulsive behavior [36]. All items were assessed in terms of likelihood of occurrence, with response options ranging from (1) "Disagree Strongly" to (4) "Agree Strongly." The subscales were calculated as separate means, with higher mean values indicating higher levels of the trait. The sensation seeking subscale consists of 12 items, which assess the tendency to seek out stimulation and excitement ($\alpha = .87$). The negative urgency subscale consists of 12 items, which assess impulsive behaviors that are related to negative affect ($\alpha = .86$).

2.2.3. Affect Lability.

Affect lability was assessed using the Affective Lability Scale-Short Form, which is an 18-item scale designed to measure fluctuations in affective states [37]. The ALS-SF has three subscales, which include anxiety and depression lability, anger lability, and depression and elation lability. The anxiety-depression lability subscale consists of 5 items, which assess fluctuations between anxiety and depression ($\alpha = .90$). The anger lability subscale consists of 5 items, which assess changes in affective states from neutral to anger ($\alpha = .89$). The depression-elation lability subscale consists of 8 items, which assess fluctuations between depression and elation ($\alpha = .88$). Response options for these items ranged from (1) "Very characteristic of me" to (4) "Very uncharacteristic of me." Separate mean values were calculated for each subscale, with higher mean values indicative of higher degrees of affect lability.

2.3. Analytic Strategy.

Using SPSS 19.0, we examined bivariate correlations among all study variables and performed a series of multiple regression and simple slope analyses. All continuous predictors were centered to facilitate interpretation of the interaction coefficients, and significant interactions were probed at the mean and +1/−1 SD of the moderator using simple slope analyses [38]. Because problematic alcohol use has been shown to differ between men and women [39], gender was included as a covariate in all analyses. Age has also

been differentially associated with problematic alcohol use [40] and was included as a covariate. We tested all potential covariates by predictor interactions to ensure that the effects of the predictors were independent of the covariates and considered retaining any interactions that were significant at $P < .01$ to guard against alpha inflation. No covariate by predictor interactions met this criterion, suggesting that the effects of the covariates were independent of those of the predictors.

3. Results

We first examined the correlations among our predictors and outcomes. Sensation seeking ($r = .13$, $P < .01$) and negative urgency ($r = .28$, $P < .01$) were both positively correlated with alcohol-related problems. Similarly, negative urgency ($r = .21$, $P < .01$) and sensation seeking ($r = .26$, $P < .01$) were positively correlated with hazardous alcohol use. Anxiety-depression lability ($r = .13$, $P < .01$), depression-elation lability ($r = .16$, $P < .01$), and anger lability ($r = .16$, $P < .01$) were positively correlated with alcohol-related problems, but not with hazardous alcohol use. Negative urgency, but not sensation seeking, was positively correlated with all the affect lability scales, with correlations ranging from .39 to .51 (all $P < .01$). Table 2 provides correlations among the predictors and outcomes.

Next, we tested whether the specific affect lability traits moderated the effects of sensation seeking and negative urgency on alcohol-related problems and hazardous alcohol use. For hazardous alcohol use, the effect of sensation seeking was moderated by anxiety-depression lability ($b = -.48$, $P = .02$). In this analysis, both gender ($b = 1.17$, $P < 0.0001$) and age ($b = 0.15$, $P = 0.02$) had significant effects on hazardous alcohol use. Simple slope analyses indicated that sensation seeking was associated with hazardous alcohol use at low levels of anxiety-depression lability ($b = 1.82$, $P < .001$), but this effect weakened for those at mean anxiety-depression lability ($b = 0.86$, $P < .001$) and was nonsignificant at high levels of anxiety-depression lability ($b = -0.09$, $P = 0.85$) (see Figure 1). Furthermore, the interaction between negative urgency and anxiety-depression lability on hazardous alcohol use approached significance ($b = -.40$, $P = .06$). Both gender ($b = 1.29$, $P < 0.0001$) and age ($b = 0.20$, $P = 0.002$)

TABLE 3: Interactions among sensation seeking, negative urgency, and affect lability on hazardous alcohol use and alcohol-related problems.

Predictors	HAU					ARP				
	b	SE	β	ΔR^2	P	b	SE	β	ΔR^2	P
SS × ADL	**−.48**	**.20**	**−.11**	**.01**	**.02**	−.29	.17	−.09	.01	.08
SS × DEL	−.47	.27	−.09	.01	.08	**−.41**	**.21**	**−.10**	**.01**	**.05**
SS × AL	−.19	.23	−.04	.00	.41	**−.47**	**.19**	**−.12**	**.02**	**.01**
NUR × ADL	**−.40**	**.22**	**−.09**	**.01**	**.06**	−.06	.17	−.02	.00	.73
NUR × DEL	−.16	.26	−.03	.00	.55	−.02	.21	−.01	.00	.91
NUR × AL	−.30	.23	−.07	.00	.18	−.18	.18	−.05	.00	.33

Note: bolded coefficients were significant at $P < .05$, and ΔR^2 refers to change in R^2 in the third step of the analyses (when the interaction term was entered). HAU: hazardous alcohol use, ARP: alcohol-related problems, SS: sensation seeking, NUR: negative urgency, ADL: anxiety-depression lability, DEL: depression-elation lability, and AL: anger lability.

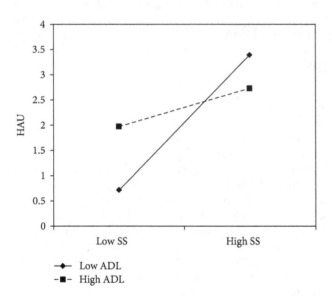

FIGURE 1: Anxiety and depression lability moderated the effect of sensation seeking on hazardous alcohol use among college students.

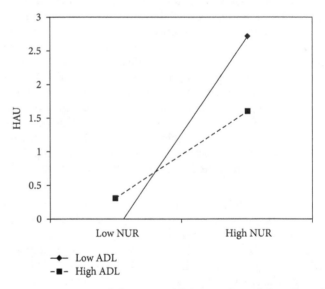

FIGURE 2: Anxiety and depression lability moderated the effect of negative urgency on hazardous alcohol use among college students.

had significant effects on hazardous alcohol use. The effects of negative urgency on hazardous alcohol use were positive and significant among those low on anxiety-depression lability ($b = 1.84$, $P < .001$) and at mean anxiety-depression lability ($b = 1.05$, $P < .001$), but not at high levels of anxiety-depression lability ($b = 0.25$, $P = 0.60$) (see Figure 2).

For alcohol-related problems, the effect of sensation seeking was moderated by anger lability ($b = -.41$, $P = .01$). Gender ($b = 0.49$, $P = 0.03$), but not age ($b = -0.01$, $P = 0.89$), had a significant effect on alcohol-related problems. Simple slope analyses indicated that sensation seeking was associated with alcohol-related problems at low levels of depression-elation lability ($b = 1.10$, $P = .02$), but the effect weakened at mean ($b = 0.22$, $P = 0.16$) and high levels of depression-elation lability ($b = -0.66$, $P = 0.18$) (see Figure 3). Furthermore, the interaction between depression-elation

lability and sensation seeking approached significance ($b = -.41$, $P = .05$). Once again, gender had a significant effect on alcohol-related problems ($b = 0.47$, $P = 0.04$), but age did not ($b = -0.002$, $P = 0.97$). Sensation seeking was associated with alcohol-related problems at low levels of anger lability ($b = 1.14$, $P = .002$), but not at mean ($b = 0.28$, $P = 0.07$) and high levels of anger lability ($b = -0.59$, $P = 0.12$) (see Figure 4). Table 3 summarizes the interaction results.

4. Discussion

Consistent with our hypotheses, our results indicated that sensation seekers and individuals high on negative urgency are at lower risk for hazardous alcohol use and alcohol-related problems, but only within the context of higher affect lability traits. These findings help explain prior inconsistencies in

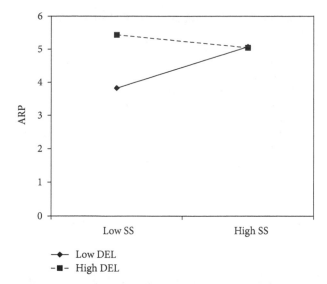

FIGURE 3: Depression and elation lability moderated the effect of sensation seeking on alcohol-related problems among college students.

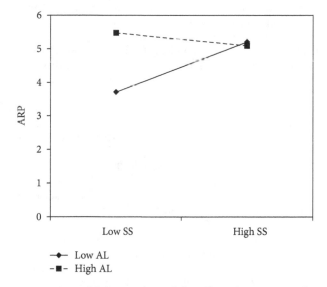

FIGURE 4: Anger lability moderated the effect of sensation seeking on alcohol-related problems among college students.

the literature [11, 14, 16] by emphasizing the importance of considering specific emotional experiences in understanding how negative urgency and sensation seeking create risk for problematic drinking. Moreover, these findings also clarify prior impulsivity-affect lability interactions [7, 23] by showing that affect lability interacts with more specific forms of impulsivity differently. Finally, these findings emphasize the importance of considering these three factors when addressing problematic drinking among college students.

It has been theorized that sensation seekers engage in risky behaviors, such as alcohol use [10], to compensate for deficiencies in emotional reactivity [24, 41]. Our findings provide some support for the notion that the concurrent experience of affect lability might compensate for these deficiencies. Specifically, college students who are high on both sensation seeking and affect lability might have less emotional reactivity deficiencies and might consequently be less likely to use alcohol to compensate for emotional reactivity deficiencies and to experience problems from alcohol use. Relatedly, although affect lability is not typically considered a protective factor, these findings suggest that problematic drinking among sensation seeking college students could be reduced by increasing emotional reactivity. However, future studies are needed to examine the extent to which emotional reactivity might protect sensation seeking college students from engaging in problematic drinking.

Furthermore, our results support prior findings indicating that the urgency-risky behavior association is strengthened by strong and stable emotions [31, 32] by showing that affective fluctuations weaken the effect of negative urgency on problematic drinking. Specifically, when college students high on negative urgency experience affective fluctuations, their current emotional states might not be stable enough to drive alcohol use behaviors. Again, although affect lability is not a protective factor, these findings indicate that one approach of reducing problematic drinking among college students high on urgency is by disrupting strong and stable emotions. Indeed, prior studies have indicated multiple therapeutic approaches that are effective for dealing with strong distressing emotions and alcohol use [42]. However, future studies are needed to examine whether disrupting strong and stable negative emotions among college students high on urgency directly lead to a reduction in problematic drinking behaviors.

Finally, we have thus far discussed affect lability as a protective factor among college students who are high on urgency and sensation seeking. However, prior studies have indicated that affectively labile individuals engage in problematic drinking as a way of coping with affective fluctuations [7, 19–21]. Based on these prior studies, affect lability does not appear to be a protective factor. At the same time, there are some features of affect lability that might confer protection against problematic drinking for certain individuals. For instance, affect lability might render sensation seeking college students more emotionally reactive and might disrupt stable negative emotions among college students high on negative urgency. Future studies should examine whether cultivating these specific features of affect lability can reduce problematic drinking among college students high on negative urgency and sensation seeking.

The current study does have some limitations, which may hamper its generalizability. First, the cross-sectional nature limits causal inferences. Second, the sample was comprised of mostly Caucasian, female, young adults. Although this sample of young adults helps attain the goal of understanding problematic alcohol use among young adults given their increased risk, it is unclear how the current results would generalize to other more diverse sample. Furthermore, the internal consistency coefficient for our measure of alcohol-related problems was low (α = .67), which may have limited our power to detect the effects of our predictors on alcohol-related problems. Additionally, the current study did not examine how affect lability might interact with other impulsivity-related traits, such as positive urgency. Finally, the interaction effects were small ($b < 3$), possibly limiting the clinical relevance of our findings and indicating that future studies should replicate these findings using college students with alcohol use disorders in order to further support clinical implications.

5. Conclusions

Overall, these results indicated that affect lability seems to alter the effects of sensation seeking and negative urgency on problematic drinking. These results suggest that we must take into account emotional stability and reactivity in order to elucidate whether sensation seeking and negative urgency are creating risk for problematic alcohol use among college students. Our results also provide some support for the development of alcohol interventions that focus on disrupting stable negative emotions and that focus on increasing emotional reactivity. Although affect lability is not necessarily a protective factor, practitioners and researchers should still consider how increasing some features of affect lability might be beneficial for college drinkers who are high on negative urgency and sensation seeking.

Conflict of Interests

There is no conflict of interests associated with the present study.

References

[1] C. Blanco, M. Okuda, C. Wright et al., "Mental health of college students and their non-college-attending peers: results from the national epidemiologic study on alcohol and related conditions," *Archives of General Psychiatry*, vol. 65, no. 12, pp. 1429–1437, 2008.

[2] R. Hingson, T. Heeren, M. Winter, and H. Wechsler, "Magnitude of alcohol-related mortality and morbidity among U.S. college students ages 18–24: changes from 1998 to 2001," *Annual Review of Public Health*, vol. 26, pp. 259–279, 2005.

[3] R. W. Hingson, W. Zha, and E. R. Weitzman, "Magnitude of and trends in alcohol-related mortality and morbidity among U.S. college students ages 18–24, 1998–2005," *Journal of Studies on Alcohol and Drugs*, no. 16, pp. 12–20, 2009.

[4] H. R. White, B. J. McMorris, R. F. Catalano, C. B. Fleming, K. P. Haggerty, and R. D. Abbott, "Increases in alcohol and marijuana use during the transition out of high school into emerging adulthood: the effects of leaving home, going to college, and high school protective factors," *Journal of Studies on Alcohol*, vol. 67, no. 6, pp. 810–822, 2006.

[5] J. R. Knight, H. Wechsler, M. Kuo, M. Seibring, E. R. Weitzman, and M. A. Schuckit, "Alcohol abuse and dependence among U.S. college students," *Journal of Studies on Alcohol*, vol. 63, no. 3, pp. 263–270, 2002.

[6] National Institute on Alcohol Abuse and Alcoholism, "Alcohol alert: young adult drinking," 2006, http://pubs.niaaa.nih.gov/publications/aa68/aa68.htm.

[7] J. S. Simons, K. B. Carey, and R. M. Gaher, "Lability and impulsivity synergistically increase risk for alcohol-related problems,"

[8] S. P. Whiteside and D. R. Lynam, "The five factor model and impulsivity: using a structural model of personality to understand impulsivity," *Personality and Individual Differences*, vol. 30, no. 4, pp. 669–689, 2001.

[9] S. Fischer and G. T. Smith, "Binge eating, problem drinking, and pathological gambling: linking behavior to shared traits and social learning," *Personality and Individual Differences*, vol. 44, no. 4, pp. 789–800, 2008.

[10] G. T. Smith, S. Fischer, M. A. Cyders, A. M. Annus, N. S. Spillane, and D. M. McCarthy, "On the validity and utility of discriminating among impulsivity-like traits," *Assessment*, vol. 14, no. 2, pp. 155–170, 2007.

[11] K. P. Lindgren, P. M. Mullins, C. Neighbors, and J. A. Blayney, "Curiosity killed the cocktail? curiosity, sensation seeking, and alcohol-related problems in college women," *Addictive Behaviors*, vol. 35, no. 5, pp. 513–516, 2010.

[12] V. Magid, M. G. MacLean, and C. R. Colder, "Differentiating between sensation seeking and impulsivity through their mediated relations with alcohol use and problems," *Addictive Behaviors*, vol. 32, no. 10, pp. 2046–2061, 2007.

[13] A. W. Stacy, M. D. Newcomb, and P. M. Bentler, "Cognitive motivations and sensation seeking as long-term predictors of drinking problems," *Journal of Social and Clinical Psychology*, vol. 12, no. 1, pp. 1–24, 1993.

[14] M. A. Cyders, K. Flory, S. Rainer, and G. T. Smith, "The role of personality dispositions to risky behavior in predicting first-year college drinking," *Addiction*, vol. 104, no. 2, pp. 193–202, 2009.

[15] S. Fischer, K. G. Anderson, and G. T. Smith, "Coping with distress by eating or drinking: role of trait urgency and expectancies," *Psychology of Addictive Behaviors*, vol. 18, no. 3, pp. 269–274, 2004.

[16] M. A. Cyders, G. T. Smith, N. S. Spillane, S. Fischer, A. M. Annus, and C. Peterson, "Integration of impulsivity and positive mood to predict risky behavior: development and validation of a measure of positive urgency," *Psychological Assessment*, vol. 19, no. 1, pp. 107–118, 2007.

[17] J. Acker, M. Amlung, J. Stojek, J. M. Murphy, and J. MacKillop, "Individual variation in behavioral economic indices of the relative value of alcohol: Incremental validity in relation to impulsivity, craving, and intellectual functioning," *Journal of Experimental Psychopathology*, vol. 3, no. 3, pp. 423–436, 2012.

[18] S. P. Whiteside, D. R. Lynam, J. D. Miller, and S. K. Reynolds, "Validation of the UPPS impulsive behaviour scale: a four-factor model of impulsivity," *European Journal of Personality*, vol. 19, no. 7, pp. 559–574, 2005.

[19] D. G. Kilpatrick, P. B. Sutker, and A. D. Smith, "Deviant drug and alcohol use: the role of anxiety, sensations seeking, and other personality variables," in *Emotions and Anxiety: New Concepts, Methods, and Applications*, M. Zuckerman and C. D. Spielberger, Eds., Lawrence Erlbaum, Oxford, UK, 1976.

[20] L. A. Rankin and J. L. Maggs, "First-year college student affect and alcohol use: paradoxical within- and between-person associations," *Journal of Youth and Adolescence*, vol. 35, no. 6, pp. 925–937, 2006.

[21] J. S. Simons and K. B. Carey, "An affective and cognitive model of marijuana and alcohol problems," *Addictive Behaviors*, vol. 31, no. 9, pp. 1578–1592, 2006.

[22] J. S. Simons, M. N. I. Oliver, R. M. Gaher, G. Ebel, and P. Brummels, "Methamphetamine and alcohol abuse and

American Journal of Drug and Alcohol Abuse, vol. 30, no. 3, pp. 685–694, 2004.

dependence symptoms: associations with affect lability and impulsivity in a rural treatment population," *Addictive Behaviors*, vol. 30, no. 7, pp. 1370–1381, 2005.

[23] J. S. Simons, K. B. Carey, and T. A. Wills, "Alcohol abuse and dependence symptoms: a multidimensional model of common and specific etiology," *Psychology of Addictive Behaviors*, vol. 23, no. 3, pp. 415–427, 2009.

[24] S. Carton, R. Jouvent, C. Bungener, and D. Widlöcher, "Sensation seeking and depressive mood," *Personality and Individual Differences*, vol. 13, no. 7, pp. 843–849, 1992.

[25] S. Lissek, J. M. P. Baas, D. S. Pine et al., "Sensation seeking and the aversive motivational system," *Emotion*, vol. 5, no. 4, pp. 396–407, 2005.

[26] S. Lissek and A. S. Powers, "Sensation seeking and startle modulation by physically threatening images," *Biological Psychology*, vol. 63, no. 2, pp. 179–197, 2003.

[27] A. Pierson, J. Le Houezec, A. Fossaert, S. Dubal, and R. Jouvent, "Frontal reactivity and sensation seeking an ERP study in skydivers," *Progress in Neuro-Psychopharmacology and Biological Psychiatry*, vol. 23, no. 3, pp. 447–463, 1999.

[28] J. S. Simons, "Differential prediction of alcohol use and problems: the role of biopsychological and social-environmental variables," *American Journal of Drug and Alcohol Abuse*, vol. 29, no. 4, pp. 861–879, 2003.

[29] M. A. Cyders and G. T. Smith, "Mood-based rash action and its components: positive and negative urgency," *Personality and Individual Differences*, vol. 43, no. 4, pp. 839–850, 2007.

[30] M. A. Cyders and G. T. Smith, "Emotion-based dispositions to rash action: positive and negative urgency," *Psychological Bulletin*, vol. 134, no. 6, pp. 807–828, 2008.

[31] M. A. Cyders and A. Coskunpinar, "Is urgency emotionality? separating urgent behaviors from effects of emotional experiences," *Personality and Individual Differences*, vol. 48, no. 7, pp. 839–844, 2010.

[32] K. A. Karyadi and K. M. King, "Urgency and negative emotions: evidence for moderation on negative alcohol consequences," *Personality and Individual Differences*, vol. 51, no. 5, pp. 635–640, 2011.

[33] C. M. Chen, M. C. Dufour, and H. Y. Yi, "Alcohol consumption among young adults ages 18-24 in the united states: results from the 2001-2002 NESARC survey," *Alcohol Research and Health*, vol. 28, no. 4, pp. 269–280, 2005.

[34] T. F. Babor, J. R. de la Fuente, J. Saunders, and M. Grant, *The Alcohol Use Disorders Identification Test: Guidelines For Use in Primary Health Care*, World Health Organization, Geneva, Switzerland, 1992.

[35] A. Coskunpinar, A. L. Dir, and M. A. Cyders, "Multidimensionality in impulsivity and alcohol use: from small to robust effects," . In press.

[36] D. Lynam, G. T. Smith, M. A. Cyders, S. Fischer, and S. A. Whiteside, "The UPPS-P: a multidimensional measure of risk for impulsive behavior," Tech. Rep., 2007.

[37] M. N. I. Oliver and J. S. Simons, "The affective lability scales: development of a short-form measure," *Personality and Individual Differences*, vol. 37, no. 6, pp. 1279–1288, 2004.

[38] J. Cohen, P. Cohen, S. G. West, and L. S. Aiken, *Applied Multiple Regression/Correlation Analysis For the Behavioral Sciences*, Erlbaum, Mahwah, NJ, USA, 3rd edition, 2003.

[39] S. Nolen-Hoeksema, "Gender differences in risk factors and consequences for alcohol use and problems," *Clinical Psychology Review*, vol. 24, no. 8, pp. 981–1010, 2004.

[40] B. C. Leigh and A. W. Stacy, "Alcohol expectancies and drinking in different age groups," *Addiction*, vol. 99, no. 2, pp. 215–227, 2004.

[41] S. Carton, "Sensation-seeking and emotional disturbances in depression: relationships and evolution," *Journal of Affective Disorders*, vol. 34, no. 3, pp. 219–225, 1995.

[42] T. C. B. Zapolski, R. E. Settles, M. A. Cyders, and G. T. Smith, "Borderline personality disorder, bulimia nervosa, antisocial personality disorder, ADHD, substance use: common threads, common treatment needs, and the nature of impulsivity," *Independent Practitioner*, vol. 30, no. 1, pp. 20–23, 2009.

11

Drug Poisoning Deaths according to Ethnicity in Utah

Ray M. Merrill,[1] Riley J. Hedin,[1] Anna Fondario,[2] Arielle A. Sloan,[1] and Carl L. Hanson[1]

[1] Department of Health Science, Brigham Young University, Provo, UT 84602, USA
[2] Violence and Injury Prevention Program, Utah Department of Health, Salt Lake City, UT 84114, USA

Correspondence should be addressed to Ray M. Merrill; ray_merrill@byu.edu

Academic Editor: Dace Svikis

This study characterizes drug-related deaths according to ethnicity in Utah during 2005–2010, based on data from the Utah Violent Death Reporting System (UTVDRS). Hispanics made up 12.1% (12.5% male and 11.7% female) of deaths. The most frequently identified drugs among decedents were opiates, then illicit drugs, benzodiazepines, over-the-counter medication, and antidepressants. Death rates for each drug were significantly greater in non-Hispanics than Hispanics. Most decedents used a combination of drugs. For each combination, rates were significantly greater for non-Hispanics than Hispanics, with an exception for opiates and illicit drugs combined, where there was no significant difference. Approximately 79% of non-Hispanics and 65% of Hispanics had one or more of the selected problems (e.g., mental, physical, or crisis related). Rates for each combination of problems were significantly greater in non-Hispanics, with the exception of crisis. Hispanics were less affected by the rise in prescription drug abuse. Hispanic decedents had a greater proportion of illegal drugs, consistent with it being more difficult to obtain prescription drugs. Hispanic decedents were less likely to have physical and mental health problems, which may be related to a smaller chance of diagnosis of such problems through the healthcare system.

1. Introduction

Drug-related death rates in the United States have steadily increased in the past decade. Deaths from drug poisonings more than doubled from 6 per 100,000 in 2000 to 12.5 per 100,000 in 2010 [1]. Since 2009, deaths due to drug poisonings have exceeded deaths from motor vehicle accidents, with males being at greater risk than females, and death rates peaking at age of 45–54 [1]. Several studies have reported increasing death rates from opioid analgesics (e.g., oxycodone, methadone, or hydrocodone) [2–7]. Since 2003, more overdose deaths have resulted from opioid analgesics than heroin and cocaine combined [6].

In 2010, the drug poisoning rate in Utah was 16.9 per 100,000, compared with 12.3 per 100,000 in the United States [8]. Utah ranked eighth highest in the nation. Recent studies have explored selected aspects of prescription opioid-related deaths in Utah [9, 10]. However, these studies have not looked at the influence of ethnicity on drug-related deaths. It has previously been observed that racial/ethnic minorities in the United States are less likely to use prescription drugs and, consequently, less likely to abuse them [11]. In the current study, we examine whether drug-related death rates are lower for Hispanics than non-Hispanics in Utah, according to age and gender. The study also explores whether differences exist in specific types of drugs implicated with the decedents and if problems experienced just prior to death differ between ethnicities. This information may help public health officials better understand and successfully intervene in reducing drug-related deaths among Hispanics and non-Hispanics.

2. Materials and Methods

A retrospective cohort study was conducted on drug overdose deaths in Utah. The Hispanic-Latino (hereafter Hispanic) population in Utah in 2012 represented 13.3% of the state's population [12]. In addition, the Hispanic population consisted of the following:

(i) 49.7% female.

(ii) 31.2% under 18 years of age.

(iii) 9.5% over 65 years old.

(iv) 66.8% of adults (18 years and older) married.

(v) Median household income of $57,783 (during 2007–2011).

(vi) 90.6% with a high school degree and 29.6% with a bachelor's degree or higher among those aged 25 years and older [12, 13].

All drug-related deaths identified for this study occurred in Utah from 2005 through 2010. Data were collected from death certificates, police reports, and reports produced by the Office of the Medical Examiner (OME) and entered into the Utah Violent Death Reporting System (UTVDRS) [14]. The OME investigates each sudden or unexpected death [15]. Police and medical examiner reports document the scene of death with pictures, detailed notes, interviews with witnesses or family members and friends of the victim, autopsies, and toxicology testing. State-level data are then pooled together in the National Violent Death Reporting System (NVDRS), a secure database implemented by the Centers for Disease Control and Prevention (CDC).

For each drug-related death in the current study, abstractors coded for selected variables, such as age, sex, ethnicity, history of mental illness, and alcohol or substance use/abuse, and also wrote a short narrative that summarized the investigative findings from medical examiner and law enforcement records. Accidental drug overdose deaths were incorporated into the UTVDRS system using the same coding manual and abstraction procedures of UTVDRS cases. To control for inconsistency among the various sources of data, abstractors participated in a coding training and a review of the coding manual. In addition, ongoing coding support was provided through the CDC, the UTVDRS team epidemiologist, and the lead abstractor. Further, the team epidemiologist reviewed each incident as it was being abstracted to check for coding errors, to ensure that endorsed circumstance variables were supported in the narrative, and to run logic queries on the data. Cases with discrepancies were flagged for further abstractor review. Further, data were analyzed by a hierarchical rule for each variable. The hierarchical rule used for our data is based on the rules set forth by the CDC. Data sources were ranked in terms of their potential reliability for each data element. For example, age of the victim was taken first from the death certificate, second from the medical examiner report, and finally from police records. When data sources had complete but discordant data, the hierarchical rule was also used for each variable. Some UTVDRS variables, including mental illness, relied on information from friends and family members when proper records were unavailable.

The process of compiling the drug overdose death data used in this study occurred during June through September 2011. There were 2,843 drug-related deaths in Utah from 2005 through 2010 (31.2% accidents, 13.3% suicides, and 55.5% undetermined intent for non-Hispanics and 25.3% accidents, 9.9% suicides, and 64.8% undetermined intent for Hispanics). Forty persons had unknown ethnicity and were therefore excluded from the current study. Institutional Review Board approval was obtained from the Utah Department of Health.

2.1. Description of Measures. The primary outcome measure was drug type. Drugs were classified as opioid analgesics (pain relievers), benzodiazepines (to relieve nervousness), antidepressants (to relieve or prevent psychic depression), illicit (e.g., cocaine, heroin, and methamphetamines), and over-the-counter.

Selected demographic variables were considered, wherein age was categorized as 0–24, 25–34, 35–44, 45–54, and 55 and older, and ethnicity was represented by Hispanics and non-Hispanics. The frequency of seven events that may have occurred just prior to the decedents drug overdose was assessed among the decedents: current mental health problem, current physical health problem, crisis in the past two weeks, alcohol problem, job problem, financial problem, and recent criminal legal problem. They were reported based on the medical examiner report and law enforcement narratives. Brief descriptions of these variables from the coding manual are as follows.

(i) Mental health problem: the victim was experiencing mental health problems that were relevant to the event.

(ii) Physical health problem: the victim was experiencing physical health problems that were relevant to the event.

(iii) Recent crisis: it identifies cases in which a very current crisis or acute precipitating event appears to have contributed to the death two weeks prior to or would have occurred within two weeks after the incident.

(iv) Alcohol problem: the victim was perceived by self or others to have a problem with, or to be addicted to, alcohol. There does not need to be any indication that the problem directly contributed to the death.

(v) Job problem: it is coded as "yes" if, at the time of the incident, the victim was either experiencing a problem at work or was having a problem with joblessness, and this appears to have contributed to the death.

(vi) Financial problem: it is coded as "yes" if, at the time of the incident, the victim was experiencing a problem such as bankruptcy, overwhelming debts, or foreclosure of a home or business, and this appears to have contributed to the death.

(vii) Recent criminal legal problem: it is coded as "yes" if, at the time of the incident, the victim was facing criminal legal problems and this appears to have contributed to the death.

2.2. Statistical Techniques. Percentages and rates were used to describe the decedents. Rates were calculated with population estimates for Hispanics and non-Hispanics obtained from the U.S. Census Bureau [16]. Poisson regression was also used to assess associations, adjusting for age and sex. Distributions of age, sex, drug type, and selected problems were compared between Hispanics and non-Hispanics and tested for statistical significance using the chi-square test. Tests of significance were based on two-sided hypothesis tests using the 0.05 level. Analysis was performed using Statistical Analysis System (SAS) software version 9.3 (SAS Institute Inc., Cary, NC, USA, 2010).

TABLE 1: Sex- and age-specific drug-related deaths in Utah according to ethnicity, 2005–2010.

Demographic	Non-Hispanic				Hispanic				Rate ratio	95% CI
	Deaths	%	Rate per 100,000	95% CI	Deaths	%	Rate per 100,000	95% CI		
Sex										
Male	1,555	58.4	22.5	21.4–23.6	82	57.7	8.3	6.5–10.1	2.72	2.28–3.40
Female	1,106	41.6	16.0	15.0–16.9	60	42.3	6.6	4.9–8.2	2.44	1.88–3.16
Age										
0–24	353	13.3	6.0	5.4–6.6	23	16.2	2.3	1.3–3.2	2.64	1.73–4.02
25–34	658	24.7	30.4	28.1–32.8	40	28.2	11.5	8.0–15.1	2.64	1.92–3.63
35–44	641	24.1	39.2	36.2–42.3	40	28.2	15.5	10.7–20.2	2.54	1.85–3.50
45–54	691	26.0	42.4	39.2–45.6	28	19.7	17.9	11.3–24.6	2.37	1.62–3.45
55+	318	11.9	12.5	11.1–13.8	11	7.7	8.1	3.3–12.8	1.55	0.85–2.82

Data source: Utah Department of Health.
Note: percentages sum to 100 across rows.

TABLE 2: Specific drug types implicated in death according to ethnicity in Utah, 2005–2010.

	Non-Hispanic				Hispanic				Rate ratio	95% CI
	Deaths	%	Rate per 100,000	95% CI	Deaths	%	Rate per 100,000	95% CI		
Opiates	1,564	58.8	11.3	10.4–12.2	71	50.0	3.7	2.3–4.9	3.04	2.39–3.85
Illicit drugs	786	29.5	5.7	4.7–6.7	72	50.7	3.8	1.7–5.8	1.50	1.18–1.91
Benzodiazepines	420	15.8	3.0	2.2–3.9	20	14.1	1.0	−0.2–2.3	2.89	1.85–4.53
Over-the-counter drugs	121	7.5	0.9	0.4–1.3	5	5.6	0.3	−0.6–1.2	2.77	1.22–6.31
Antidepressants	200	4.6	1.4	1.0–1.9	8	4.2	0.4	−0.7–1.5	3.44	1.70–6.98

Data source: Utah Department of Health.
Note: percentages reflect the decedents having the selected drug type involved in their death.

3. Results

During 2005 through 2010, the percent of the Utah population that was Hispanic was 12.1 (12.5 for males and 11.7 for females). Among Hispanics, racial classifications were 92.1% White, 2.3% Black, 4.0% American Indian/Alaska Native, and 1.5% Asian or Pacific Islander. Corresponding classifications for non-Hispanics were 94.0%, 1.3%, 1.3%, and 3.5%. The percent of the Utah population who were Hispanic steadily increased during 2005 through 2010, from 11.5 to 13.4 in males and from 10.5 to 12.7 in females. The increasing percentages occurred across the following age groups: 13.1 to 16.0 (22.3%) in ages 0–24, 13.5 to 14.0 (3.3%) in ages 25–34, 11.9 to 15.0 (26.4%) in ages 35–44, 7.5 to 10.1 (34.8%) in ages 45–54, and 4.6 to 5.5 (20.6%) in ages 55 years and older.

Drug-related overdose deaths are presented according to ethnicity in Table 1. The distribution of males and females was not significantly different between non-Hispanic and Hispanic decedents (chi-square $P = 0.8708$). In addition, the age distribution did not significantly differ between the ethnic groups (chi-square $P = 0.1641$). Approximately 58% of decedents were male and about 75% were aged from 25 to 54 years. The death rate (per 100,000) attributed to drug poisoning was 19.2 for non-Hispanics compared with 7.4 for Hispanics (Rate ratio = 2.59, 95% CI = 2.18–3.06). The higher rate ratio observed in non-Hispanics was more pronounced in males than females and became insignificant in the oldest age group.

The most frequently identified drugs among decedents were opiates, followed by illicit drugs, benzodiazepines, over-the-counter medication, and finally antidepressants (Table 2). The distribution of the selected drug types shown in the table significantly differed between non-Hispanics and Hispanics (chi-square $P = 0.0004$). Non-Hispanic decedents reflected a greater percentage of opiates and a lower percentage of illicit drugs compared with Hispanics. Rates of death associated with each drug type were significantly greater in non-Hispanics than in Hispanics.

Most decedents used a combination of drugs (83.7%), with the more common combinations of drug types shown for non-Hispanic and Hispanic decedents in Figure 1. Opiates only, illicit drugs only, and then opiates and benzodiazepines only were the most common in non-Hispanics, whereas illicit drugs only, opiates only, and then opiates and illicit drugs only were the most common in Hispanics. For each combination of drugs shown in Figure 1, rates were significantly greater for non-Hispanics than Hispanics (indicated by the non-overlapping 95% confidence intervals), with an exception for opiates and illicit drugs only, where there was no significant difference.

Selected problems were considered among the decedents (Table 3). The distribution of problems did not significantly differ between non-Hispanics and Hispanics (chi-square $P = 0.7736$). Approximately 79% of non-Hispanics and 65% of Hispanics had one or more of these problems. The most

TABLE 3: Selected problems among drug-related deaths according to ethnicity in Utah, 2005–2010.

	Non-Hispanic				Hispanic				Rate ratio	95% CI
	Deaths	%	Rate per 100,000	95% CI	Deaths	%	Rate per 100,000	95% CI		
Current mental health problem	1,374	50.9	9.9	9.4–10.5	53	37.3	2.8	2.0–3.5	3.57	2.71–4.70
Current physical health problem	1,010	37.6	7.3	6.8–7.7	44	31.0	2.3	1.6–3.0	3.16	2.34–4.28
Crisis in past two weeks	635	23.8	4.6	4.2–4.9	33	23.2	1.7	1.1–2.3	2.65	1.87–3.76
Alcohol problem	381	14.3	2.8	2.5–3.0	15	10.6	0.8	0.4–1.2	3.50	2.09–5.86
Recent criminal-legal problem	142	5.2	1.0	0.9–1.2	5	3.5	0.3	0.0–0.5	3.91	1.60–9.55
Job problem	102	3.7	0.7	0.6–0.9	2	1.4	0.1	0.0–0.3	7.03	1.73–28.48
Financial problem	73	2.7	0.5	0.4–0.6	3	2.1	0.2	0.0–0.3	3.35	1.06–10.64

Data source: Utah Department of Health.
Note: percentages reflect the decedents having the selected problem.

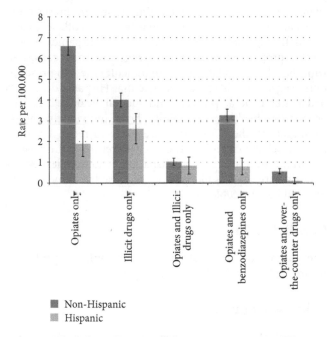

FIGURE 1: Selected combination of drug types among non-Hispanic and Hispanic decedents in Utah, 2005–2010.

common problems were mental, physical, or crisis-related. Non-Hispanics compared with Hispanics had significantly higher rates for each of the selected problems. Combinations of mental problems, health problems, and crisis within the two weeks prior to death are presented in Figure 2. Rates of mental problems only were the greatest, then a combination of mental and physical health problems, and then physical health problems only. Rates for each combination of problems shown in Figure 2 were significantly greater in non-Hispanics than Hispanics, with the exception of crisis only.

4. Discussion

The results showed significantly higher rates of drug-related deaths among non-Hispanics than Hispanics from 2005 through 2010 in Utah (2.7 times for males and 2.4 times for females). A US study involving 2003–2007 data found the drug-related death rate to also be greater in non-Hispanic whites compared with Hispanics (1.4 times in males and 1.3 times in females) [11]. In 2010, a national study found the ratio of non-Hispanic whites compared with Hispanics to be 2.8 [1].

A national trend analysis of pharmaceutical opioid-related overdose deaths compared with other substance-related overdose deaths showed that from 1999 through 2009 the death rate related to pharmaceutical opioids increased fourfold and that opioids were responsible for the greatest relative increase in overdose death rates [5]. Other studies have also identified the rising rate of opioid-related deaths [2, 3, 6, 7, 9]. The number of opioid analgesic overdoses has been shown to be proportional to the amount and dose of the drug prescribed [17]. Although the current study showed that opioid use was common among both non-Hispanic and Hispanic decedents, it was less likely present in Hispanics (58.8% versus 50.0%). Another study found that in New York City, from 1990 to 2006, drug-related deaths involving analgesics were less likely in Hispanics [7].

Not only did Hispanic decedents have lower use of opiates, but they also had lower use of benzodiazepines, over-the-counter drugs, and antidepressants. A surveillance study in the United States previously showed that racial/ethnic minorities are less likely to use prescription drugs and, thus not as likely to abuse them [11]. A 2011 report showed that 40% of Hispanics compared with 10% of white non-Hispanics and 18% of other non-Hispanics in Utah did not have health insurance coverage [18]. It has also been suggested that some Hispanic immigrants lack the cultural and language fluency to navigate the healthcare system [19].

Studies indicate that the rate of drug-related deaths is greater among males than females and increases in successive age groups through 45–54 and then decreases thereafter [1, 20]. We observed this same pattern among both non-Hispanics and Hispanics in Utah. In addition, the higher drug-related death rates among non-Hispanics were seen in both males and females and across the age span. Hence,

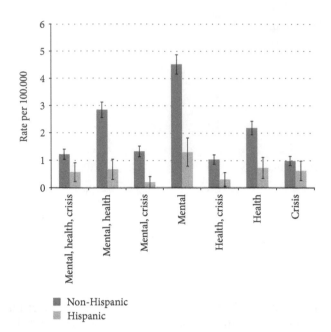

FIGURE 2: Selected combination of problems among non-Hispanic and Hispanic decedents in Utah, 2005–2010.

greater limitation to prescription drugs among Hispanics appears to similarly exist between both sexes and across the age groups.

Non-Hispanics had higher rates of death from not just legal drugs but illegal drugs as well. In a study covering 2002–2011 in the United States, the highest level of illegal drug use in the past month among individuals aged 12 and older was in Blacks, then Whites, then Hispanics, and lastly Asians [21]. Nevertheless, the current study found that among those who died from a drug overdose, opiates had the greatest presence in non-Hispanics and illicit drugs had the greatest presence in Hispanics, which is consistent with a lack of prescription drug access among Hispanics in the state.

Some research supports the hypothesis that Hispanics who migrate to the USA tend to have better health behaviors, are healthier, and are less likely to return to their native country [22, 23], which is consistent with our findings. For example, 37.6% of non-Hispanic compared with 31.0% of Hispanic decedents had a current physical health problem. In addition, 50.9% of non-Hispanic compared with 37.3% of Hispanic decedents had a current mental health problem. This is consistent with The First Surgeon General's Report on Mental Health, which indicated that Hispanic Americans born in the United States had similar overall rates of mental illness compared to those of Whites but that Hispanic immigrants born in Mexico or living in Puerto Rico had lower rates of mental illness than Hispanic Americans born in the United States [24].

A limitation of this study results from the inherent uncertainties of death investigations. However, as described in the Methods, several steps were taken to minimize errors in the data (e.g., extensive training of abstractors and quality checks). Second, the state of Utah has a high percentage of illegal immigrants, many of whom are of Hispanic origin who

come to Utah to work [25]. Some of these individuals may not be recorded in the death records for the state. Third, ethnic misclassification may lead to an underestimation of 25–35% of Aboriginal and Hispanic drug-related deaths nationally [11]. Finally, the Utah population upon which this study is based has a comparatively high level of opiate drug and antidepressant use and a low level of illicit drug use, which should be considered when generalizing the results.

5. Conclusion

The rate of drug-related death is significantly greater among non-Hispanics than Hispanics in Utah. The large difference is explained, in part, by Hispanics being less affected by the rise in prescription drug abuse, perhaps because of lower access to healthcare and prescription drugs.

The higher drug-related death rates among non-Hispanics occur in both males and females and across the age spans, indicating that greater limitations to prescription drugs among Hispanics are similar between both sexes and across the age span. Among decedents, Hispanics have a greater proportion with illegal drugs involved, consistent with their having relatively more difficult access to prescription drugs. There is some evidence that Hispanic decedents had better general physical and mental health. This may be because healthier non-native born individuals choose to migrate to the USA, are more likely to retain healthier lifestyle behaviors, and are less likely to return to their native country. It may also be that Hispanics, who have less access to healthcare, are less likely to be diagnosed with mental and physical health problems.

Conflict of Interests

The authors declare that there is no conflict of interests regarding the publication of this paper.

Acknowledgment

This publication was supported by Cooperative Agreement Numbers CE001697 and CE001612 from the Centers for Disease Control and Prevention. Its contents are solely the responsibility of the authors and do not necessarily represent the official views of the Centers for Disease Control and Prevention.

References

[1] "National Center for Health Statistics data on drug poisoning deaths, National Center for Health Statistics," 2012, http://www.cdc.gov/nchs/data/factsheets/factsheet_drug_poisoning.htm.

[2] S. Galea, J. Ahern, K. Tardiff et al., "Racial/ethnic disparities in overdose mortality trends in New York City, 1990–1998," Journal of Urban Health, vol. 80, no. 2, pp. 201–211, 2003.

[3] D. K. Wysowski, "Surveillance of prescription drug-related mortality using death certificate data," Drug Safety, vol. 30, no. 6, pp. 533–540, 2007.

[4] L. J. Paulozzi, "Statement on trends in unintentional drug overdose deaths before senate judiciary subcommittee on crime

and drugs," 2008, http://www.hhs.gov/asl/testify/2008/03/t20080312g.html#.UebmR5WHofE.

[5] S. Calcaterra, J. Glanz, and I. A. Binswanger, "National trends in pharmaceutical opioid related overdose deaths compared to other substance related overdose deaths: 1999–2009," *Drug and Alcohol Dependence*, vol. 131, no. 3, pp. 263–270, 2012.

[6] L. Paulozzi, G. Baldwin, G. Franklin et al., "CDC grand rounds: prescription drug overdoses—a U.S. epidemic," *Morbidity and Mortality Weekly Report*, vol. 61, no. 1, pp. 10–13, 2012.

[7] M. Cerdá, Y. Ransome, K. M. Keyes et al., "Prescription opioid mortality trends in New York City, 1990–2006: examining the emergence of an epidemic," *Drug and Alcohol Dependence*, vol. 132, no. 1-2, pp. 53–62, 2013.

[8] "Death rates for drug poisoning, by state of residence, United States, Centers for Disease Control and Prevention," 2010, http://www.cdc.gov/nchs/pressroom/states/drug_deaths_2010.pdf.

[9] E. M. Johnson, W. A. Lanier, R. M. Merrill et al., "Unintentional prescription opioid-related overdose deaths: description of decedents by next of kin or best contact, Utah, 2008-2009," *Journal of General Internal Medicine*, vol. 28, no. 4, pp. 522–529, 2013.

[10] R. M. Merrill, E. Johnson, A. Sloan, and W. A. Lanier, "Characterizing unintentional nonillicit and illicit drug-related deaths," *Journal of Drug Issues*, vol. 43, no. 2, pp. 144–153, 2013.

[11] L. J. Paulozzi, "Drug-induced deaths—United States, 2003–2007," *Morbidity and Mortality Weekly Report*, vol. 60, pp. 60–61, 2011.

[12] "Utah people quickfacts, U.S. Census Bureau," 2013, http://quick-facts.census.gov/qfd/states/49000.html.

[13] "Demographics, Centers for Disease Control and Prevention," 2010, http://apps.nccd.cdc.gov/BRFSS/list.asp?cat=DE&yr=2010&qkey=745&state=All.

[14] "National violent death reporting system web site [Internet], Centers for Disease Control and Prevention," 2011, http://www.cdc.gov/violenceprevention/nvdrs/index.html.

[15] "The medical examiner act, Utah Department of Health," 2009, http://health.utah.gov/ome/act.html.

[16] Surveillance, Epidemiology, and End Results (SEER) Program, SEER*Stat Database: Incidence-SEER 9 Regs Research Data, (1973–2010) "Katrina/Rita Population Adjustment"-Linked to County Attributes-Total U.S., 1969–2011 Counties, National Cancer Institute, DCCPS, Surveillance Research Program, Surveillance Systems Branch, http://www.seer.cancer.gov/.

[17] L. J. Paulozzi, D. S. Budnitz, and Y. Xi, "Increasing deaths from opioid analgesics in the United States," *Pharmacoepidemiology and Drug Safety*, vol. 15, no. 9, pp. 618–627, 2006.

[18] Indicator report—Health insurance coverage, Utah Department of Health, 2012, http://ibis.health.utah.gov/indicator/view/HlthIns.Eth.html.

[19] H. M. González, M. N. Haan, and L. Hinton, "Acculturation and the prevalence of depression in older Mexican Americans: baseline results of the Sacramento area Latino study on aging," *Journal of the American Geriatrics Society*, vol. 49, no. 7, pp. 948–953, 2001.

[20] M. J. Wunsch, K. Nakamoto, G. Behonick, and W. Massello, "Opioid deaths in rural Virginia: a description of the high prevalence of accidental fatalities involving prescribed medications," *American Journal on Addictions*, vol. 18, no. 1, pp. 5–14, 2009.

[21] Substance Abuse and Mental Health Services Administration, "Results from the 2011 National Survey on Drug Use and Health: Mental Health Findings," NSDUH Series H-45, HHS Publication (SMA) 12-4725, Substance Abuse and Mental Health Services Administration, Rockville, Md, USA, 2012.

[22] L. Blue and A. Fenelon, "Explaining low mortality among US immigrants relative to native-born Americans: the role of smoking," *International Journal of Epidemiology*, vol. 40, no. 3, pp. 786–793, 2011.

[23] A. F. Abraído-Lanza, B. P. Dohrenwend, D. S. Ng-Mak, and J. B. Turner, "The Latino mortality paradox: a test of the "salmon bias" and healthy migrant hypotheses," *American Journal of Public Health*, vol. 89, no. 10, pp. 1543–1548, 1999.

[24] U.S. Department of Health and Human Services U.S. Department of Health and Human Services, Substance Abuse and Mental Health Services Administration, Center for Mental Health Services, National Institutes of Health, National Institute of Mental Health, Rockville, MD, 1999.

[25] J. Passel and D. Cohn, "Unauthorized immigrant population: national and state trends," 2010, http://www.pewhispanic.org/2011/02/01/unauthorized-immigrant-population-brnational-and-state-trends-2010/.

12

Therapist's Gender and Gender Roles: Impact on Attitudes toward Clients in Substance Abuse Treatment

Tytti Artkoski and Pekka Saarnio

School of Social Sciences and Humanities, 33014 University of Tampere, Finland

Correspondence should be addressed to Pekka Saarnio; pekka.saarnio@uta.fi

Academic Editor: Gallus Bischof

The purpose of the present study was to investigate the impact of therapist's gender and gender roles on attitudes toward clients. Attitudes toward motivational interviewing were also a focus as MI can be hypothesized to be feminine rather than masculine in nature. The subjects (N = 246) were Finnish substance abuse therapists. Their attitudes toward clients were measured using a vignette task. Results indicated that female therapists were significantly more positive toward clients than were male therapists. Although females were significantly more feminine than males, they saw themselves as masculine as the males did. The more feminine the therapist was, the more s/he preferred MI. In the future, an examination of this kind should be combined with measurement of treatment processes and outcomes.

1. Introduction

The effects of various treatments on outcome have been studied extensively both in psychotherapy and substance abuse treatment [1, 2]. The investigation of between-therapist variation in outcome has been infrequent, although it has proved an important factor in both disciplines [3, 4].

Other little-studied factors are the gender and gender roles of the therapist and their impact on treatment effectiveness [5]. Gender role is a key concept in our study. It refers to the set of attitudes and behaviors socially expected of the members of a particular gender [6]. According to Bem's [7] theory, a traditionally gender-typed person is highly attuned to the cultural definitions of gender-appropriate behavior and uses such definitions as the ideal standard against which her or his own behavior is to be evaluated. Masculinity and femininity are gender roles of the traditional type. Androgyny, in turn, is considered to be a modern gender role. It means that a person is both masculine and feminine; these traits are not mutually exclusive.

Research on psychotherapy has indicated that therapy effectiveness may be predicted on the basis of gendered factors [8]. In the substance abuse field, there is evidence that therapist's attitudes toward clients vary according to the client's gender. DeJong et al. [9] demonstrated that therapists were more confrontational and critical with male clients, while female clients received more empathy and support. The male clients were seen by the therapists as threatening, in which case the attitudes became confrontational, while female clients were seen as submissive, which led to empathetic attitudes. These attitudes were due to stereotypical gender roles common in society. The therapist's own gender had no impact on the attitudes toward clients in the study by DeJong et al.

By contrast, findings on mental health professionals have indicated that males generate more stereotypical attitudes toward clients than do females [10, 11]. These findings corroborate a study by Bernstein and Lecomte [12] reporting that psychotherapist's gender is an important factor for attitudes toward clients, males being more stereotypical than females.

A small study by Saarnio et al. [13] showed that the clients of male therapists dropped out of inpatient substance abuse treatment significantly more frequently than did the clients of female therapists (20 versus 10%). Five therapists of each gender and 105 clients took part. Unfortunately, a more detailed examination of the findings was not possible because no in-session data were collected.

However, one possible explanation is that female therapists were more adept at avoiding alliance ruptures that easily lead to dropping out. This explanation is supported by a recent Finnish study which found that female therapists in substance abuse treatment were significantly more empathetic and friendly toward clients than were their male colleagues [14]. Moreover, avoidance of excessive directiveness was considered more important by female therapists than by males.

There is evidence that therapist empathy is an essential factor in substance abuse treatment [15]. Empathy is significant for the working alliance and thus for the continuity of treatment [16]. Miller et al. [17] demonstrated that therapist empathy explained as much as 67% of variance in treatment outcome; in other words, the more empathetic the therapist, the better the outcome.

Miller et al. [18] showed experimentally that the therapist's style affects the client's drinking after treatment. From among two experimental groups, the therapists in one group were instructed to work in a directive-confrontational style and the therapists in the other group in a client-centered style. The therapists in the second group followed the principles of the motivational interviewing (MI) in which emphasis is placed on a positive attitude toward the client, especially empathy [19]. The directive-confrontational style caused significantly more opposition than did the client-centered style. The treatment results can be summed up as follows: the more the therapist confronted, the more the client drank one year after the treatment.

MI can be hypothesized to be feminine rather than masculine in nature as in it avoidance of confrontation and excessive directiveness play important roles. It would be interesting to find out whether there are between-therapist differences in attitudes toward MI due to gender or gender roles. The hypothesis is wholly explorative in nature.

The purpose of the present study was to investigate the impact of therapist's gender and gender roles on attitudes toward clients with different genders and sexual orientations. Attitudes toward MI were also a focus. These were formulated as three questions:

(1) are there differences in masculinity, femininity, or androgyny between male and female therapists?

(2) are there between-therapist differences due to gender or gender roles in attitudes toward clients?

(3) are gender or gender roles connected with attitudes toward MI?

2. Method

2.1. Subjects. The subjects ($N = 246$) were Finnish substance abuse therapists employed by the A-Clinic Foundation. The A-Clinic Foundation has treated clients with various addictions since 1955, and today it provides about 40% of the substance abuse treatment in Finland.

An electronic questionnaire was sent via the Internet to counselors, social workers, nurses, physicians, psychologists, and team leaders ($N = 546$). Regardless of job title, they all had the same task, therapy with clients. Therefore, for simplicity, they are called as therapists. The response rate was 45.1%. Unfortunately, we did not get any information on nonrespondents. This was due to an anonymous procedure in data collection.

Out of those participating in the study, 29.7% were men ($n = 73$) and 70.3% women ($n = 173$). The gender distribution was similar to that of the total personnel of the A-Clinic Foundation (22.2% men and 77.8% women). The age of the subjects varied between 24 and 63 years ($M = 44.0$; $SD = 10.0$), while the women ($M = 42.8$; $SD = 9.9$) were significantly ($t_{244} = 3.3$; $P = 0.001$) younger than the men ($M = 47.2$; $SD = 9.5$).

On average, the female therapists had a higher level of professional education than the male therapists, even though the males had acquired university degrees more often than their female colleagues (Table 1). Among therapists in team leader position, men were more common than women. Compared to men, the women more often worked as nurses. Every tenth subject had a history of personal recovery of substance abuse.

Male therapists reported more often being homosexual than did female therapists. According to a population-based Finnish study, the proportion of individuals with gay, lesbian, or bisexual identities has been estimated to be 2.5% of males and 1.9% of females in the year 2007 [20].

2.2. Materials. The first part of the questionnaire contained 18 items eliciting background information. The question on MI was formulated as follows: "In motivational interviewing one avoids directly telling the client what to do. How important do you consider this principle to be in substance abuse treatment?" The subjects were requested to use a five-point scale (1 = not so important $\cdots$ 5 = very important).

The different gender roles of the subjects, which in this study included masculinity, femininity, and androgyny, were measured by the Bem Sex-Role Inventory (BSRI) [21]. For this purpose, a short version of the BSRI consisting of 30 items was translated into Finnish by an expert translator. Backtranslation was not used as there were only single adjectives to translate.

Each item, such as "I am gentle" or "I am assertive," was rated on a seven-point scale (1 = never or almost never true $\cdots$ 7 = almost or almost always true). Both masculine and feminine traits were measured by ten items. In addition, ten neutral fillers were included.

The androgyny score is the difference between an individual's femininity and masculinity. A high positive score indicates femininity and a high negative score indicates masculinity; the closer the score is to zero, the more androgynous the person is.

The alpha reliabilities of masculinity and femininity in the present study were of the same level as in the original study [7]: 0.78 (0.86) and 0.81 (0.81). It was not possible to calculate the alpha reliability for androgyny.

Despite having been developed over 30 years ago, the BSRI continues to be extensively used in both research and clinical work. In addition, its psychometric properties

TABLE 1: Background information on therapists by gender. Comparison used χ^2 test.

	Men (n = 73)		Women (n = 173)		
	n	%	n	%	P
Marital status					ns
Single	13	17.8	22	12.7	
Cohabiting	15	20.5	46	26.6	
Married	38	52.2	80	46.3	
Divorced or separated	5	6.8	21	12.1	
Widowed	2	2.7	4	2.3	
Sexual orientation					0.01
Heterosexual	66	90.5	167	96.5	
Bisexual	2	2.7	5	2.9	
Homosexual	5	6.8	1	0.6	
Professional education					0.001
Brief professional education	2	2.7	1	0.6	
School level	16	21.9	16	9.2	
College or polytechnic	31	42.5	119	68.8	
University	24	32.9	37	21.4	
Job title					0.008
Counselor	25	34.2	52	30.1	
Social worker	11	15.1	33	19.1	
Nurse	6	8.2	44	25.4	
Physician or psychologist	7	9.6	7	4.0	
Team leader	24	32.9	37	21.4	
Experience in substance abuse treatment					0.05
Under 5 years	14	19.2	59	34.1	
5–15 years	33	45.2	71	41.0	
Over 15 years	26	35.6	43	24.9	
Technical orientation					ns
Cognitive therapies	9	12.3	19	11.0	
Motivational interviewing	4	5.5	11	6.3	
Solution-focused	15	20.5	27	15.6	
System theoretical	3	4.1	2	1.2	
Psychodynamic	2	2.7	6	3.4	
Community treatment	14	19.2	22	12.7	
Eclectic	22	30.2	84	48.6	
None of these	4	5.5	2	1.2	
Lengthy therapy training*					ns
Yes	25	34.2	53	30.6	
No	48	65.8	120	69.4	
Personal recovery of substance abuse					0.001
Yes	14	19.2	10	5.8	
No	59	80.8	163	94.2	

*At least two years of intensive therapy training.

are considered valid [22]. However, recent studies have reanalyzed and questioned the BSRI's factor structure and validity [23, 24].

The attitudes of the therapists toward clients were measured with a vignette task, in which the subject had to associate adjectives with three different fictional client cases. The cases differed from each other only as regards the client's gender and sexual orientation. The first case was a heterosexual male with a substance use disorder. The second vignette had to do with a heterosexual female, and the third vignette concerned a homosexual male.

The vignette rating made use of 50 adjectives extracted from the Adjective Check List (ACL), which is commonly used to measure personality traits [25]. Half of adjectives were negative and half positive in meaning. The subjects selected six adjectives for each vignette.

Like the BSRI, the ACL has a wide range of uses and applications in both research and clinical work. In addition, the validity of the ACL has been found to be high [25].

2.3. Procedure. The study was approved by the A-Clinic Foundation's Ethics Committee. The electronic questionnaire was sent to the therapists via the Internet. The participation of the therapists was voluntary and anonymous.

The statistical analyses were carried out using SPSS software (version 16.0). The χ^2 test, t-test, correlations, and analyses of variance (ANOVA, repeated measures, and MANOVA) were used. Effect sizes were calculated with Cohen's d, defined as the difference between the means of female and male therapists, divided by the pooled standard deviation of these groups.

3. Results

3.1. Gender and Gender Roles. First, the results on gender roles measured by the BSRI were compared between male and female therapists. The raw scores were not converted to t-scores because they were based on normative data over 30 years old. In addition, the results were not compared to those of other populations.

The male therapists received a slightly higher mean score for masculinity (M = 4.9; SD = 0.6) than the female therapists (M = 4.8; SD = 0.6). According to the t-test, the difference was not statistically significant (t_{244} = 0.7; P = 0.5). Effect size was small (d = 0.1).

As for femininity, the means between males (M = 5.2; SD = 0.6) and females (M = 5.5; SD = 0.6) differed significantly (t_{244} = 2.6; P = 0.01) from each other. The male therapists were less feminine than the females. However, effect size was small (d = 0.3).

As regards the androgynous gender role, the male (M = 0.3; SD = 0.8) and female therapists (M = 0.6; SD = 0.8) differed significantly (t_{244} = 2.5; P = 0.01) from each other. Effect size was small (d = 0.3). The mean score of female therapists deviated more from zero than that of men, so the male therapists were more androgynous than the women.

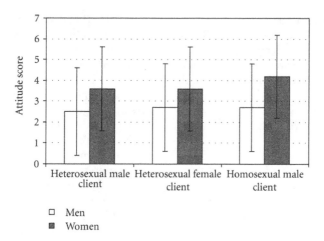

FIGURE 1: Means and standard deviations (±) for men ($n = 73$) and women ($n = 173$) in attitudes toward clients as measured by the vignette task. Total number of positive adjectives was used as an attitude score.

TABLE 2: Interactions of gender with marital status and length of therapy training on attitudes toward cases in the vignette task ($N = 246$). Analysis used ANOVA.

	F	Df	P
Heterosexual male client			
Gender × marital status	6.9	1,242	0.009
Gender × length of therapy training	2.0	1,242	0.16
Heterosexual female client			
Gender × marital status	4.8	1,242	0.03
Gender × length of therapy training	6.4	1,242	0.01
Homosexual male client			
Gender × marital status	5.8	1,242	0.02
Gender × length of therapy training	5.2	1,242	0.02

3.2. Attitudes toward Clients.

In the next section of the questionnaire, the therapists had to select six adjectives that best described the client in each of the three vignettes. Gender roles were not significantly connected with the ratings. Instead, gender as such was a significant factor: female therapists had a more positive attitude than the males toward all cases (Figure 1). A repeated analysis of variance indicated that the difference between the columns was significant ($F_{1,244} = 19.8$; $P = 0.000$).

On the basis of the t-test, the difference between genders was greatest in attitudes toward the homosexual male client ($t_{244} = 5.4$; $P = 0.000$) and smallest in attitudes toward the heterosexual female client ($t_{244} = 3.1$; $P = 0.002$). The genders also differed significantly ($t_{244} = 4.0$; $P = 0.000$) from each other in their attitudes toward the heterosexual male client. Effect sizes for vignettes were medium to large ($d = 0.8$; 0.6; 1.1).

When controlling for background variables described in Table 1, the one-way analysis of variance revealed three variables on the basis of which the therapists differed significantly from each other as regards their attitudes toward the vignettes: professional education, job title, and technical eclecticism. When these variables and gender were used as independent variables and the combined score of the vignettes as a dependent variable in MANOVA, only technical eclecticism ($F_{3,235} = 3.1$; $P = 0.03$) and gender ($F_{3,235} = 7.4$; $P = 0.000$) remained significant. Eclectic therapists were more positive toward vignettes when compared with single-method therapists.

In addition, ANOVA indicated that the therapist's marital status and length of therapy training interacted significantly with gender on the attitudes toward the vignettes (Table 2). Single men had more positive attitudes toward all vignettes than men in pair relationships. For women the inverse was true: female therapists in a pair relationship had a more positive attitude than single women toward all cases. As for lengthy therapy training, the attitudes of the male therapists who had completed lengthy training were more positive, while among the female therapists such training weakened the positive client images.

3.3. Attitudes toward MI.

The study also focused on the connections between gender, gender roles, and attitude toward MI. Femininity had a significant positive correlation ($r = 0.18$; $P < 0.01$) with attitude toward MI: as the therapist's femininity increased, so did the preference for MI. Masculinity and androgyny did not correlate significantly with the attitude score.

MI was slightly more important for female therapists ($M = 4.0$; $SD = 0.7$) than in males ($M = 3.8$; $SD = 0.7$). However, they did not differ significantly ($t_{244} = 1.3$; $P = 0.2$) from each other. Effect size was small ($d = 0.2$). When controlled for, MI usage per se was not significantly connected with preference for MI.

4. Discussion

The present study investigated the impact of therapist's gender and gender roles on attitudes toward clients. Attitudes toward motivational interviewing were also a focus.

On average, the female therapists were significantly more feminine than the male therapists. However, masculinity was at the same level in both genders. The degree of androgyny was higher among the male therapists than among the females.

Female therapists were significantly more positive than male therapists in their attitudes toward all the cases in the vignette task. This finding indirectly supports Saarnio's [14] conclusion: "On the grounds of personality and interpersonal functioning, female therapists were keener on working according to motivational interviewing" (page 1470).

Our finding differs from the conclusion of DeJong et al. [9] that therapist's gender has no impact on attitudes toward clients. On the contrary, the vignette task result corroborates the findings for mental health professionals, indicating between-gender differences in attitudes toward clients [10–12].

Client's gender was not a relevant factor for therapist's attitudes: the vignette task scores were at the same level for both male and female cases. This finding also differs from the result of DeJong et al. [9] that depending on the client's gender, substance abuse therapists will prefer different attitudinal stances.

As to why the female therapists had the most positive attitudes toward the homosexual male client, no answer can be given on the basis of the present study. However, in an international comparison, there were population-level differences between the genders in attitudes toward homosexuals, particularly in the Nordic countries [26]. Women were more positive toward homosexuals.

The topic is an important one, since some studies have indicated that homosexuals may have a higher risk of substance use disorders than heterosexuals [27]. In addition, it has been demonstrated that homosexuals have difficulties in entering substance abuse services [28]. These findings could be taken into account in therapist training, especially for men.

We hypothesized MI to be feminine rather than masculine in nature as in it avoidance of confrontation and excessive directiveness play important roles. The results indicated that gender as such had no significant association with the therapist's attitude toward MI, while a significant correlation was found between femininity and the attitude score: the more feminine therapist was, the more s/he preferred MI. To the best of our knowledge, there are no studies available on this subject.

Our findings showed that eclectic therapists were more positive toward clients when compared with single-method therapists. This may be considered as an indication of more expertise among the eclectic therapists. We also found that therapist's marital status and length of therapy training interacted significantly with gender on attitudes toward the vignettes. However, these interactions were explorative in nature, and no parallel information was available. It is therefore difficult to discuss them without the risk of speculation. A more detailed analysis of this topic is desirable.

There were certain limitations in the present study. One of them was the modest response rate. Although the questionnaires sent via the Internet had a high degree of anonymity, more responses might have been obtained if data had been gathered through personal contacts. Second, while the BSRI has been used extensively, there are questions and limitations as to how valid its underlying factors currently are [23, 24]. Third, the assessment of attitudes toward clients could partly have been confounded by socially desirable responding [29]. Tourangeau and Yan [30] concluded in their review that responses to questions on sexual orientation, in particular, are often based on social expectations. Fourth, attitudes toward MI were only measured by a single item. Consequently, the measurement was not optimally reliable.

What the findings mean for practical substance abuse treatment remains open. In the future, an examination of this kind should be combined with the measurement of treatment processes and outcomes. Are there differences between female and male therapists in the continuity and outcome of substance abuse treatment? What do the gender roles matter for everyday treatment practice? These are necessary steps before we can draw sound conclusions on gendered effects in this field.

Conflict of Interest

The authors declare that they have no conflict of interests. The authors alone are responsible for the content and writing of the paper.

References

[1] M. Lambert and B. Ogles, "The efficacy and effectiveness of psychotherapy," in *Handbook of Psychotherapy and Behavior Change*, M. Lambert, Ed., pp. 139–193, Wiley, New York, NY, USA, 2004.

[2] D. Raistrick, N. Heather, and C. Godfrey, *Review of the Effectiveness of Treatment for Alcohol Problems*, NTA, London, UK, 2006.

[3] L. Beutler, M. Malik, S. Alimohamed, T. Harwood, H. Talebi, S. Noble et al., "Therapist variables," in *Handbook of Psychotherapy and Behavior Change*, M. Lambert, Ed., pp. 227–306, Wiley, New York, NY, USA, 2004.

[4] L. M. Najavits, P. Crits-Christoph, and A. Dierberger, "Clinicians' impact on the quality of substance use disorder treatment," *Substance Use and Misuse*, vol. 35, no. 12–14, pp. 2161–2190, 2000.

[5] A. J. Blow, T. M. Timm, and R. Cox, "The role of the therapist in therapeutic change: does therapist gender matter?" *Journal of Feminist Family Therapy*, vol. 20, no. 1, pp. 66–86, 2008.

[6] C. Philpot, "Socialization of gender roles," in *Handbook of Family Development and Intervention*, W. Nichols, M. Pace-Nichols, D. Becvar, and A. Napier, Eds., pp. 85–108, Wiley, Hoboken, NJ, USA, 2000.

[7] S. L. Bem, "The measurement of psychological androgyny," *Journal of Consulting and Clinical Psychology*, vol. 42, no. 2, pp. 155–162, 1974.

[8] S. F. Greenfield, A. J. Brooks, S. M. Gordon et al., "Substance abuse treatment entry, retention, and outcome in women: a review of the literature," *Drug and Alcohol Dependence*, vol. 86, no. 1, pp. 1–21, 2007.

[9] C. A. J. DeJong, W. Van den Brink, and J. A. M. Jansen, "Sex role stereotypes and clinical judgement: how therapists view their alcoholic patients," *Journal of Substance Abuse Treatment*, vol. 10, no. 4, pp. 383–389, 1993.

[10] A. L. Aslin, "Feminist and community mental health center psychotherapists' expectations of mental health for women," *Sex Roles*, vol. 3, no. 6, pp. 537–544, 1977.

[11] A. Maslin and J. L. Davis, "Sex-role stereotyping as a factor in mental health standards among counselors-in-training," *Journal of Counseling Psychology*, vol. 22, no. 2, pp. 87–91, 1975.

[12] B. L. Bernstein and C. Lecomte, "Therapist expectancies: client gender, and therapist gender, profession, and level of training," *Journal of Clinical Psychology*, vol. 38, no. 4, pp. 744–754, 1982.

[13] P. Saarnio, M. Tolonen, K. Heikkilä, S. Kangassalo, M. L. Mäkeläinen, P. Niitty Uotila et al., "Päihdeongelmaisten selviytyminen hoidon jälkeen," *Sosiaalilääketieteellinen Aikakauslehti*, vol. 35, no. 4, pp. 207–219, 1998.

[14] P. Saarnio, "Big five personality traits and interpersonal functioning in female and male substance abuse therapists," *Substance Use and Misuse*, vol. 45, no. 10, pp. 1463–1473, 2010.

[15] T. Moyers and W. Miller, "Is low therapist empathy toxic?" *Psychology of Addictive Behaviors*, In press.

[16] B. Nielsen, A. S. Nielsen, and O. Wraae, "Factors associated with compliance of alcoholics in outpatient treatment," *Journal of Nervous and Mental Disease*, vol. 188, no. 2, pp. 101–107, 2000.

[17] W. R. Miller, C. A. Taylor, and J. A. C. West, "Focused versus broad-spectrum behavior therapy for problem drinkers," *Journal of Consulting and Clinical Psychology*, vol. 48, no. 5, pp. 590–601, 1980.

[18] W. R. Miller, R. G. Benefield, and J. S. Tonigan, "Enhancing motivation for change in problem drinking: a controlled comparison of two therapist styles," *Journal of Consulting and Clinical Psychology*, vol. 61, no. 3, pp. 455–461, 1993.

[19] W. Miller and S. Rollnick, *Motivational Interviewing. Helping People Change*, Guilford Press, New York, NY, USA, 2012.

[20] O. Kontula, *Between Sexual Desire and Reality. The Evolution of Sex in Finland*, Population Research Institute, Helsinki, Finland, 2009.

[21] S. Bem, *Bem Sex-Role Inventory: Professional Manual*, Consulting Psychologists Press, Palo Alto, Calif, USA, 1981.

[22] C. L. Holt and J. B. Ellis, "Assessing the current validity of the Bem Sex-Role Inventory," *Sex Roles*, vol. 39, no. 11-12, pp. 929–941, 1998.

[23] A. Colley, G. Mulhern, J. Maltby, and A. M. Wood, "The short form BSRI: instrumentality, expressiveness and gender associations among a United Kingdom sample," *Personality and Individual Differences*, vol. 46, no. 3, pp. 384–387, 2009.

[24] R. M. Hoffman and L. DiAnne Borders, "Twenty-five years after the Bem Sex-Role Inventory: a reassessment and new issues regarding classification variability," *Measurement and Evaluation in Counseling and Development*, vol. 34, no. 1, pp. 39–55, 2001.

[25] H. Gough and A. Heilbrun, *The Adjective Check List Manual*, Consulting Psychologists Press, Palo Alto, Calif, USA, 1980.

[26] J. Kelley, "Attitudes towards homosexuality in 29 nations," *Australian Social Monitor*, vol. 4, pp. 15–22, 2001.

[27] D. A. Bux, "The epidemiology of problem drinking in gay men and lesbians: a critical review," *Clinical Psychology Review*, vol. 16, no. 4, pp. 277–298, 1996.

[28] B. N. Cochran and A. M. Cauce, "Characteristics of lesbian, gay, bisexual, and transgender individuals entering substance abuse treatment," *Journal of Substance Abuse Treatment*, vol. 30, no. 2, pp. 135–146, 2006.

[29] D. Paulhus, "Socially desirable responding: the evolution of a construct," in *The Role of Constructs in Psychological and Educational Measurement*, H. Braun, D. Jackson, and D. Wiley, Eds., pp. 49–69, Lawrence Erlbaum Associates, Mahwah, NJ, USA, 2002.

[30] R. Tourangeau and T. Yan, "Sensitive questions in surveys," *Psychological Bulletin*, vol. 133, no. 5, pp. 859–883, 2007.

13

Measuring Problematic Mobile Phone Use: Development and Preliminary Psychometric Properties of the PUMP Scale

Lisa J. Merlo,[1] Amanda M. Stone,[2,3] and Alex Bibbey[2,4]

[1] Department of Psychiatry, University of Florida, P.O. Box 100183, Gainesville, FL 32610-0183, USA
[2] University of Florida, Gainesville, FL 32610, USA
[3] Department of Emergency Medicine, Orlando Regional Medical Center, Orlando, FL 32806, USA
[4] Department of Radiology, Duke University, Durham, NC 27705, USA

Correspondence should be addressed to Lisa J. Merlo; lmerlo@ufl.edu

Academic Editor: Dace Svikis

This study aimed to develop and assess the psychometric properties of an English language measure of problematic mobile phone use. Participants were recruited from a university campus, health science center, and other public locations. The sample included 244 individuals (68.4% female) aged 18–75. Results supported a unidimensional factor structure for the 20-item self-report Problematic Use of Mobile Phones (PUMP) Scale. Internal consistency was excellent ($\alpha = 0.94$). Strong correlations ($r = .76$, $P < .001$) were found between the PUMP Scale and an existing scale of cellular phone dependency that was validated in Asia, as well as items assessing frequency and intensity of mobile phone use. Results provide preliminary support for the use of the PUMP Scale to measure problematic use of mobile phones.

1. Introduction

Mobile phones (a.k.a., cellular telephones) have many perceived benefits, including increased accessibility and social connection, efficiency in the workplace, convenience, and improved safety. However, in recent years, there has been increasing public interest in the negative consequences of mobile phone use. In one Saudi Arabian study, 44.4% of participants related common health complaints such as headache, trouble concentrating, memory loss, hearing loss, and fatigue to their mobile phone use [1]. Another Saudi Arabian study suggested that 3%-4% of mobile phone users exhibit problems such as tension, fatigue, sleep disturbance, and dizziness related to their mobile phone use, and over 20% complain of headaches [2]. Accidents caused by distracted driving [3, 4] have been highlighted as a public health concern. In addition, anecdotal observation and media reports suggest that the number of self-professed "cell phone addicts" and compulsive users of "crack-berries" and other smartphones has increased as mobile phones have become ubiquitous. Public recognition of this phenomenon is reflected in the many websites and blogs addressing the issue, as well as

numerous articles in the popular press describing cell phone addiction. Though stories have appeared in publications such as the *New York Times* [5], the *Los Angeles Times* [6], and http://www.forbes.com/ [7] for many years, the academic literature surrounding problematic mobile phone use remains fairly limited, even when compared to other "behavioral addictions" such as pathological gambling, problematic internet use, and problem video gaming [8–10].

While "addiction" is a term commonly used and arguably overused in society, the conceptualization of addiction remains controversial even among researchers and clinicians who specialize in substance use disorders and addictive behaviors. Indeed, the *Diagnostic and Statistical Manual of Mental Disorders, Fourth Edition—Text Revision [DSM-IV-TR]* [11] did not include a condition called "addiction." Rather, it described substance abuse and substance dependence as distinct psychiatric disorders, and failed to include discussion of addictive behaviors that do not involve substance use. Furthermore, the recently released *Diagnostic and Statistical Manual of Mental Disorders, Fifth Edition (DSM-5)* describes "substance use disorders" using the following 11 criteria: (1) use in larger quantities or over longer amounts of time than initially intended, (2) a desire to cut down or control use, (3) spending a great deal of time obtaining, using, or recovering from the substance, (4) craving, (5) recurrent substance use resulting in a failure to fulfill major role obligations, (6) continued use despite social/interpersonal problems, (7) neglect of other important activities because of substance use, (8) use in situations in which it is physically hazardous, (9) continued use of the substance despite adverse physical or psychological consequences associated with use, (10) tolerance, and (11) withdrawal symptoms [12].

Though the *DSM-IV-TR* and *DSM-5* do not include any disorders related to the problematic use of technology, pathological gambling is included in *DSM-IV* as a diagnosable condition under the category of impulse control disorders not elsewhere classified [11], and in *DSM-5* as the first "behavioral addiction." Even though pathological gambling does not involve the use of a chemical substance, the similarities between the diagnostic criteria for substance use disorders and pathological gambling are striking. In general terms, both may be described as disorders involving loss of control over a compulsive, time- and resource-consuming behavior, which persists in the face of adverse consequences, with continued escalation of the behavior and/or withdrawal symptoms from reduction of the behavior.

Similarly, it was suggested as early as 1982 (i.e., well before the widespread use of mobile phones) that pathological use of technology may exist in the form of "technodependence" [13]. The constructs of internet addiction and problem video gaming are gaining both clinical and empirical support [10, 14]. In addition, though problematic mobile phone use has not, to date, been recognized as a diagnosable condition, experts in the field are debating its inclusion as one [15]. While evidence is scarce regarding a true "addiction" to mobile phones, data from recent studies suggest that some mobile phone users exhibit serious problematic behaviors analogous to the diagnostic criteria for substance use disorders or pathological gambling. These symptoms include preoccupation with mobile phone-based communication, excessive time or money spent on mobile telephones/communication plans, use of cellular devices in socially inappropriate or even physically dangerous situations (e.g., "texting" while driving an automobile), adverse effects on relationships, increased frequency or duration of mobile phone communication, and anxiety when separated from one's telephone or when without an adequate cellular signal [16–19]. Given these findings, it seems plausible that the consequences and psychological dependence seen in problematic mobile phone use (like pathological gambling and problematic internet and video game use) seem to parallel substance use and dependence and may be important to consider as a potential diagnostic entity and target of intervention.

In order to evaluate the extent to which problematic mobile phone use may be related to other addictive behaviors, research is needed to clarify the construct. To date, research on problematic mobile phone use has been limited by the lack of validated diagnostic criteria or standardized assessment measures. For this study, we operationally defined "problematic mobile phone use" as any pattern of mobile phone use resulting in subjective distress or impairment in important

areas of functioning. Given that some individuals have legitimate reason to use their mobile phone very frequently (e.g., for work obligations) and are able to do so without negative consequences, we believed it was important to distinguish "problematic" use from "very frequent" use. We expected rates of mobile phone use to be higher among individuals who exhibited symptoms of problematic mobile phone use, just as substance abusers generally tend to use substances in greater quantities/frequencies than nonabusers. However, as with substance use disorders, we did not feel that high frequency use should be considered a symptom of the condition. For this study, quantity of use was not included as a component of "problematic mobile phone use," except that individuals' subjective assessment of their use as excessive and troublesome was considered.

The purpose of the present study was to develop an English language measure of problematic mobile phone use symptoms, based on adaptations of the *DSM-5* substance use disorder criteria. The study followed a similar methodology to that utilized in previous studies regarding behavioral addictions [10, 20]. Specifically, our overarching hypotheses for this study included the following.

(1) Symptoms of problematic mobile phone use can be measured reliably and validly using a self-report questionnaire.

(2) Scores on the preliminary measure of problematic mobile phone use developed for this study will correlate significantly with an existing measure of cellular phone "dependency," which was validated on Asian samples.

(3) Symptoms of problematic mobile phone use will correlate positively with frequency and intensity of mobile telephone usage.

2. Method

All procedures were approved by the University of Florida Institutional Review Board. Participants were recruited for this study using several methods. First, flyers advertising the study were posted around the university campus, the health science center, and in public locations including a mobile phone store. Individuals who were interested in study participation called the research team to obtain a survey packet or to arrange a time to complete the survey. Second, university students were recruited for the study via announcements made in various undergraduate and graduate level courses. Questionnaires were passed out with a self-addressed, stamped envelope for participants to return the survey to the research team. Third, other participants learned of the study via word-of-mouth and made contact with members of the research team in order to participate. All surveys were completed anonymously. Completion of the full study questionnaire required 20–30 minutes, and no compensation was provided to study participants.

2.1. Participants. Data were collected from 244 individuals (68.4% female) who ranged in age from 18 to 75 years old

TABLE 1: Pearson correlations between PUMP Scale, CPDQ, CUQ, and self-assessment items.

Item	PUMPS total score	P
CPDQ[a] total score	.755	<.001
CUQ[b,c]		
How frequently do you typically use the email function on your phone?	.225	<.001
How frequently do you typically use the internet feature of your phone?	.312	<.001
How frequently do you use the games feature of your cell phone?	.203	.002
How often do you talk on the phone while driving?	.411	<.001
How often do you write text messages or emails while driving?	.612	<.001
Self-assessment questions		
I sometimes think that I might be "addicted" to my cell phone.	.733	<.001
I use my cell phone more often than other people I know.	.609	<.001
Friends or family members have commented to me about my cell phone use.	.626	<.001

[a]CPDQ refers to the cell phone dependency tendency questionnaire.
[b]CUQ refers to the cell phone use questionnaire.
[c]All CUQ item responses ranged from 1= never to 6= constantly.

(M = 29.8 years old, SD = 14.1 years). Participants were self-identified as Caucasian (74.4%), Hispanic/Latino (11.3%), Asian/Pacific Islander (9.2%), African American/Black (2.5%), or Other (2.5%). The sample included university students (37.7%), individuals employed full-time (32.6%), individuals employed part-time (17.4%), and individuals who were not currently employed or in school (12.2%). Annual income was reported by 86.5% of the sample and ranged from $0 to $190,000 ($M$ = $24,562, SD = $35,587).

2.2. Measures

2.2.1. Problematic Use of Mobile Phones (PUMP) Scale. A pool of 69 potential items for the PUMP Scale was developed by the first author based upon (1) informal interviews with several self-identified "cell phone addicts" who contacted the first author to discuss their mobile phone usage, (2) adaptation of the *DSM-IV* criteria for substance use disorders, and (3) review of existing measures assessing consequences of excessive internet use. These items were reviewed by 4 undergraduate research assistants for clarity but were not specifically pretested to assess psychometric properties before the questionnaires were distributed. After reviewing the proposed criteria for substance use disorders in the *DSM-5* [21], which was not yet published, the first and second authors together selected 22 items for inclusion in the scale. Item selection was guided by the rational method, with the authors together choosing the 2 items that best reflected each of the 11 substance use disorder criteria proposed by the *DSM-5* Task Force on Substance-Related Disorders. All items were rated on a 5-point scale ranging from 1 = "strongly disagree" to 5 = "strongly agree." Scale analysis was utilized to assess psychometric properties of the individual items and the scale as a whole. Further description of the scale is included in the results section.

2.2.2. Cellular Phone Dependence Tendency Questionnaire (CPDQ: [22]). The CPDQ was originally developed in Japan, to assess cellular phone "dependency" among Japanese university students. It was later translated from Japanese to Thai and was used to study high school and university students in Thailand [18]. Kawasaki and colleagues also published an English translation of the CPDQ in the report of their research [18]. For the present study, some items from this English translation were reworded slightly to more closely match the accepted local vernacular. The CPDQ is a 20-item self-report measure. Though it taps the domain of "cell phone addiction," the CPDQ was not developed on the basis of either *DSM-IV* or *DSM-5* criteria for substance use disorders and does not include items that would be considered reflective of "abuse" criteria per *DSM-IV-TR* guidelines. Rather, items solely assess respondents' perceived dependence on their cellular phone (e.g., "I would feel worse if I lost my cellular phone than if I lost my wallet" and "I send text messages even during work or class"). Items are rated on a 4-point scale ranging from "not true at all" to "true." The CPDQ has demonstrated good reliability and validity in non-English-speaking populations [18, 19, 22]. In addition, internal consistency for the current sample was excellent (α = .91).

2.2.3. Cellular Phone Usage Questionnaire (CUQ). The CUQ is a compilation of items assessing specific mobile phone usage patterns. It was developed for the present study as a general measurement of mobile phone use and does not attempt to distinguish excessive usage or identify consequences or symptoms associated with mobile phone use. Items assess the amount of time spent utilizing various components of cellular phones (e.g., phone minutes, text messaging, emailing, internet access, and video game play). Items are rated on a 6-point scale ranging from "never" to "constantly." Participants also completed 3 self-assessment questions regarding perceptions of their mobile phone usage. Items are included in Table 1.

3. Results

All statistical analyses were conducted using PASW 17.0. In order to address isolated cases of missing data, mean substitution was utilized for subscales in which at least 80% of the data were complete.

TABLE 2: PUMP Scale item analysis.

Item	M (SD)	Range	Corrected item total correlation	Alpha if item deleted
When I decrease the amount of time spent using my cell phone I feel less satisfied. *(Tolerance)*	1.61 (.96)	1–5	.68	.933
Tolerance—I need more time using my cell phone to feel satisfied than I used to need. *(Tolerance)*	1.53 (.84)	1–5	.65	.933
When I stop using my cell phone, I get moody and irritable. *(Withdrawal)*	1.43 (.83)	1–5	.72	.933
It would be very difficult, emotionally, to give up my cell phone. *(Withdrawal)*	2.36 (1.36)	1–5	.62	.934
The amount of time I spend using my cell phone keeps me from doing other important work. *(Longer time than intended)*	1.70 (.99)	1–5	.74	.932
I have thought in the past that it is not normal to spend as much time using a cell phone as I do. *(Longer time than intended)*	1.73 (1.06)	1–5	.57	.934
I think I might be spending too much time using my cell phone. *(Great deal of timespent)*	1.67 (1.09)	1–5	.72	.932
People tell me I spend too much time using my cell phone. *(Great deal of time spent)*	1.60 (1.08)	1–5	.74	.931
When I am not using my cell phone, I am thinking about using it or planning the next time I can use it. *(Craving)*	1.86 (1.07)	1–5	.75	.931
I feel anxious if I have not received a call or message in some time. *(Craving)*	2.23 (1.23)	1–5	.67	.932
I have ignored the people I'm with in order to use my cell phone. *(Activities given up or reduced)*	2.09 (1.28)	1–5	.72	.931
I have used my cell phone when I knew I should be doing work/schoolwork. *(Activities given up or reduced)*	2.73 (1.56)	1–5	.68	.933
I have used my cell phone when I knew I should be sleeping. *(Use despite physical or psychological problems)*	2.66 (1.64)	1–5	.64	.934
When I stop using my cell phone because it is interfering with my life, I usually return to it. *(Use despite physical or psychological problems)*	1.85 (1.10)	1–5	.67	.933
I have gotten into trouble at work or school because of my cell phone use. *(Failure to fulfill role obligations)*	2.00 (1.38)	1–5	.56	.935
At times, I find myself using my cell phone instead of spending time with people who are important to me and want to spend time with me. *(Failure to fulfill role obligations)*	1.65 (.96)	1–5	.74	.932
I have used my cell phone when I knew it was dangerous to do so. *(Use in physically hazardous situations)*	2.45 (1.41)	1–5	.55	.935
I have almost caused an accident because of my cell phone use. *(Use in physically hazardous situations)*	2.13 (1.32)	1–5	.51	.936
My cell phone use has caused me problems in a relationship. *(Use despite social or interpersonal problems)*	1.53 (1.02)	1–5	.43	.936
I have continued to use my cell phone even when someone asked me to stop. *(Use despite social or interpersonal problems)*	1.69 (1.15)	1–5	.56	.934

Note: item responses ranged from 1 = strongly disagree to 5 = strongly agree.

3.1. Mobile Phone Use Patterns. Participants reported having a mobile phone for an average of 7.29 years (SD = 3.73, range = 0–20 years). The majority of respondents (88.8%) reported having a personal cellular phone with a monthly contract, 6.6% reported having a personal cellular phone with a prepaid contract, and 1.2% reported sharing a cellular phone with at least one other person. Of the sample, 3.3% of respondents denied having a cellular phone.

3.2. Reliability Analysis. The items of the proposed PUMP Scale were subjected to scale analysis. Results demonstrated that the 2 items assessing the DSM criterion "desire to cut down" (i.e., "I would feel relieved if I was somewhere that my cell phone did not work" and "I sometimes wish I could get rid of my cell phone") had extremely low item total correlations (.05 and .15, resp.). After first considering their theoretical importance, it was decided that these items should be deleted

TABLE 3: PUMP Scale item frequencies.

Item	Strongly disagree %	Disagree %	Neutral %	Agree %	Strongly agree %
When I decrease the amount of time spent using my cell phone I feel less satisfied.	62.8	23.0	5.9	7.5	0.8
I need more time using my cell phone to feel satisfied than I used to need.	64.0	23.8	7.5	2.9	0.8
When I stop using my cell phone, I get moody and irritable.	73.2	16.7	4.6	5.0	0.4
It would be very difficult, emotionally, to give up my cell phone.	39.7	18.4	13.8	20.9	6.7
The amount of time I spend using my cell phone keeps me from doing other important work.	59.4	20.9	10.9	8.4	0.4
I have thought in the past that it is not normal to spend as much time using a cell phone as I do.	57.7	18.8	11.7	8.8	1.3
I think I might be spending too much time using my cell phone.	65.7	15.5	7.9	8.4	2.5
People tell me I spend too much time using my cell phone.	70.3	12.6	6.7	7.9	2.5
When I am not using my cell phone, I am thinking about using it or planning the next time I can use it.	50.2	26.8	12.1	8.8	2.1
I feel anxious if I have not received a call or message in some time.	39.8	20.7	19.5	16.6	3.3
I have ignored the people I'm with in order to use my cell phone.	47.3	20.7	13.7	12.4	5.8
I have used my cell phone when I knew I should be doing work/schoolwork.	36.9	10.4	12.0	23.7	17.0
I have used my cell phone when I knew I should be sleeping.	43.2	7.5	10.0	19.1	20.3
When I stop using my cell phone because it is interfering with my life, I usually return to it.	56.1	14.2	20.9	6.3	2.1
I have gotten into trouble at work or school because of my cell phone use.	59.1	10.3	8.3	15.7	6.6
At times, I find myself using my cell phone instead of spending time with people who are important to me and want to spend time with me.	59.0	25.5	7.9	6.3	1.3
I have used my cell phone when I knew it was dangerous to do so.	39.4	14.9	12.9	25.3	7.1
I have almost caused an accident because of my cell phone use.	47.9	17.8	14.9	12.4	7.0
My cell phone use has caused me problems in a relationship.	74.0	11.2	5.0	8.3	1.7
I have continued to use my cell phone even when someone asked me to stop.	67.2	11.6	10.0	7.5	3.7

from the final scale, as they did not appear to fit the overall construct of problematic mobile phone use. The final PUMP Scale demonstrated excellent internal consistency (20 items, $\alpha = .94$). Removal of any item would have resulted in a negative impact on the scale alpha. Items included in the final PUMP Scale are listed in Table 2.

3.3. *Factorial Validity.* A principal components analysis was utilized to assess the factor structure of the 20-item PUMP Scale. Results supported a one-factor solution, with factor loadings for all items ≥.48. The one-factor solution explained 49.05% of the variance, meeting Carmines and Zeller's criterion [23]. Analysis of the Scree plot also supported a

one-factor solution [24], with the eigenvalue of the first component (9.86) far exceeding the eigenvalue of the second component (1.45), which was not significantly different from the remaining eigenvalues.

3.4. *Convergent and Discriminant Validity Data.* Scores on the PUMP Scale ranged from 20 to 82 ($M = 38.40$, SD = 16.11) out of a possible score of 100. Frequency counts for each item response are listed in Table 3. PUMP scores were compared to scores on the Cellular Phone Dependency Tendency Questionnaire (CPDQ), the Cell Phone Use Questionnaire (CUQ), and the self-assessment items. Results are listed in Table 1. It is noteworthy that PUMP Scale total scores were not associated with the length of time the individual has owned a mobile phone (Pearson $r = -.08$, ns) or with the amount of money spent per month for mobile phone minutes (Pearson $r = -.04$, ns). However, PUMP Scale scores were positively correlated with the amount of time spent engaging in any form of mobile phone use (see Table 1), as well as the amount of money spent for text messaging service ($r = .27, P < .001$). As seen in Table 1, PUMP Scale scores also correlated positively with perceptions of excessive mobile phone usage, including self-reported feelings of "addiction" to the mobile phone.

4. Discussion

The purpose of the present study was to develop and validate a self-report measure of problematic mobile phone use (i.e., "cell phone addiction") for English-speaking respondents, based on criteria utilized for other addictive behaviors. Results indicated that problematic mobile phone use can be measured via self-report. The Problematic Use of Mobile Phones (PUMP) Scale demonstrated a single-factor structure, with excellent internal consistency. It also displayed convergent validity when compared to an existing measure of cellular phone dependency [the CPDQ [22]], items measuring the frequency and intensity of cellular phone use behaviors (the CUQ), and self-reported feelings of "addiction" to the mobile phone. These data provide preliminary support for the use of the PUMP Scale in research examining problematic mobile phone use in English-speaking samples.

Items included on the PUMP Scale instrument covered a wide range of symptoms. Most participants did not report symptoms, but it is noteworthy that a significant minority of respondents endorsed experiencing harm to their relationships, finances, and safety as a result of excessive phone use or use in inappropriate circumstances. Some respondents also acknowledged subjective loss of control over escalating phone use, as well as withdrawal-like symptoms when unable to use their phone. Finally, individuals who reported more symptoms of problematic mobile phone use on the PUMP Scale were more likely to endorse feeling "addicted" to their cellular phone. These findings support the popular construct of problematic mobile phone use (sometimes referred to as "cell phone addiction") and suggest that this area merits further study.

When considering these findings, it is important to acknowledge some limitations of the present study. First, like many instrument development studies, the sample was relatively small ($N = 244$) and was comprised of individuals recruited through convenience. Many of the participants were recruited from a college campus, and some were recruited from a mobile phone store, which may have introduced selection bias. Thus, the generalizability of results to the population as a whole may be limited. Future validation efforts should include larger, more diverse samples that are randomly selected. Second, the use of self-report, particularly regarding past behaviors and experiences, may have introduced biases due to faulty recall, social desirability, or shared methods variance. Obtaining more objective measures (i.e., mobile phone records, collateral reports) would strengthen the data. Third, no "gold standard" measure (i.e., accepted

formal diagnostic criteria) exists for problematic mobile phone use. Therefore, it was not possible to assess the operating characteristics of the PUMP Scale. Future research is needed to identify the cut-point(s) of the PUMP Scale for the purpose of detecting clinically significant symptoms.

It must also be emphasized that the construct of problematic mobile phone use is not yet well-studied or supported in the literature. The merits and implications of considering this construct should be further explored and developed. Clearly, some individuals use their mobile phones more than others, but the reasons for this may be multifaceted. Job requirements, safety issues, and family and social factors all may contribute. However, "problematic mobile phone use" appears to extend beyond frequency of use, to the extent that mobile phone use produces social, occupational, and psychological distress; it may be useful to identify these symptoms as potential targets for prevention and intervention. More research is needed to support the results of the current study. Finally, future studies should elucidate the mechanisms underlying problematic mobile phone use, in order to determine whether it exists as a primary phenomenon or alternatively is a symptom of other underlying pathology (e.g., anxiety disorders, impulse control deficits, personality factors). The long-term goal of research into problematic mobile phone use should be to effectively identify and treat problem users or those at risk for problematic use and ultimately to maximize communication utility of mobile technology while minimizing resulting dysfunction.

Acknowledgment

Lisa J. Merlo's work was supported in part by National Institute on Drug Abuse (NIDA) Training Grant no. T32-DA-07313-10 (PI: Linda B. Cottler).

References

[1] M. M. Khan, "Adverse effects of excessive mobile phone use," *International Journal of Occupational Medicine and Environmental Health*, vol. 21, no. 4, pp. 289–293, 2008.

[2] T. Al-Khlaiwi and S. A. Meo, "Association of mobile phone radiation with fatigue, headache, dizziness, tension and sleep disturbance in Saudi population," *Saudi Medical Journal*, vol. 25, no. 6, pp. 732–736, 2004.

[3] C. Laberge-Nadeau, U. Maag, F. Bellavance et al., "Wireless telephones and the risk of road crashes," *Accident Analysis and Prevention*, vol. 35, no. 5, pp. 649–660, 2003.

[4] A. T. McCartt, L. A. Hellinga, and K. A. Bratiman, "Cell phones and driving: review of research," *Traffic Injury Prevention*, vol. 7, no. 2, pp. 89–106, 2006.

[5] M. Richtel, "Drivers and legislators dismiss cellphone risks," *The New York Times*, July 2009.

[6] S. Brink, "Disconnect for R & R? That's LOL," *Los Angeles Times*, p. 14F, May 2007.

[7] W. Tanaka and S. Terry-Cobo, "Cellphoneaddiction," June 2008, http://www.forbes.com/2008/06/15/cellphone-addict-iphone-tech-wireless08-cx_wt0616addict.html.

[8] H. R. Lesieur and S. B. Blume, "The South Oaks Gambling Screen (SOGS): a new instrument for the identification of

Pathological gamblers," *American Journal of Psychiatry*, vol. 144, no. 9, pp. 1184–1188, 1987.

[9] L. A. Nichols and R. Nicki, "Development of a psychometrically sound internet addiction scale: a preliminary step," *Psychology of Addictive Behaviors*, vol. 18, no. 4, pp. 381–384, 2004.

[10] R. A. Tejeiro Salguero and R. M. Bersabé Morán, "Measuring problem video game playing in adolescents," *Addiction*, vol. 97, no. 12, pp. 1601–1606, 2002.

[11] American Psychiatric Association, *Diagnostic and Statistical Manual of Mental Disorders (DSM-IV-TR)*, American Psychiatric Association, Washington, DC, USA, 4th edition, 2000.

[12] American Psychiatric Association, *Diagnostic and Statistical Manual of Mental Disorders (DSM-5)*, American Psychiatric Association, Washington, DC, USA, 5th edition, 2013.

[13] C. Brod, "Managing technostress: optimizing the use of computer technology," *The Personnel Journal*, vol. 61, no. 10, pp. 753–757, 1982.

[14] S. Byun, C. Ruffini, J. E. Mills et al., "Internet addiction: meta-synthesis of 1996–2006 quantitative research," *Cyberpsychology and Behavior*, vol. 12, no. 2, pp. 203–207, 2009.

[15] M. Choliz, "Mobile phone: a point of issue," *Addiction*, vol. 105, no. 2, pp. 373–374, 2010.

[16] A. Bianchi and J. G. Phillips, "Psychological predictors of problem mobile phone use," *Cyberpsychology and Behavior*, vol. 8, no. 1, pp. 39–51, 2005.

[17] C. Jenaro, N. Flores, M. Gómez-Vela, F. González-Gil, and C. Caballo, "Problematic internet and cell-phone use: psychological, behavioral, and health correlates," *Addiction Research and Theory*, vol. 15, no. 3, pp. 309–320, 2007.

[18] N. Kawasaki, S. Tanei, F. Ogata et al., "Survey on cellular phone usage on students in Thailand," *Journal of Physiological Anthropology*, vol. 25, no. 6, pp. 377–382, 2006.

[19] M. Toda, K. Monden, K. Kubo, and K. Morimoto, "Mobile phone dependence and health-related lifestyle of university students," *Social Behavior and Personality*, vol. 34, no. 10, pp. 1277–1284, 2006.

[20] L. Widyanto and M. McMurran, "The psychometric properties of the internet addiction test," *Cyberpsychology and Behavior*, vol. 7, no. 4, pp. 443–450, 2004.

[21] American Psychiatric Association, *DSM-5 Development: Substance-Use Disorders*, 2010, http://www.dsm5.org/ProposedRevision.aspx?rid=431, Archived by WebCite, http://www.webcitation.org/5r3EW4O87.

[22] M. Toda, K. Monden, K. Kubo, and K. Morimoto, "Cellular phone dependence tendency of female university students," *Japanese Journal of Hygiene*, vol. 59, no. 4, pp. 383–386, 2004 (Japanese).

[23] E. Carmines and R. Zeller, *Reliability and Validity Assessment*, Sage, London, UK, 1979.

[24] F. Lord, *Applications of Item Response Theory to Practical Testing Problems*, Lawrence Erlbaum Associates, Hillsdale, NJ, USA, 1980.

14

Controlling Chaos: The Perceptions of Long-Term Crack Cocaine Users in Vancouver, British Columbia, Canada

Steven Persaud,[1,2] **Despina Tzemis,**[1] **Margot Kuo,**[1] **Vicky Bungay,**[3] **and Jane A. Buxton**[1,2]

[1] *Communicable Disease Prevention and Control, British Columbia Centre for Disease Control, 655 West 12th Avenue, Vancouver, BC, Canada V5Z 4R4*
[2] *School of Population and Public Health, University of British Columbia, 2206 East Mall, Vancouver, BC, Canada V6T 1Z3*
[3] *School of Nursing, University of British Columbia, 302-6190 Agronomy Road, Vancouver, BC, Canada V6T 1Z3*

Correspondence should be addressed to Jane A. Buxton; jane.buxton@bccdc.ca

Academic Editor: Brian Conway

People who smoke crack cocaine are described as chaotic and more likely to engage in risky sex, polysubstance use and contract infectious diseases. However, little is known about how individuals perceive smoking crack as compared to other forms of cocaine use, especially injection. We explored the lived experience of people who smoke crack cocaine. Six gender-specific focus groups ($n = 31$) of individuals who currently smoke crack in Vancouver, Canada, were conducted using a semi-structured interview guide. Focus groups were transcribed and analyzed by constant comparative methodology. We applied Rhodes' risk environment to the phenomenological understanding that individuals have regarding how crack has affected their lives. Subjects reported that smoking rather than injecting cocaine allows them to begin "controlling chaos" in their lives. Controlling chaos was self-defined using nontraditional measures such as the ability to maintain day-to-day commitments and housing stability. The phenomenological lens of smoking crack instead of injecting cocaine "to control chaos" contributes a novel perspective to our understanding of the crack-smoking population. This study examines narratives which add to prior reports of the association of crack smoking and increased chaos and suggests that, for some, inhaled crack may represent efforts towards self-directed harm reduction.

1. Introduction

Smoking crack cocaine is a relatively neglected public health problem in Canada in comparison to injection drug use (IDU), despite indications that crack use in Canada is increasing. The Vancouver Injection Drug Users Study found that crack use in a group of injection drug users in Vancouver almost doubled from about 31% in 1997 to over 60% in 2004; and daily crack smoking in this population rose from <10% in 1996 to 40% in 2002/05 period [1].

Canadian data also provides evidence of high prevalence of crack use among drug user populations. A recent surveillance report of 794 people who inject drugs across Canada indicated that 52.2% of the total sample had also used crack cocaine in the last 6 months [2]. Another Canadian cohort of illicit opioid users in five cities indicated that 54.6% (371/679) of baseline participants had smoked crack in the 30 days prior to the survey. However, there was considerable regional variation, with crack use reported ranging from 86.2% in Vancouver to 2.4% in Quebec City [3]. On the other hand, in a study of people who smoked crack in Vancouver only 39% of those who smoked crack also reported injecting drugs [4]. In Canada, many services for people who use drugs are targeted to people who inject; therefore, people who only smoke crack may not be linked with appropriate health and social services.

Compared to other drug using populations, people who use crack cocaine are described as a particularly chaotic population. Crack using populations are more likely than nondrug using populations to engage in illegal activities, to experience homelessness and health problems; yet they are less likely to access health and social services [5]. While cocaine users in general are at elevated risk of risky sexual practices, the crack house environment has been implicated in increased "sex for crack" exchanges and unprotected sexual encounters [6, 7]. DeBeck et al. (2009) reported that crack smokers smoke a median of 4 times per day [1]. Results of a population-based study revealed that recent-onset crack cocaine smokers were about twice as likely to experience cocaine dependence, as compared to recent-onset cocaine HCl powder users who did not smoke crack [8]. Crack smoking also involves particular risks and harms, including HIV incidence [1], potential HCV and tuberculosis transmission, and agranulocytosis from crack cocaine containing levamisole [9–14].

Vancouver's downtown eastside (DTES) has a longstanding reputation as Canada's poorest urban area. Through a historical trajectory of diminishing housing options, an increase in single-room occupancy rentals and a mass influx of marginalized individuals have led to a disproportionate concentration of individuals with mental illness, addiction, and an HIV/AIDS epidemic termed by the local health board as a "public health emergency" [15, 16].

Although harm reduction interventions such as needle/syringe distribution and a supervised injection site are available in the DTES neighborhood, the majority of evidence-based public health responses to problematic drug use in British Columbia (BC) are not tailored for people who smoke crack cocaine and their unique needs. Plastic mouthpieces, push sticks, and, recently, brass screens are provided by the provincial harm reduction program. However, glass stems are not currently available through this program [17].

Crack cocaine use is a growing concern in Canada with many associated harms. Yet, there is no clear understanding of the perception of harms related to the type of cocaine (powder cocaine versus crack cocaine) and mode of administration (snorting, smoking, and injecting) by people who use crack. The psychosocial determinants and factors related to crack cocaine initiation, continuation, and the trajectory of substance use by mode of administration have not been well identified either. To assist in developing appropriate services there is an urgent need to learn more through a qualitative study of people who smoke crack.

To this end, this study sought to investigate the lived experience of crack smokers, especially in comparison to injected cocaine and other drugs in the context of the DTES. This contributes to our still limited understanding of this population with the ultimate aim to provide health service providers and policy makers with information to better design, plan, and implement prevention programs at an individual and community level.

This study was informed by two theoretical frameworks: phenomenology and Rhodes' risk environment. The phenomenological framework elucidates data from participants, treating their subjective perceptions as real insofar as it shapes their worldview and behaviors. This individual understanding of events and behaviors is significant in interpreting the meaning that people attribute to various things, and therefore, why they respond in certain ways. It "seeks to understand the lived experiences of individuals and their intentions within their 'life world'"[18].

The risk environment framework, first applied by Rhodes (2005) to explain the factors affecting HIV risk, describes the "space, whether social or physical in which a variety of factors exogenous to the individual interact to increase vulnerability" [19]. This holistic understanding of the complex interplay of what Zinberg terms "set and setting" [20] or intrinsic attitudes and structural factors that contribute to overall risk is useful in identifying potential areas of harm reduction.

2. Methods

A semi-structured interview guide was developed in collaboration with stakeholders including local service agencies and people who use drugs. Due to the overwhelming response usually seen with general recruitment strategies such as fliers, participants were purposively selected, based on ability to meet study criteria and lived experience, by the 2 organizations located in the Vancouver DTES neighborhood. One organization is a peer-support agency for people who use drugs, and another is a shelter and multiservice centre for women in survival sex work. Stakeholders at each of these agencies were instructed to approach potential participants with informational material and contact information of the study investigators if they chose to participate. Participants were 19 years old or older, able to speak and understand English, smoke crack at least 3 times per week in the past year, and provided written consent for participation prior to focus groups. Ethics approval was received from the University of British Columbia Behavioral Ethics Board, and standard ethical research practices, including voluntary consent, confidentiality, and minimal risk of harm to participants, were maintained.

2.1. Focus Groups. In total, 10 male and 21 female participants were recruited, and 6 semi-structured focus groups were conducted (2 male, 4 female), each comprised of 5-6 participants and 2 coinvestigators. One coinvestigator facilitated discussion, and the other took field notes. Focus groups were conducted at the respective recruiting agencies between June and November 2011. These focus groups were 1 hour long and were recorded and transcribed for data analysis. A 20$ honorarium was given to participants. The use of gender-specific focus groups allowed for frank discussion between participants, as both men and women were able to discuss gender norms openly and comment on interactions with the opposite gender with relative safety. In discussing topics with other crack users, participants were also able to highlight both areas of consensus and norms, as well as individual opinions, providing a distinction which would have been difficult using individual interviews.

2.2. Data Analysis. Transcripts were cleaned of any identifying data and were loaded into qualitative analysis software QSR NVivo 8 [21]. They were then reviewed by the two coinvestigators facilitating the focus groups for content and orientation. An initial line-by-line free coding was conducted using a constant comparative approach, in keeping with grounded theory research [22]. Themes and conceptual categories were identified and constantly compared to each other in order to develop codes, which represented both areas of commonalities between and within groups, as well as unique or opposing information.

TABLE 1: Demographic information of study participants*.

Variable	Totals (%) $N = 31$
Sex n (%)	
Female	21 (67.7)
Male	10 (32.3)
Age years	
Mean (range)	47.15 (27–64)
Ethnicity n (%)	
Caucasian	11 (35.5)
Aboriginal	19 (61.3)
Other	1 (3.2)
Duration of crack use years	
Mean (range)	10.4 (3–25)
Injection drug use n (%)	
Currently use	26 (83.9)
Ever used injection drugs	31 (100)

*Four focus groups were conducted at a support agency for people who use drugs (2 male, both $n = 5$; 2 female, both $n = 5$). Two focus groups were conducted at a multiservice centre for women in survival sex work ($n = 5$, $n = 6$).

Themes and impressions were then discussed between researchers, and an axial coding was then conducted for more focused themes and more insight into findings. This process involved a higher level of coding which compares and organizes themes according to a theoretical framework to better conceptualize their relative significance, hierarchy, or relation to established theory. In our case, Rhodes' risk environment was used to describe codes relating to the various perceptions of risk, and a phenomenological lens explained what role smoking crack represented in participants' lives. Member checking was conducted in the form of poster presentations at the same agencies, confirming central themes. Member checking included 5 participants who took part in the focus groups and 12 other individuals who were users of the service.

3. Results

Demographic information of study participants is found in Table 1. Though the proportion of aboriginal participants is quite high, this is representative of the DTES population, which includes between 10 and 14% aboriginal individuals, [15] compared with the national average of 3.8% [23]. The two theoretical frameworks yielded a number of themes through two conceptual ideas: the phenomenological notion of controlling chaos and Rhodes' risk environment. The first sought to identify participants' own perceptions regarding smoking crack, what it meant to them and how it affected their daily lived experience. The latter described the social, economic, and physical risks unique to smoking crack. Findings presented here represent only those themes with strong consensus and little to no dissent from both within and between the different focus groups, as identified through transcripts, field observations of nonverbal cues, and comparative analysis.

3.1. Phenomenological Lens: Controlling Chaos. In the midst of an admittedly chaotic lived experience, smoking crack represented both internal and practical efforts by users to exert control and autonomy over their drug use and other aspects of daily life. It effectively represented them "controlling chaos", as manifested in examples of the subjective experience, means of reducing harm, and reprioritizing drug use within the context of other daily needs. Participants constantly referred to the chaos that previously defined their lives, and how they were better able to control it now that they smoked rather than injected.

> *Female Participant: we're past the part where we're in the chaos … I'm not living the same lifestyle anymore.*

3.2. Subjective Experience. Many participants viewed crack cocaine use as improvements in their stability and control. This theme was confirmed in 5 of 6 focus groups:

> *Male Participant: So this [crack] sort of keeps me, you know, keeps me away from doing anything worse that I could do.*

> *Female Participant: I'm a functioning user. I don't miss things because of dope [crack]. I still have to pay my rent … dope comes last.*

One of the most explicit examples of controlling chaos came from the subjective high of the drug itself. Smoked crack was described as more gradual in onset, especially when compared to the instantaneous rush of IV cocaine use. Similarly, the sustained drug effect is much more vivid when injecting than smoking.

> *Female Participant: Oh, an injection hits you right away, it's—it gives you the—wham!*

> *Female Participant: To the cliff's edge right now.*

It is important to note that unlike a consistently intense experience with injecting, the high of smoking crack was widely variable and highly dependent on the agents added, either to add inert bulk to the drug (wax) or as an adulterant with additional effects (levamisole [13], methamphetamine). In this way, users give up a measure of certainty of their high. However, the delayed onset makes it easier to temper some of the impulsive and risky actions, including high-risk sexual activity that is often associated with drug use.

While some participants described feeling less paranoia than with injecting, particularly with respect to police interaction, others were aware of more "tweaking" and other side-effects of the additives. Many users said that they would still prefer the high and subjective experience of injecting and choose to smoke for other reasons. For many, it is due to the perceived improvements in overall stability and control.

> *Male Participant: when I compare injecting to smoking the pipe, injecting was more intense, more expensive, more time consuming. It was always on my mind. It was harder for me to shut*

*it down out of my mind when I was injecting ...
I just finally decided that I had more control over
the drug by smoking.*

Male Participant: when I do inject, yeah, everything's just—spur of the moment.

3.3. Drug Use Trajectory. Participants were also able to contextualize crack smoking with respect to other drugs. The majority smoke crack either in addition to injecting cocaine or as a replacement for this. For many, this change was out of necessity as they could no longer find viable injection sites or fear of contracting infections after having contracted HCV from injection. Others were introduced by a partner or spouse, and many decided that it was safer or associated with less stigma. Nevertheless, delineating a common trajectory of drug use is difficult. General consensus among study participants was that many new users start with inhalation without ever injecting, and one's drug route of choice is highly individualistic.

*Female Participant: I think everybody's different
...Anything starts any way, it's 2011, anything goes
now.*

3.4. Polysubstance Use. The significance of polysubstance use can be explained within the phenomenological framework of controlling chaos. In an intentional way of attempting to reduce drug use, several participants reported using beer or marijuana to stave off cravings between highs. This allows them to go longer without smoking crack and to reduce their overall use.

*Male Participant: And that's where the pot comes
into play because that replaces—takes away the
craving of me wanting more. So the pot helps me to
be able to maintain when I can't afford any more
crack*

*Female Participant: That's what I do. I use a little
bit of weed with my crack ... yeah, it kind of helps
me cope with the—crave the—you know*

*Female Participant: I find that I usually smoke less
rock if I have the weed [be]cause it helps with the
jonesing or takes the crave down.*

3.5. Reprioritizing. Injection use is described as an everpresent concern, where users are constantly thinking about their next high. Conversely, smoking has allowed some users enough reprieve to focus on other pursuits without the constant and pervasive craving. In this way, the role of crack in the daily lives of users seems to allow for more stability. While using IV drugs, participants reported their drug use taking priority over basic needs such as shelter and food. In contrast, smoking crack seemed to be lower on their list of priorities, often coming second to housing, food, or family relationships. This enabled participants to maintain obligations to employers, relationships with family and friends,

and self-care and finances issues which were frequently and spontaneously raised when participants described their level of stability or chaos.

*Female Participant: My bills are all paid. I don't
owe money. I don't do crime anymore. I keep
my appointments, you know, all stuff. So it's like
people going out and having a glass of wine
at lunchtime and bringing home a six-pack or
something. I like to take home—when I go home
in the evening, I like to take a little—like, 20 piece
or something home and then watch TV.*

*Female Participant: I still do all my jobs that—my
little volunteer stuff that I'm supposed to do-*

*Male Participant: for me it is a lot easier to accomplish cutting myself off the rock for a substantial
amount of time so that I am eating proper, sleeping
proper and taking better care of myself. And it's
given me back a lot of my self-respect and respect
for others, too.*

3.6. Risk Environment. The risks of crack smoking are multifactorial and involve characteristics of the drug itself, the social environment, especially as it pertains to gender inequalities, and the physical elements of place.

3.7. Infection and Safety. Though many acknowledged an understanding that infection is still a reality, participants readily agreed that smoking is a safer way of consuming drugs than injecting. Frequent anecdotes of cellulitis, phlebitis, and other soft tissue infections, as well as HCV transmission with previous IDU, cause many participants to assert that smoking is the safer alternative. In addition, the gradual onset of smoking drugs could help reduce overdose events; most respondents maintain that their risk of overdose is much less than when they inject.

*Male Participant: Injecting is everything ... I seen
some really bad infections that opened, like, you
know, where you could see inside the arm ...*

Despite a fundamental knowledge of how disease is spread through smoking crack, participants still reported sharing crack pipes, doing so much more frequently than they would with needles.

Male Participant: Pipes are shared a lot.

*Female Participant: People know—can I borrow
your pipe, can I borrow your pipe? And ... gives
them a toke up.*

3.8. Quality. Some of the biggest health concerns relate to cutting agents and uncertain drug quality, as well as the respiratory complications of inhaling Brillo, used as a screen to avoid inhaling crack. Moreover, the wide range of quality and variation in cutting agents mean that there is rarely any certainty about what and how much one is smoking in any given rock. Many, though not all, focus group participants were aware of levamisole being used as a cutting agent and the health effects of agranulocytosis that may result, accepting this and other cutting agents as a dangerous but unavoidable consequence of the variable quality of crack. The same is true of adulterants such as methamphetamine which, when added, may cause tweaking, paranoia, and unpredictable behavior.

> *Male Participant: when it first came out, like, when you knew rock was fucking rock, it was real. And you used to get high. Now it's just fucking pills and baking soda.*

3.9. Social Environment. Though crack pipes are more likely to be shared, most describe the high as being an antisocial experience and say that they are more likely to smoke alone or seek solitude when smoking crack, worried that someone will ruin their high, interrupt the experience, or judge them for tweaking.

> *Male Participant: it's not a social event when you're getting high ... it's a selfish drug, isn't it.*

> *Female Participant: it tends to make me isolate even more, because I'm in there and it's like to leave is, like, a—that's a major, major feat.*

3.10. Gender and Sex. Crack users do not associate smoking with an increase in risky behaviours as compared to injected cocaine, and in fact, associate injecting with more spontaneity. Specifically with respect to risky sexual practices, participants believe that smoking crack is an inhibitor of spontaneous sex, both genders agreeing that most men cannot achieve an erection and consider it a futile endeavor.

> *Female Participant: They can't get it up. I'm saying, it's just too much ... when I'm doing the crack, I do not even want the sex.*

However, despite the clearly unproductive effects of crack on sexual activity, some women also describe men wanting to initiate sexual encounters. Interestingly, although male users claim that they rarely attempt sexual encounters, female users highlighted it as a frequent request and shared anecdotes of crack-for-sex transactions.

> *Female Participant: A lot of the guys that I smoked with, they always wanted something in return sexually.*

There is a highly gendered element to the use of smoked crack, especially evident in the stories of how participants began smoking crack. Men often describe a highly individualistic choice weighing factors such as cost, availability, inability to find injectable veins, and fear of infection.

> *Male Participant: If I had veins now I'd be doing powder again. So this sort of keeps me, you know, keeps me away from doing anything worse that I could do.*

Conversely, the vast majority of women began smoking crack or switched from injecting to smoking either with a male partner or family member or at the request of a partner or spouse.

> *Female Participant: I moved to Vancouver and started smoking crack [be]cause my spouse at the time didn't want me fixing down here [be]cause he thought maybe I might O.D. ... so he made me start smoking crack.*

The contrasting experiences of different genders as well as the further marginalization of female crack smokers [24] are seen in one male participant's comments of sharing crack as a means of achieving power and companionship.

> *Male Participant: I like sharing with the opposite sex. Gets me that power, what you really want to call it, because you feel like you got something that somebody wants ... because of my age [60 years], the un-security of saying okay, ... you're wanted.*

3.11. Housing and Place. A common theme highlighted by study participants was the need for a safe place. Individuals unanimously agree that given the choice, they would much rather smoke inside as they are less likely to be assaulted or have a high ruined by paranoia. The ability to smoke crack in one's own home leads to a more controlled, safer experience. Several anecdotes outline altercations in crack houses where a user became violent with other occupants, they were harassed by police, or of vulnerability to street crime.

> *Female Participant: And if you don't want us smoking in our safe haven, which was looking out for us and us looking out for each other ... you're putting me and my sisters looking out in the alleyways at 3:00 in the morning, for a safe place to—which leads us, you know, to guys raping us, to robbing us, to getting us set up. Just because the neighbourhood wants to feel better.*

> *Female Participant: ... especially women. But it also happens to guys. They're out in the back alley and they're getting robbed, getting punched out ... if you're in a place, a safe place, you have people around, that's not going to happen.*

> *Female Participant: if it's legalized [inhalation room], you know, you do not have to worry.*

Safe housing has additional significance to participants as both a sign of their increasing stability, as well as a protective factor in the control and moderation that they seek to achieve over their drug use. The following quote illustrates a belief that was reiterated by almost all participants; stable housing contributes to increased stability in life and drug use.

> *Male Participant: I have a place to live now for a little over two years and that makes a tremendous difference on my usage. I'm able to keep more of a handle on my usage before it starts getting way out of control. And it—because I have a home now there's other things that are higher priority for me.*

Despite the highly reclusive experience of crack smoking, some participants identified a supervised inhalation site as the most helpful strategy to assist with harm reduction. This was widely supported by all participants, with no participant disagreeing that this would be a beneficial strategy. This location would give users an indoor location to smoke, safe from harassment and police interference often experienced on the street, as well as worry about being disturbed. As well, they would have access to resources for health education and other social resources.

> Male Participant: [a] safe injection site but for smoking crack … somewhat social, but also to learn, right, to learn more of the addiction and to learn—and remind myself that there are caring people who care and that there ways out, you know. Because sometimes I do forget and I feel that I'm trapped in this addiction forever, right.

4. Discussion

This study represents a novel application of two theoretical frameworks to illuminate the experiences of those who use crack. Drug use has been well studied; however, while a great deal of the literature assumes a measure of equivalence between injection and inhalation, we have found crack inhalation to be notably different from other methods of cocaine consumption.

4.1. Controlling Chaos. The meaning that individuals who smoke crack attribute to their drug use adds an important voice to the discourse surrounding crack smoking. Studies such as Hatsukami and Fischman [25] describe crack users as leading especially chaotic lives and being at increased risk of engaging in unsafe sexual practices, polysubstance use, and contracting HIV or HCV. Our findings suggest that our participants view it in a different light. They report qualities of smoked crack that allow them to mitigate this chaos, including the subjective experience, and addictive potential.

Our findings both confirm and challenge the current understanding of increased polysubstance use. While they confirm previous reports of a higher likelihood of polysubstance use, [26] our findings suggest an alternative interpretation of the significance of this. Instead of representing more chaos in the crack smoker's life, our study participants describe their use of these other drugs as an intentional effort to reduce their crack consumption. Notably, our sample was comprised of a number of older individuals, many of whom had prior injection drug use and had transitioned to crack smoking. While these findings may not hold true in less seasoned drug users or with respect to other drug use trajectories, this population described a novel understanding and perception of crack which should be at least considered when attempting to explain the significance of these often observed behaviors. Instead of a measure of chaos, polysubstance use is a means of decreasing frequency of crack use—effectively, a harm reduction strategy. While many studies have confirmed this polysubstance use, very few seek to explain its meaning, and while the assumption of increasing chaos may be largely

true, this study proposes an alternative view based on the beliefs and perceptions of the participants themselves.

This phenomenological contextualization of smoking crack certainly leads to unexpected conclusions regarding its subjective meaning, but even more significant are its implications for the greater discourse on smoking crack. Much of our understanding of the instability of smoking crack is evaluated through metrics such as HIV and HCV transmissions, risky sexual practices, polysubstance use, and dependence on cocaine. Throughout the transcripts, however, efforts to elucidate participants' level of stability were constantly met with declarations of bills paid on time, relationships and obligations maintained, and permanent housing and employment sustained. Thus, when asked to self-report their control, individuals who smoke crack used not only a different set of metrics to measure this but also a fundamentally different dimension.

Our understanding of the chaos or control experienced by crack users may be ignoring important qualitative measures of maintaining obligations and social roles. Previous qualitative studies support our findings that an important self-identified measure of whether an individual is a stable or unstable user relates largely to subjective priority-setting and interrelational factors [27]. By reframing our notion of control through these self-identified metrics, we gain a more holistic and accurate picture of the lived experience of individuals who smoke crack.

4.2. Risk Environment. As speculated and previously observed, the social, political, economic, and physical risk environments within which individuals who smoke crack reside are rife with potential harms, many of which are singular to crack use.

Despite its favorable comparison to IDU, the real threat of infectious disease transmission is not overlooked by participants. Nevertheless, they still report sharing crack pipes, a clear route of transmission of disease [1, 28]. This mirrors previously observed trends, where one estimate was that over 47% of Vancouver crack smokers reported sharing a crack pipe in the previous 6 months [28]. Most of the attention surrounding crack use has been in relation to the transmission of HCV and HIV. Clearly, this is a serious risk, both due to the disproportionate prevalence in this population, and the persistence of HCV on crack pipes and oral sores common to crack smokers [9]. There are a number of potential reasons for sharing pipes: it may be a product of the greater drug culture and the norms surrounding sharing of drugs, which may be supported by the insight that many new users were initiated into crack smoking by sharing a pipe with someone else. It may be a form of risk compensation, with the understood reduction in transmission risk emboldening individuals to share more readily. However, the most commonly repeated reason is related to the fear of crack pipes being confiscated and destroyed by police. The threat of police harassment, combined with the personal cost of crack pipes, may be creating a disincentive to carrying one's own pipe. As Leonard et al. demonstrated, increasing the accessibility of harm reduction supplies is effective in reducing the sharing of drug smoking paraphernalia [29], suggesting that a way of mitigating both the social risks of police harassment and physical risks of infection lies in facilitating harm reduction supply distribution with the cooperation of law enforcement.

The implications of substantially variable strength and quality of crack are major concern. Much of the instability surrounding crack is blamed on the unpredictability of a given high. The addition of methamphetamine and other drug adulterants causes tweaking and paranoia, which adds an element of danger in communal use and may be an inciting factor in the desire for solitary consumption. While participants had no clear suggestion for how to mitigate this risk, identifying it is an important first step. Concerns about increasing risky sexual practices are not borne out in our findings. Women certainly describe trading sexual favors for the use of a crack house, drugs or materials, and as part of the experience of sharing drugs with a partner. Maranda et al. [30] highlight an association between increased sexual partners and crack use as justification for the folk belief that it increases libido. However, crack is clearly not portrayed in our findings as a sexually stimulating drug, and sexual activity may be related more to the gendered power differentials prevalent in this population.

Certainly, the marginalization associated with smoking crack seems to disproportionately affect females. Focus group data seems to support a different trajectory into smoking crack, associated with more external influence and perhaps even coercion. Women recruited from an organization helping survival sex workers understandably had more to say on this matter; however, recruitment from the broader population of women who use crack also endorsed a sexual dimension very different than that of male participants.

4.3. Housing and Place. Housing was noted to be an important factor in increasing the overall stability and control over users' addiction,= as well as mitigating many of the inherent dangers of smoking crack. The significance of safety and stability lends further support to the housing first philosophy that stable housing is a precursor to, and not a consequence of, addictions treatment [31]. Also, the strong support for a supervised inhalation site and access to resources from a group which, by their own admission prefer isolation, speaks to the benefit which they see in such a facility.

4.4. Harm Reduction Strategies. A number of harm reduction strategies were identified by participants, both directly and by virtue of the obstacles to safer inhalation. Most notably, a supervised inhalation site was ubiquitously supported. According to DeBeck et al., 71% of surveyed crack smokers would use such a facility, and it could serve as a distribution site for safe inhalation supplies and a means to connect people who smoke crack cocaine to health and social service providers [32]. Though men also suggested the benefit of a safe inhalation facility, women seemed especially emphatic when speaking of the risks surrounding the lack of safe space. Handlovsky et al. [33] also found housing and the concept of safe places to be a key determinant of harm-reduction in female crack smoking populations.

Similarly, users described various strategies for reducing crack use, largely by mitigating cravings with alcohol and cannabis. Beyond the health effects of reducing crack use, the agency exercised in rationing crack may be empowering and encouraging. A significant risk characteristic in crack smoking is the uncertainty surrounding drug quality and cutting agents. Employing initiatives aimed at improving quality and consistency of crack cocaine would allow for a much more predictable high and reduce the risk of immune compromise from levamisole.

4.5. Limitations. For logistical reasons, the sample of study participants was recruited from individuals already using the two support service organizations. This poses a potential bias, as users connected to peer support agencies may represent a subset of drug users who have greater access to resources or are at a specific place in terms of their drug use trajectory. This may yield insight into why there is an abundance of previous injection use amongst study participants despite the claim that there is no clear escalation from one method to the other and that many new users begin by smoking crack. Additionally, the median age of our sample population was 47 years and may reflect a longer drug use career, implying higher chance of damaged veins, maturity, and a specific trajectory that is not representative of the greater crack smoking population. Were it feasible, a broader demographic range may reveal disparate trends between newer cocaine users and those who have been using it for several decades.

5. Conclusion

Smoking crack is, in fact, very different than other forms of cocaine in both subjective experience and impact on the lives of users. Employing a phenomenological framework yielded many insights into the lived experience of crack inhalation, but more importantly, contributed the qualitative dimension of meaning to previously documented observations regarding populations who smoke crack. Through this lens, we posit that for some, especially those with long-standing drug use careers, smoking crack may represent an increase in efforts to control chaos, and the observed polysubstance abuse is a mechanism for reducing overall crack consumption. The conclusions of this study are not intended to describe the entirety of crack using populations, but rather to highlight an alternative understanding that illustrates one of the many ways that some individuals view crack use as compared with injected cocaine and other drugs.

Moreover, the measures by which individuals define their own level of control or stability incorporate metrics which are often neglected by much of the literature when describing the same. By exploring the qualitative perceptions and understanding of observed trends in drug use, further studies can explore the meaning that people who use drugs attribute to their behaviors.

Additionally, the significant variability in drug quality, constant threat of violence, further marginalization of women, and lack of a safe place to get high all pose concerns from a health standpoint and offer opportunities to create relevant harm reduction initiatives to address them.

Conflict of Interests

The authors declare that they have no conflict of interests.

Acknowledgments

The authors would like to thank the following people from the BC Centre for Disease Control for their contribution to the study: Ellison Richmond and Lianping Ti. The authors would like to thank Siavash Jafari for his insights and contribution to the paper. This research was funded by the BC Harm Reduction Program at the BC Centre for Disease Control.

References

[1] K. DeBeck, T. Kerr, K. Li et al., "Smoking of crack cocaine as a risk factor for HIV infection among people who use injection drugs," *CMAJ*, vol. 181, no. 9, pp. 585–589, 2009.

[2] Public Health Agency of Canada, "I-Track: enhanced surveillance of risk behaviours among people who inject drugs," Phase 1 Report, Surveillance and Risk Assessment Division, Centre for Infectious Disease Prevention and Control, Public Health Agency of Canada, August 2006.

[3] B. Fischer, J. Rehm, S. Brissette et al., "Illicit opioid use in Canada: comparing social, health, and drug use characteristics of untreated users in five cities (OPICAN Study)," *Journal of Urban Health*, vol. 82, no. 2, pp. 250–266, 2005.

[4] J. Johnson, L. Malchy, T. Mulvogue et al., "Lessons learned from the score project: a document to support outreach and education related to safer crack use," Final Report for Safer Crack Outreach, Research and Education Project, June 2008.

[5] J. Buxton, "Vancouver Drug Use Epidemiology," Vancouver Site Report of the Canadian Community Network on Drug Use (CCENDU), 2007.

[6] J. A. Inciardi, "Crack, crack house sex, and HIV risk," *Archives of Sexual Behavior*, vol. 24, no. 3, pp. 249–269, 1995.

[7] P. A. Cavazos-Rehg, E. L. Spitznagel, M. Schootman et al., "Risky sexual behaviors and sexually transmitted diseases: a comparison study of cocaine-dependent individuals in treatment versus a community-matched sample," *AIDS Patient Care and STDs*, vol. 23, no. 9, pp. 727–734, 2009.

[8] C.-Y. Chen and J. C. Anthony, "Epidemiological estimates of risk in the process of becoming dependent upon cocaine: cocaine hydrochloride powder versus crack cocaine," *Psychopharmacology*, vol. 172, no. 1, pp. 78–86, 2004.

[9] B. Fischer, J. Powis, M. F. Cruz, K. Rudzinski, and J. Rehm, "Hepatitis C virus transmission among oral crack users: viral detection on crack paraphernalia," *European Journal of Gastroenterology and Hepatology*, vol. 20, no. 1, pp. 29–32, 2008.

[10] J. Caranci, "TB outbreak tied to crack users," Alberni Valley Times, Port Alberni, BC, Canada, October 2007.

[11] J. Buxton, "Canadian Community Epidemiology Network on Drug Use (CCENDU)," Vancouver Site Report, 2007.

[12] S. Tortu, J. M. McMahon, E. R. Pouget, and R. Hamid, "Sharing of noninjection drug-use implements as a risk factor for Hepatitis C," *Substance Use and Misuse*, vol. 39, no. 2, pp. 211–224, 2004.

[13] L. Knowles, J. A. Buxton, N. Skuridina et al., "Levamisole tainted cocaine causing severe neutropenia in Alberta and British Columbia," *Harm Reduction Journal*, vol. 6, article 30, 2009.

[14] J. A. Buchanan, R. J. Oyer, N. R. Patel et al., "A confirmed case of agranulocytosis after use of cocaine contaminated with levamisole," *Journal of Medical Toxicology*, vol. 6, no. 2, pp. 160–164, 2010.

[15] J. McGuire, "Vancouver's downtown eastside: a community in need of balance," Strathcona Business Improvement Association, 2012http://strathconabia.comwp-content/uploads/2012/08/DTES-A-Community-in-Need-of-Balance.pdf.

[16] Vancouver/Richmond Health Board, "Action plan to combat HIV/AIDS in the downtown Eastside—media backgrounder," October 1997.

[17] Toward the Heart, BC Centre for Disease Control, Vancouver, Canada, 2010, http://towardtheheart.com/ezine/.

[18] J. M. Morse and P. A. Field, *Qualitative Research for Health Professionals*, Sage, Thousand Oaks, Calif, USA, 1995.

[19] T. Rhodes, "Risk environments and drug harms: a social science for harm reduction approach," *International Journal of Drug Policy*, vol. 20, no. 3, pp. 193–201, 2009.

[20] N. Zinberg, *Drug, Set, and Setting: The Basis for Controlled Intoxicant Use*, Yale University Press, New Haven, Conn, USA, 1984.

[21] "NVivo qualitative data analysis software," QSR International Pty Ltd., version 7, 2006.

[22] B. G. Glaser and A. Strauss, *The Discovery of Grounded Theory: Strategies for Qualitative Research*, Aldine, Chicago, Ill, USA, 1967.

[23] Statistics Canada, *Aboriginal Statistics at a Glance*, Statistics Canada, Ottawa, Canada, 2010.

[24] C. W. Lejuez, M. A. Bornovalova, E. K. Reynolds, S. B. Daughters, and J. J. Curtin, "Risk factors in the relationship between gender and crack/cocaine," *Experimental and Clinical Psychopharmacology*, vol. 15, no. 2, pp. 165–175, 2007.

[25] D. K. Hatsukami and M. W. Fischman, "Crack cocaine and cocaine hydrochloride: are the differences myth or reality?" *Journal of the American Medical Association*, vol. 276, no. 19, pp. 1580–1588, 1996.

[26] L. Malchy, V. Bungay, and J. Johnson, "Documenting practices and perceptions of "safer" crack use: a Canadian pilot study," *International Journal of Drug Policy*, vol. 19, no. 4, pp. 339–341, 2008.

[27] D. German and C. E. Sterk, "Looking beyond stereotypes: exploring variations among crack smokers," *Journal of Psychoactive Drugs*, vol. 34, no. 4, pp. 383–392, 2002.

[28] L. Ti, J. Buxton, E. Wood, R. Zhang, J. Montaner, and T. Kerr, "Difficulty accessing crack pipes and crack pipe sharing among people who use drugs in Vancouver, Canada," *Substance Abuse: Treatment, Prevention, and Policy*, vol. 6, no. 1, article 34, 2011.

[29] L. Leonard, E. DeRubeis, and N. Birkett, "City of Ottawa public health: safer crack use initiative evaluation report," 2006, http://www.ohrdp.ca/wpcontent/uploads/pdf/Final_Crack_Report_ES_f.pdf.

[30] M. J. Maranda, C. Han, and G. A. Rainone, "Crack cocaine and sex," *Journal of Psychoactive Drugs*, vol. 36, no. 3, pp. 315–322, 2004.

[31] D. K. Padgett, V. Stanhope, B. F. Henwood, and A. Stefancic, "Substance use outcomes among homeless clients with serious mental illness: comparing housing first with treatment first programs," *Community Mental Health Journal*, vol. 47, no. 2, pp. 227–232, 2011.

[32] K. DeBeck, J. Buxton, T. Kerr, J. Qi, J. Montaner, and E. Wood, "Public crack cocaine smoking and willingness to use a supervised inhalation facility: implications for street disorder," *Substance Abuse: Treatment, Prevention, and Policy*, vol. 6, no. 1, article 4, 2011.

[33] I. Handlovsky, V. Bunjay, J. Johnson, and J. C. Philips, "The process of safer crack use among women in vancouver's downtown eastside," *Qualitative Health Research*, vol. 23, no. 4, pp. 450–462, 2013.

15

The AC-OK Cooccurring Screen: Reliability, Convergent Validity, Sensitivity, and Specificity

Andrew L. Cherry[1] **and Mary E. Dillon**[2]

[1] *School of Social Work, University of Oklahoma, Tulsa Campus, Tulsa, OK 74135, USA*
[2] *University of Central Florida, Orlando, FL 32816, USA*

Correspondence should be addressed to Andrew L. Cherry, alcherry@ou.edu

Academic Editor: Ingmar Franken

The principal barriers to universal screening for the cooccurring disorders of mental illness and substance abuse are training, time, cost, and a reliable and valid screen. Although many of the barriers to universal screening still remain intact, the lack of a cooccurring screen that is effective and can be administered in a cost efficient way is no longer an obstacle. This study examined the reliability, factor structure, and convergent validity of the 15-item AC-OK Cooccurring Screen. A total of 2,968 AC-OK Cooccurring Screens administrated to individuals who called or went to one of the nine participating mental health and substance abuse treatment facilities were administrated and analyzed. Principal axis factor (PAF) analysis was used in the confirmatory factor analysis to identify the common variance among the items in the scales while excluding unique variance. Cronbach's Alpha was used to establish internal consistency (reliability) of each subscale. Finally, the findings from the AC-OK Cooccurring Screen were compared to individual scores on two standardized reference measures, the addiction severity index and the Client assessment record (a measure of mental health status) to determine sensitivity and specificity. This analysis of the AC-OK Cooccurring Screen found the subscales to have excellent reliability, very good convergent validity, excellent sensitivity, and sufficient specificity to be highly useful in screening for cooccurring disorders in behavioral health settings. In this study, the AC-OK Cooccurring Screen had a Cronbach's Alpha of .92 on the substance abuse subscale and a Cronbach's Alpha of .80 on the mental health subscale.

1. Introduction

The knowledge that the cooccurring disorders of addiction or mental illness are widespread in the treatment population and are more complicated to treat has long been the accepted reality among practitioners and researchers. These assumptions are well founded. Estimates based on the 2009 National Survey on Drug Use and Health in the United States suggest that among the 45.1 million adults 18 years of age or older who experienced a mental illness in the year before the survey 8.9 million adults (19.7%) met criteria for substance dependence or abuse (a cooccurring disorder) in that period compared with 6.5% (11.9 million adults) who did not have mental illness in the past year. Based on these numbers, an important finding for alcohol and drug treatment programs is that among the 20.0 million adults who were identified with

a substance use disorder, 4 out of 10 (43%) will also have a mental illness that will need to be treated.

Currently, the recommended approach for treating a person with a cooccurring disorder is an Integrated Treatment model. The objective is to treat both disorders simultaneously. Although identified as an evidence-based treatment by SAMHSA, this does not mean that parallel or sequential treatment is less effective. At this point in time, the results of randomized controlled trials to determine the effectiveness of the Integrated Treatment model are "equivocal but encouraging" [1]. Even so, program administrators have recognized the disadvantages of separate treatment systems and are attempting to increase integrative approaches [2]. Above all, integrated treatment is designed to increase effectiveness by minimizing obstacles experienced by individuals who are seeking care for cooccurring disorders [3]. In a context where there is a need to identify people with a cooccurring disorder, for example, by programs exclusively treating addiction and programs exclusively treating mental health disorders, a screen for cooccurring would also contribute to more attention being paid to both disorders.

2. The Need for an Integrated Screening Tool

A formidable challenge to implementing treatment for people with a cooccurring disorder is the lack of a practical way of screening people for this comorbid disorder, as Lehman [4] pointed out the lack of screening and assessment for cooccurring disorders was an important barrier that prevented less than effective treatment reaching people with a cooccurring disorder. One approach that can be used to identify people with a cooccurring disorder is to conduct two assessments (one to identify a substance use disorder and one to detect a mental health disorder) on everyone who asks for help with a behavioral health disorder [5]. Although effective, this is an expensive strategy. Training staff to administer a large battery of tests, the time involved in administering and interpreting multiple assessments, and the lack of funders who are willing to pay for a large battery of assessments on everybody that seeks treatment make this approach cost prohibitive for most agencies. Given these realities, an *integrated screening tool* that will identify people who likely have a cooccurring disorder is sorely needed. An *integrated screening tool* is defined as a brief measure that can identify both an addition and mental health problem. An *integrated screening tool* is not intended to assess or diagnose, or determine the severity of the disorder, "but only whether or not the person is likely to have a disorder and indicates when additional assessment is needed" [6].

Consequently, rather than completing two assessments on each person who seeks behavioral health services, it is more cost effective to use a rapidly administered screen to identify people who are most likely to have a cooccurring disorder and then do an assessment on only those individuals [6, 7].

The literature search conducted to identify screening instruments found journals and monographs from the United States, Canada, Australia, and England that addressed issues of screening and assessing for a cooccurring disorder. A monograph published by the Population Health Division, Australian Government Department of Health and Ageing, provided a detailed review for usable measures and screens related to substance abuse and mental disorders. It covers the measures described in a matrix and several others used internationally [8]. Another monograph was the *Best Practices: Concurrent Mental Health and Substance Use Disorders* [9]. As well, the monograph, TIP 42, *Substance Abuse Treatment for Persons with Cooccurring Disorders* also reviews instruments available for screening and assessment [5].

Among the scales found in the literature that could be used as a screen, the majority were time consuming to administer and nearly all required specific clinical skills and training and covered only one disorder (i.e., mental health, or substance abuse). While there are few scales specifically

designed to identify people with a cooccurring disorder, the Dartmouth Assessment of Lifestyle Instrument (DALI) is a notable exception [10]. The DALI is a substance abuse measure in the public domain that has 18 questions. It is specifically designed to detect problematic alcohol and marijuana use among people who are *inpatient at a mental health facility*. It does not address mental health issues. The DALI uses weighted items that must be scored. Unlike the AC-OK Cooccurring Screen (AC, Andrew Cherry; OK, Oklahoma), some training is needed to effectively administer this measure.

The CAGE-AID is another instrument that is being used in the mental health field to identify people with a mental health disorder that have a substance use problem [11]. Although not designed to screen for both mental illness and drug use, the CAGE-AID was validated with a sample of people with severe mental illness. In this case, the CAGE-AID performed better than other approaches such as clinical variables, laboratory tests, and collateral reports. A serious limitation, however, is that the CAGE-AID collects information related to *lifetime* rather than *current* substance use problems. This tends to be a limitation when the purpose of the screen is to determine the need for an assessment to determine a cooccurring disorder. In contrast, the AC-OK Cooccurring Screen can be rapidly administered, is easy to interpret, and takes little or no training to administer.

The Comprehensive Addictions and Psychological Evaluation (CAAPE) is another comprehensive diagnostic assessment interview that assesses for substance misuse and mental health disorders designed to assess for cooccurring disorders. The criteria for each diagnosis are based on the DSM-IV TR. This is a fairly extensive questionnaire that covers 14 mental health and substance abuse conditions [12].

The need to screen for a cooccurring disorder is strongly supported by the literature. Yet, there are no integrated screening tools available that are specifically designed to identify people who are likely to have a cooccurring disorder of mental illness and substance abuse. The AC-OK Cooccurring Screen was designed to meet that need. The following provides the psychometric information from the analysis of the AC-OK Cooccurring Screen.

3. Development of the AC-OK Cooccurring Screen

The AC-OK Cooccurring Screen is a version of an earlier screen described in more detail elsewhere [13]. This was a pilot study with 200 volunteer participants. The results of the pilot showed very good psychometric statistics for the items and structure, and provided valuable data that was used to refine the version presented here, the AC-OK Cooccurring Screen. This screen was designed to be a "hot button screen." Hypothetically, if a person asking for treatment services answers "yes" to at least one question in both the mental health and substance abuse subscales, that person would then be administered an assessment battery to determine if the person has a cooccurring disorder.

The original set of questions for the screen came from an advisory group consisting of experts in psychometrics (instrument construction), professionals in both private and public practice from the fields of mental health, and substance abuse. Additionally, people who represented advocacy groups and service recipients were on the committee.

The AC-OK Cooccurring Screen identifies four broad spectrum disorders listed in the DSM-IV TR (i.e., substance use, psychoses, mood disorders, and anxiety spectrum Disorder). The AC-OK Cooccurring Screen is designed to collect self-report information from people seeking either mental health or substance abuse treatment services. Self-report information on substance abuse and mental health is typically considered reliable and valid unless the context in which the questions are asked has potential negative consequences for the person such as loss of job, arrest, and hospitalization [14].

4. Methodology

The definition of a person with a cooccurring disorder that underpins the AC-OK Cooccurring Screen is: "…individuals who have at least one psychiatric disorder as well as an alcohol or drug use disorder. While these disorders may interact differently in any one person (e.g., an episode of depression may trigger a relapse into alcohol abuse, or cocaine use may exacerbate schizophrenic symptoms) at least one disorder of each type can be diagnosed independently of the other" [15].

After IRB approval was received from both the researcher's University and the State Agency of Mental Health and Substance Abuse Treatment, data collection was carried out over a six-month period by nine different agencies. Limited data was solicited from people not admitted for treatment to be in compliance with the Health Insurance Portability and Accountability Act (HIPAA) rules and to protect the identity of any person inquiring about treatment services.

5. Participants

Those who participated in the pilot of the AC-OK Cooccurring Screen were individuals who called or went to one of nine southwestern behavioral health agencies seeking help for what they believed was a mental health or a substance misuse problem. The AC-OK Cooccurring Screen was integrated into the intake process at the nine agencies. Five agencies specialized in mental health treatment and four agencies specialized in addiction treatment. There were a total of 2,968 screens completed. Of those, 1,714 people (58%) who completed the screen entered a treatment facility. For people who did not enter treatment, there is no information beyond the individual's responses to the screen, and the agency that did the screening. There were 2,267 screens completed at the mental health agencies, and 701 screens completed at the substance abuse treatment centers.

These participants were not a homogeneous group. The heterogeneity, however, is not a result of a failure of the sampling technique or the sample drawn, but is a natural reflection of the people seeking help from these behavioral health agencies (no selection bias present). The nine agencies that participated in this study were selected (based on statewide treatment data) because they represented both urban and rural treatment populations. Based on the following analysis and the large number of people screened, the results of the analysis should be strongly reflective of a large group of people seeking help for a mental health, a substance abuse, or a cooccurring disorder.

5.1. Age, Gender, and Those Admitted and Not Admitted. The average age of people seeking treatment in this population was 35.7 years with a standard deviation of 10.87 years. The participants ranged in age from 18 to 75 years old. Some 50% were between 18 and 35 years of age. Of those who completed the screen, 56.3% were male and 43.7% were females.

5.2. Data Collected on Those Admitted and Not Admitted. The only data collected on people asking for help and who were not admitted were gender, age, and agency where the screen was completed, and the person's responses to the screen questions. If the person screened was later admitted to a treatment program additional deidentified admission information was added to the screen information collected on the individual.

5.3. Comparing People Not Admitted to People Who Were Admitted on Age and Gender. When those *not* admitted to treatment are compared to those who were admitted to treatment, the average age for both groups is virtually the same. The average age of those *not* admitted was 35.87 years with a standard deviation of 11.08 years. They ranged in age from 18 to 75 years of age. The average age for those admitted was 35.52 years with a standard deviation of 10.63 years. They ranged in age from 18 to 72 years of age. By gender among those *not* admitted, 56.8% were males and 43.2% were females. Among those admitted, 55.9% were males and 44.1% were females.

They were no significant differences between age and gender among people in the two groups. Age was tested using the t-test ($t = -.958$, df $= 3593.44$, $P < .339$). Gender differences were tested using the chi-square test for significance ($\chi^2 = .247$, df $= 1$, $P < .601$).

Based on the data gathered from this population of people who called or went to a mental health or substance abuse treatment agency for service during this study period, statistical tests were used to determine the reliable, convergent validity, and discriminate validity, sensitivity, and specificity of the two screen subscales. The overarching aim of the analysis was to determine how well the AC-OK Cooccurring Screen subscales can be expected to screen out people with only one disorder and screen in people who possibly have both disorders.

The first step in the analysis was to do a confirmatory factor analysis. Confirmatory factor analysis is a theory-testing approach. Confirmatory factor analysis begins with a hypothesis that specifies which items will be correlated with which factors [16]. In this study, confirmatory factor analysis was used to verify or invalidate the construct of the

15 questions that were hypothesized to form two dimensions; one of mental illness items and one of substance abuse items.

The preferred extraction method when conducting a confirmatory factor analysis is Principal Axis Factor (PAF) analysis, because this method identifies the common variance among the variables, excluding unique variance. Appropriate factor loadings above .50 are defined as supporting the construct validity of the scale.

The second step employed Cronbach's Alpha to measure the internal consistency (reliability) of each of the two subscales. Finally, the AC-OK Cooccurring Screen was compared to two standardized references the Addiction Severity Index (ASI) and the Client Assessment Record (CAR).

The ASI was designed to gather information from people who request alcohol or drug abuse treatment on seven areas of life: medical, employment/support, drug and alcohol use, legal, family history, family/social relationships, and psychiatric problems. The Client Assessment Record (CAR) is a clinical assessment of problems, strengths, and functioning related to one's mental health. The CAR is designed to provide the clinician with a comprehensive overview of an individual's capacity to function in the community. It measures depression, anxiety, mania, attention, thought, disrespect, issues, suicide, self-care, dangerousness, security, family, role, issues, substance, and legal on six (6) levels of functioning. The ASI and CAR are used by the agencies to determine the severity of addiction and mental illness and the need to be admitted for treatment.

6. Results

Principal Axis Factoring (PAF) was used to confirm the association among items in the subscales. First, the screen data was converted to a tetrachoric correlation matrix [17]. In this analysis, tetrachoric correlation coefficients are used because the responses on the screen items are binary (yes, 1; no, 2). A tetrachoric correlation between items with binary responses estimates the correlation as if the two responses ("yes" and "no") were continuous measures [18]. In this analysis the tetrachoric correlations are considered a special case of latent trait modeling. As a result, an analysis of a tetrachoric correlation tends to give a more precise view of the latent structure that underlies the response characteristics of a scale using items with binary responses [19–21].

Next, to evaluate the appropriateness of using a factor analysis procedure with this matrix of tetrachoric correlations, the Bartlett's Test of Sphericity was used. This test suggests that the data met the basic assumption of sphericity ($\chi^2 = 52040.98$, df = 105, $P < .000$). In other words, the correlations in the data matrix are not due to sampling error.

The Kaiser Measure of Sample Adequacy (KMO) was the second test used to check the appropriateness for employing a factor analysis procedure with this data. The resulting KMO for the mental health scale was .914. Kaiser considered KMO's in the .80's as "meritorious" [22]. These tests suggest that the data are adequate for using in a PAF Analysis.

Once it was established that the data from the screen items could be used in a factorial procedure, the structure of

TABLE 1: Varimax rotated solution with factorial loadings and percentage of variance for the AC-OK Co-occurring screen ($N = 2,969$).

Items	Factor I	Factor II
SA2	**.943**	
SA1	**.920**	
SA6	**.920**	
SA9	**.915**	
SA15	**.913**	
SA13	**.882**	
MH3		**.867**
MH4		**.742**
MH7		**.732**
MH8		**.706**
MH10		**.668**
MH11		**.656**
MH12		**.650**
MH14		**.618**
MH5		**.559**
Rotated sum of squared loading: percentage of variance	35.218	30.431

* The bold numbers indicate that the associated questions are in a factor representing one of two subscales: mental health and substance abuse.

the tetrachoric correlation matrix was investigated using PAF as the guiding extraction criteria. In this analysis, the screen items with factor loadings of .50 were selected because they are more likely to produce stable and reliable subscales [23–25]. The PAF analysis extracted two factors. Table 1 presents the Varimax rotated factor loadings. The two-factor solution accounted for 65.65% of the variance. The factor analysis in Table 1 shows that the questions from the screen make up two clear and compelling dimensions, mental illness, and substance abuse.

7. Reliability Analyses

Once the items in each domain were confirmed by the PAF analysis, the Cronbach's Alpha coefficient was used to determine the degree of response consistency among those screened who answered the items on the two subscales. Using the items in the two subscales (the set of questions developed by committee and the same questions identified in the two factors produced by the PAF analysis) a Cronbach's Alpha coefficient was computed for each of the two subscales. The results of these analyses are presented in Table 2.

For the nine items that make up the mental health screen, the mean score was 12.82 with a standard deviation of 2.62 with a 95% confidence interval ranging from 12.74 to 12.90. The median score was 12 (mode = 11) with scores ranging from 9 to 18. Finally, the distribution of scores was slightly skewed (0.399; SE = 0.41) with a kurtosis of −0.80 (SE = 0.82). An examination of the corrected item-total correlations suggests that all nine items are moderately correlated to the total score. In the analysis, corrected item-total correlations

TABLE 2: Descriptive statistics and item analysis for the 15-item AC-OK Co-occurring screen ($N = 2,968$).

Item	M	SD	Corrected Item correlation	Alpha if Deleted
SA2	1.46	0.50	.79	.85
SA1	1.45	0.50	.76	.86
SA6	1.39	0.49	.76	.86
SA9	1.52	0.50	.76	.86
SA15	1.50	0.50	.76	.86
SA13	1.36	0.48	.39	.91
MH3	1.18	0.39	.55	.77
MH4	1.49	0.50	.53	.77
MH7	1.32	0.47	.53	.77
MH8	1.44	0.50	.52	.77
MH10	1.67	0.47	.45	.78
MH 11	1.30	0.46	.48	.77
MH12	1.36	0.48	.44	.78
MH14	1.61	0.49	.43	.78
MH5	1.46	0.50	.41	.78

Note: alphas for mental health = .922; substance abuse screen = .795.

range from a low of .42 to a high of .55 with a final Alpha of .795. Moreover, if any item is removed from the scale the Cronbach's Alpha Coefficient will be reduced.

For the six items reflecting the substance abuse subscale, the mean score is 8.69 with a standard deviation of 2.37 with a 95% confidence interval ranging from 8.61 to 8.76. The median score was 8.00 (mode = 6.00) with scores ranging from 6.00 to 12.00. Finally, the distribution of scores was not skewed (0.19; SE = 0.04) with a kurtosis of −1.61 (SE = 0.08). Examination of the corrected item-total correlations among the substance abuse items suggests that all six items are strongly correlated to the total score. In this analysis, corrected item-total correlations range from .73 to .81. The final Cronbach's Alpha coefficient was .922. If any item is removed from the scale the Cronbach's Alpha Coefficient will be reduced.

Given the results of both the PFA and item analysis of the screen's two subscales, the psychometric stability of the screen is reasonably positive, indicating a moderate to high level of reliability. The substance abuse screen has excellent reliability (α = .92). The mental health screens has good reliability (α = .80). Test-retest reliability has not been established. The client data had to be deidentified per HIPPA requirements, which made it impossible to use test-retest methodology in this study.

8. Convergent and Discriminant Validity

After finding that the two subscales in the AC-OK Cooccurring Screen had excellent to good reliability, the validity of the AC-OK Cooccurring Screen was tested. Pearson correlation coefficients were used to test the levels of convergent and discriminant validity. In this analysis, the two subscales of

the screen are correlated with the reference scales (i.e., the Addiction Severity Index and the Client Assessment Record).

The substance abuse treatment agencies that participated in this study were required by state law to use the Addiction Severity Index (ASI) to determine if an individual should be admitted for treatment. The ASI uses a 10-point scale to rate severity based on historical and current information. It is designed to be administered in a semistructured interview that takes approximately an hour [26]. The reliability alpha for the ASI ranges from .56 to .85. The ASI-psych is a subscale of the ASI that gathers information and severity of psychiatric problems. The ASI-psych reliability alpha ranges in the low .90s. The ASI psychometrics with substance abuse populations have been well established over many years. The primary focus of the ASI is on substance use. However, it also contains a section on psychological problems and functioning. Extensive training materials are available for the ASI. It takes a relatively low level of skill to administer. It is easily scored and relatively inexpensive. Trained lay interviewers are needed to administer the ASI [27]. The subscale of the ASI that measures the severity of psychopathology (ASI-psy) is used as a reference scale to the measure of mental health.

The CAR scales are not designed to be administered as standalone scales. Their reliability depends in part on being embedded in the CAR assessment interview. Reliabilities across CAR scales are reported to ranging from .67 to .87. The CAR-substance use scale reliability alpha ranges from .70 to .80. The clinician needs to be trained in the administration of the CAR. Typically, the information needed to complete the CAR is gathered by the clinician from a face-to-face semiinterview with the client [28]. The subscale of the CAR, the substance use scale (CAR-sa), measures the extent to which a person used addictive drugs. The CAR-sa is used as a reference scale to measure alcohol and other drug abuse.

The correlations between the reference scales, the two AC-OK Cooccurring Screen subscales and the ASI-psy and the CAR-sa are presented in Table 3. As expected, a substantial and significant correlation was found between the AC-OK Cooccurring Screen mental health measure and the ASI-psy (r = .56; P < .001). Additionally, a substantial and significant correlation was found between the AC-OK Cooccurring Screen substance abuse measure and the CAR-sa (r = .59; P < .001). These correlations represent concurrent validity between the AC-OK Screen and the ASI-psy and the CAR-sa. The correlations (interpreted like any Pearson correlation of this magnitude) show a moderate level of convergent validity providing support that the AC-OK Screen is a reliable and valid brief screen for detecting possible co-occurring disorders.

9. Screen Sensitivity and Specificity

The AC-OK Cooccurring Screen was designed to be used in behavioral health settings. This is important because in a setting where a large number of people are expected to have a cooccurring disorder (i.e., mental health and substance abuse treatment settings), the goal is to miss as few people with the disorder as possible. In those settings, the *sensitivity* of a

TABLE 3: Correlations between AC-OK Co-occurring Screen and the reference scales.

	CAR SA	ASI Psy
AC-OK COD-MH	.18**	.56**
	n = 1,275	n = 525
AC-OK COD-SA	.59**	.28**
	n = 1,275	n = 525

** Correlation is significant at the 0.01 level (2 tailed).

screen is stressed. On the other hand, where a small number of people with a cooccurring disorder are expected to request services (i.e., a general medical practice setting) the goal is to identify as few false positives as possible. In these settings *specificity* is stressed.

The purpose of the AC-OK Cooccurring Screen is twofold. Its primary purpose is to identify people that may have a cooccurring disorder (sensitivity). Secondly, it is designed to identify people who most likely do *not* have cooccurring disorder, people who do *not* need a comprehensive assessment for a cooccurring disorder (specificity).

Sensitivity is defined as the probability of a screen testing positive, when in fact the person being screened has the disorder (the true positive rate). Likewise, high sensitivity suggests that a negative screen score indicates that an assessment is not needed.

Specificity is defined as the probability that a negative screen test is negative because the person does not have the disorder (the true negative rate). Conversely, high specificity suggests that a positive screen score strongly suggests that an assessment is needed. Overall accuracy of the screen is determined by the combination of sensitivity and specificity [6].

The AC-OK Cooccurring Screen based on this group of participants had a higher level of *sensitivity* than *specificity*. As a result, the AC-OK Cooccurring Screen produced a fair number of false positives (people identified by the Screen who did not have a cooccurring disorder). This is acceptable, however, because in mental health and substance abuse treatment agencies, the goal is to miss as few people as possible with a cooccurring disorder.

The sensitivity of the AC-OK Cooccurring Screen is excellent. It missed only 7 out of 177 people (96% correctly identified) who were later found to have a cooccurring disorder using the ASI-psy. Among people assessed with the CAR-sa and found to have a cooccurring disorder, the Screen missed 48 out of 507 people (90.5% correctly identified) (see Table 4).

The new Screen's specificity is fair. The Screen identified approximately 72% of all people screened as needing a comprehensive assessment to determine if the person had a cooccurring disorder. The number of people in this population with a cooccurring disorder was estimated to be 35% [29]. This lower level of specificity suggests that about 50% of the people identified as having a potential cooccurring disorder by the AC-OK Cooccurring Screen will actually have the disorder (see Table 4). The level of specificity could be improved but when specificity increases sensitivity decreases.

10. Discussion

The data collected to determine the reliability, convergent and discriminant validity, sensitivity, and specificity of the AC-OK Cooccurring Screen strongly suggests that the psychometric stability of the screen is reasonably positive, indicating a moderate to high level of reliability. The substance abuse screen has the best reliability (α = .92). The mental health screen has good reliability (α = .80). In terms of *sensitivity*, the AC-OK Cooccurring Screen can be expected to identify about 70% of those being screened as needing to be assessed for a cooccurring disorder. Of this number, the AC-OK Cooccurring Screen missed about 7% of people who could be identified as having a cooccurring disorder if they were fully assessed for both a mental health and substance use disorder.

One limitation of the analysis is that AC-OK COD was not compared to the SCID (Structured Clinical Interview for DSM-IV Axis I Disorders), the gold standard for establishing specificity and sensitivity diagnoses such as a cooccurring disorder. Instead it was compared to two assessments measures used by the treatment facilities to determine severity and need for admission to treatment. Furthermore, another limitation might be the lack of strong correlations between the AC-OK COD and the two-reference scale. The lack of strong correlations in this case, however, was not because of the predictive value of the screen but because the purpose of the screen and the *two reference measures* are very different. The screen is used to detect the presence of a cooccurring disorder while the ASI-psy and the CAR-sa are used to detect the present of a disorder and to determine the severity. Another reason is the time it takes to administer two assessment tools. While psychosocial assessments like the ASI (for addiction) and the CAR (for mental health disorders) take an hour each to administer, the AC-OK Screen which takes less than five minutes to administer and score will still add 10 to 15 minutes to each client intake. For some programs this will be a financial burden.

An issue to keep in mind when using this screen (and for that matter other screens and assessments) especially for people presenting with substance abuse problems is that some symptoms (i.e., hallucinations, paranoia, and depression) caused by intoxication or withdrawal can subside or disappear after a period of abstinence.

Nevertheless, Authors of [30] suggested that failing to identify substance use and cooccurring mental health disorders can result in a misdiagnose and less than effective pharmacological interventions, neglect of appropriate substance abuse treatments, and inappropriate treatment planning and referral. Indeed, a best practice for providing services to people with a cooccurring disorder includes time sensitive screening of all people seeking help for a mental health or substance abuse disorder.

Screening for the single disorders such as substance abuse, mental illness, and trauma has a rich history of success. The AC-OK Cooccurring Screen is a screening tool with 15 questions that can efficiently identify people who are likely to have a cooccurring disorder. It can be easily incorporated into an agency's intake process and can be completed in five minutes or less. Moreover, the screen is easy to score. A "yes"

TABLE 4: Specificity and sensitivity AC-OK Co-occurring Screen agreement compared to two reference measures.

Specificity		
The probability of the screen being positive when the person has the disorder		
AC-OK Co-occurring Screen	ASI-psy	CAR-sa
Correct	170/96%	459/90.5%
Missed	7/4%	48/9.5%
Sensitivity		
The probability of the screen being negative when the person does *not* have the disorder.		
(i) The AC-OK Co-occurring Screen identified approximately 72% of all people screened as needing an assessment to determine if the person had a co-occurring disorder.		
(ii) The estimated number of people in this population needing treatment for a co-occurring was 35%.		
(iii) The disadvantage of a lower level of sensitivity is that only half of the people being screened will be assessed as having a co-occurring disorder.		

answer on any question in the related subscales would signal the need for an assessment in that area. Based on the results of this study, the AC-OK Cooccurring Screen is reliable and valid and has high levels of sensitivity and specificity.

The AC-OK Cooccurring Screen could also have potential to identify people who need to be assessed for a possible cooccurring disorder whether the person presents at a mental health facility or at a substance abuse treatment facility. It could also be helpful at a shelter for victims of domestic violence, in jails and detention settings, in medical clinics, in emergency rooms, and in other settings to determine if a person needed to be fully assessed for a cooccurring disorder.

Although many of the barriers to universal screening for a cooccurring disorder are still intact (training, time, cost, and an infrastructure where everybody seeking mental health or substance abuse services is screened), the lack of a cooccurring screen that is effective and can be administered economically for detecting people who need a comprehensive assessment for a cooccurring disorder is no longer a barrier.

Questions Used in the AC-OK Cooccurring Screen

(1) Have you been preoccupied with drinking alcohol and/or using other drugs?

(2) Have you experienced problems caused by drinking alcohol and/or using other drugs, and kept using alcohol and/or other drugs?

(3) Have you experienced serious depression (felt sadness, hopelessness, loss of interest, change in appetite, change in sleep pattern, or difficulty going about your daily activities)?

(4) Have you experienced thoughts of harming yourself?

(5) Have you ever been hit, slapped, kicked, emotionally or sexually hurt, or threatened by someone?

(6) Have you drunk alcohol and/or used other drugs more than you intended?

(7) Have you experienced a period of time when your thinking speeds up and you have trouble keeping up with your thoughts?

(8) Have you experienced a traumatic event and since had repeated nightmares/dreams and/or anxiety which interferes with you leading a normal life?

(9) Have you needed to drink more alcohol and/or use more drugs to get the same effect you used to get with a less amount?

(10) Have you attempted suicide?

(11) Have you had periods of time where you felt that you could not trust family or friends.

(12) Have you been prescribed medication for any psychological or emotional problem?

(13) Have you drank alcohol and/or used other drugs to alter the way you feel?

(14) Have you experienced hallucinations (heard or seen things others do not hear or see)?

(15) Have you tried to stop drinking alcohol and/or using other drugs, but could not?

Disclosure

Do not copy any part of this document without permission from Dr. A. L. Cherry, the Oklahoma Endowed Professor of Mental Health, School of Social Work, University of Oklahoma, Tulsa. The AC-COD Screen and the AC-OK Screen are copyrighted scales. Commercial use of the AC-COD Screen or the AC-OK Cooccurring Screen is prohibited. However, *these screens are available without charge to researchers, clinicians, and agencies serving people with a cooccurring disorder* with the compliments of the authors. Go to the following webpage to download a copy: http://faculty-staff.ou.edu/C/Andrew.L.Cherry-1.Jr/AC-CODScreenPg.htm.

Acknowledgments

This study was conducted in conjunction with a SAMHSA COSIG project. Thanks to the Oklahoma Department of Mental Health and Substance Abuse Services and the nine agencies that participated in piloting the AC-OK-COD

Screen. They are Bill Willis CMHC, Family and Children's Services, Gateway to Prevention and Recovery, Grand Lake M.H.C., Norman Alcohol and Drug Treatment Center, Norman Alcohol Information Center, OK County Crisis Intervention Center, Tulsa Center for Behavioral Health, and 12 & 12. This project was supported by funding awarded by the Oklahoma Department of Mental Health and Substance Abuse Services (ODMHSAS) by SAMHSA. Points of view in this document are those of the authors and do not necessarily represent the official position or policies of ODMHSAS.

References

[1] J. Horsfall, M. Cleary, G. E. Hunt, and G. Walter, "Psychosocial treatments for people with co-occurring severe mental illnesses and substance use disorders (dual diagnosis): a review of empirical evidence," *Harvard Review of Psychiatry*, vol. 17, no. 1, pp. 24–34, 2009.

[2] S. Sterling, F. Chi, and A. Hinman, "Integrating care for people with co-occurring alcohol and other drug, medical, and mental health conditions," *Alcohol Research and Health*, vol. 33, no. 4, pp. 338–349, 2011.

[3] C. M. Chowa, D. Wiemana, B. Cichockia, H. Qvicklunda, and D. Hiersteinera, "Mission impossible: treating serious mental illness and substance use co-occurring disorder with integrated treatment: a meta-analysis ," *Mental Health and Substance Use.* In press.

[4] A. F. Lehman, "Heterogeneity of person and place: assessing co-occurring addictive and mental disorders," *American Journal of Orthopsychiatry*, vol. 66, no. 1, pp. 32–41, 1996.

[5] SAMHSA, *Substance Abuse Treatment for Persons with a Co-Occurring Disorder: A Treatment Improvement Protocol*, TIP 42, U.S. Department of Health and Human Services, Washington, DC, USA, 2005.

[6] S. Sacks, "Brief overview of screening and assessment for co-occurring disorders," *International Journal of Mental Health Addiction*, vol. 6, no. 1, pp. 7–19, 2008.

[7] R. W. Kanwischer, "Principles and practice for the screening, diagnosis, and assessment of persons with co-occurring mental illness and substance abuse," *Journal of Social Work Practice in the Addictions*, vol. 5, no. 1, pp. 29–51, 2001.

[8] S. Dawe, N. J. Loxton, L. Hides, D. J. Kavanagh, and R. P. Mattick, *Review of Diagnostic Screening Instruments for Alcohol and Other Drug Use and Other Psychiatric Disorders*, Monograph no. 48, The National Drug Strategy, Commonwealth Department of Health and Ageing, Canberra, Australia, 2002.

[9] Health Concerns, *Best Practices—Concurrent Mental Health & Substance Use Disorders*, Minister of Public Works and Government Services, Ottawa, Canada, 2002.

[10] S. D. Rosenberg, R. E. Drake, G. L. Wolford et al., "Dartmouth assessment of lifestyle instrument (DALI): a substance use disorder screen for people with severe mental illness," *American Journal of Psychiatry*, vol. 155, no. 2, pp. 232–238, 1998.

[11] D. Mayfield, G. McLeod, and P. Hall, "The CAGE questionnaire: validation of a new alcoholism screening instrument," *American Journal of Psychiatry*, vol. 131, no. 10, pp. 1121–1123, 1974.

[12] S. M. Gallagher, P. E. Penn, A. J. Brooks, and J. Feldman, "Comparing the CAAPE, a new assessment tool for co-occurring disorders, with the SCID," *Psychiatric Rehabilitation Journal*, vol. 30, no. 1, pp. 63–65, 2006.

[13] A. L. Cherry, M. E. Dillon, C. M. Hellman, and L. D. Barney, "The AC-COD screen: rapid detection of people with the co-occurring isorders of substance abuse, mental illness, domestic violence, and trauma," *Journal of Dual Diagnosis*, vol. 4, no. 1, pp. 35–53, 2008.

[14] K. B. Carey and C. J. Correia, "Severe mental illness and addictions: assessment considerations," *Addictive Behaviors*, vol. 23, no. 6, pp. 735–748, 1998.

[15] SAMHSA, *Report to Congress on the Prevention and Treatment of Co-Occurring Substance Abuse Disorders and Mental Disorders, Substance Abuse and Mental Health Services Administration*, U. S. Department of Health and Human Services, Center for Mental Health Services, Washington, DC, USA, 2005.

[16] J. Stevens, *Applied Multivariate Statistics for the Social Sciences*, Lawrence Erlbaum Associates, Mahwah, NJ, USA, 3rd edition, 1996.

[17] J. S. Uebersax, "The tetrachoric and polychoric correlation coefficients. Statistical Methods for Rater Agreement," 2006, http://ourworld.compuserve.com/homepages/jsuebersax/tetra.htm.

[18] F. Drasgow, "Polychoric and polyserial correlations," in *Encyclopedia of Statistical Sciences*, L. Kotz and N. L. Johnson, Eds., vol. 7, pp. 69–74, Wiley, New York, NY, USA, 1988.

[19] J. B. Carroll, "The nature of the data, or how to choose a correlation coefficient," *Psychometrika*, vol. 26, no. 4, pp. 347–372, 1961.

[20] G. V. Glass and J. C. Stanley, *Statistical Methods in Education and Psychology*, Prentice Hall, Englewood Cliffs, NJ, USA, 1970.

[21] L. L. Thurstone, *Multiple-Factor Analysis*, University of Chicago Press, Chicago, Ill, USA, 1947.

[22] H. F. Kaiser, "An index of factorial simplicity," *Psychometrika*, vol. 39, no. 1, pp. 31–36, 1974.

[23] R. B. Cattell, "The screen test for the number of factors," *Multivariate Behavioral Research*, vol. 1, pp. 245–276, 1996.

[24] E. Guadagnoli and W. F. Velicer, "Relation of sample size to the stability of component atterns," *Psychological Bulletin*, vol. 103, no. 2, pp. 265–275, 1988.

[25] W. R. Zwick and W. F. Velicer, "Comparison of five rules for determining the number of components to retain," *Psychological Bulletin*, vol. 99, no. 3, pp. 432–442, 1986.

[26] A. T. McLellan, "The Addiction severity index (ASI)," University of Pennsylvania's Center for the Studies of Addiction, 1980, http://www.tresearch.org/ASI.htm.

[27] P. A. McDermott, A. I. Alterman, L. Brown, A. Zaballero, F. C. Snider, and J. R. McKay, "Construct refinement and confirmation for the addiction severity index," *Psychological Assessment*, vol. 8, no. 2, pp. 182–189, 1996.

[28] D. B. Altschul, J. Wackwitz, A. S. Coen, and D. Ellis, "Colorado client assessment record interrater reliability study," Final Report, Mental Health Services, Denver, Colo, USA, 2011, http://john-uebersax.com/stat/tetra.htm .

[29] A. L. Cherry, L. G. Byers, M. E. Dillon, and L. Barnett, "OK-End of year 3 evaluation report," 2006, http://faculty-staff.ou.edu/C/Andrew.L.Cherry-1.Jr/okcosig_project.htm

[30] R. E. Drake, K. T. Mueser, R. E. Clark, and M. A. Wallach, "The course, treatment, and outcome of substance disorder in persons with severe mental illness," *American Journal of Orthopsychiatry*, vol. 66, no. 1, pp. 42–51, 1996.

16

Everyday Prospective Memory and Executive Function Deficits Associated with Exposure to Second-Hand Smoke

Thomas M. Heffernan and Terence S. O'Neill

Collaboration for Drug and Alcohol Research (CDAR), Division of Psychology, Department of Psychology, Northumbria University, Newcastle upon Tyne NE1 8ST, UK

Correspondence should be addressed to Thomas M. Heffernan; tom.heffernan@northumbria.ac.uk

This study explored whether exposure to second-hand smoke (SHS) has a detrimental impact upon everyday memory in two groups of non-smokers; one which reported regular exposure to SHS and one that reported never having been exposed to SHS. Thirty-four non-smokers who reported having been regularly exposed to SHS (SHS group) and 34 non-smokers who reported never having been exposed to SHS (non-SHS group) were compared on self-reports of prospective memory (PM: remembering future intentions and/or activities) and executive function (EF: those processes involved in attention, multitasking and decision-making). The Prospective and Retrospective Memory Questionnaire (PRMQ) assessed everyday PM lapses; the Executive Function Questionnaire (EFQ) assessed self-reported problems in EF; a drug-use questionnaire and a mood questionnaire were also administered. Two univariate ANCOVAs were applied to the PM and EF data, controlling for between-group differences in age, weekly alcohol use, anxiety and depression scores, and self-reported retrospective memory scores. The SHS group reported significantly more lapses on the PRMQ and more deficits on the EFQ than the non-SHS group. These findings provide new insights into PM and EF deficits associated with prolonged exposure to SHS in a group of non-smokers. Possible explanations and suggestions for future research are also considered.

1. Introduction

Second-hand smoke (SHS) refers to a situation where one person inhales another person's smoke either by exposure to side stream smoke (smoke emitted from the end of a cigarette, pipe, or cigar) or mainstream smoke (the smoke that is exhaled by the smoker directly). Previous research has suggested that exposure to second-hand smoke (SHS) not only has a detrimental effect upon health, including cardiovascular disease [1, 2], but also is associated with poorer cognitive performance in children, adolescents, and adults (3–6). For example, children exposed to SHS show reduced vocabulary and reasoning abilities [3], as well as more general cognitive and intellectual deficits [4]. In addition, recent work has shown a strong relationship between exposure to SHS and impairments in reading, mathematics, and visuospatial skills in children and adolescents [5] and poorer cognitive function in adults [6, 7]. In the first of

these adult studies [6], participants included in the study had no history of smoking or using any tobacco product, and had no history of cardiovascular disease or dementia. Based on their self-reported long-term exposure to SHS tobacco smoke (having lived with a smoker for 3 decades) the study found that those exposed to SHS were about 30% more likely to develop dementia over a period of six years when compared with those who reported never having been exposed. In the second of these adults studies [7] participants who had no history of smoking any tobacco product were measured on exposure to SHS using cotinine biomarker assays. In a cross-sectional design, participants exposed to different levels of SHS were compared on cognitive measures including processing speed and executive function. The findings from the study revealed that exposure to increasingly higher levels of SHS corresponded with greater deficits in cognitive function. From this research it can be concluded that exposure to SHS in never-smoked groups equates to deficits in cognitive function. These deficits have been linked to risk factors, such as cardiovascular disease, associated with SHS in the past [8, 9]. These data suggest that exposure to SHS may be causally associated to impairments in a range of cognitive processes. However, what is not clear is whether exposure to second-hand smoke is associated with impairments in everyday cognition, of which *prospective memory* and *executive function* are two good examples.

Prospective memory (PM) is an important aspect of day-to-day memory function and refers to the process of remembering to do things at some future point in time [10]. For example, remembering to attend an appointment at a clinic, remembering to carry out a task such as paying a bill on time or remembering to take ones medication on time are all examples of PM. Executive function (EF) is an umbrella term that is used to describe a collection of processes making up the central executive component of the working memory model [11, 12] and includes planning, task coordination, impulse control, and attention. PM is thought to be critical to independent living [13] and a compromised EF is likely to lead to confusion, poor planning, and other executive problems on everyday tasks, so developing a greater understanding of how both these sets of processes might be affected by exposure to potentially harmful substances, such as SHS exposure.

There is good evidence that performance on PM tasks relies on prefrontal systems in the brain and on the integrity of related EF [14–18]. Frontally mediated EF is believed to play key roles in a range of processes, including planning a task, monitoring one's environment, the inhibition of extraneous responses, and cognitive flexibility [19–21]. For example, research has shown that when high demands are placed on EF (using a dual-task paradigm) executive processes (measured using the Tower of London task, the Stroop task, and the Wisconsin Card Sorting Task) predicted performance on the more complex dual-task PM paradigms, but not on simple (single) PM task paradigms [20]. This supports the notion that frontal/executive functions are intimately related to PM performance. Furthermore, evidence from brain-imaging studies also highlights strong links between PM and EF [19, 22]. Given that prolonged exposure to SHS is linked to deficits in EF [7] and based on the links between PM and EF discussed here, it is feasible to hypothesise that prolonged exposure to SHS in a never-smoked group may lead to impairments in both EF and PM in the same cohort, when compared with a group who have never smoked and whom have not been exposed to SHS. The issue of what physical harm exposure to SHS has upon the individual is gaining international interest [23], yet despite this there is very little in the way of systematic research into what impact SHS exposure has upon everyday cognition in nonsmoking adults. The current study seeks to address this by comparing two groups of nonsmokers (individuals who had never smoked): one of which reported regular exposure to SHS and one that reported never having been exposed to SHS, upon self-reports of PM and EF. Since other drug use can independently impede PM performance [24, 25] and given that variations in mood can negatively affect cognition [26, 27], these were measured and included

in the main analysis as covariates. Finally, since retrospective memory (RM) deficits have been found in those exposed to SHS and given the RM is related to both PM and EF [19], self-reported RM was also gauged and included as a covariate.

2. Method

2.1. Participants. An original sample of 150 individuals attending a university in the North East of England was recruited. From this original sample, 82 were omitted on the basis that they reported using an illegal substance (e.g., cannabis, ecstasy), were or had been smokers, and/or were heavy drinkers or had drunk any alcohol within the last 48 hours, and/or had reported a psychiatric illness (e.g., depression, substance dependence). Of the remaining 68 participants, 34 were non-smokers who reported that they had been regularly exposed to second-hand smoke (SHS) either in a home or social situation (the SHS group) and 34 were nonsmokers who had reported never having been exposed to SHS (the non-SHS group). In the SHS group (29 females, 5 males; mean age = 20.2 years, S.D.: 2.73) 70% of them reported that their exposure to SHS came from the home which they shared with smokers and 30% reported that their exposure came from a social setting within which they sat with smokers in a partially confined "smoking hut/area" outside a pub/restaurant/bar. This group reported that they were exposed to SHS for an average of 13.8 hours per week, S.D.: 16.9, and had been exposed in this way for an average of 6.14 years, S.D.: 6.04. They also reported that they drank on average 10.2 units of alcohol per week, S.D.: 7.60, had been drinking for an average of 4.00 years, S.D.: 2.39, and had not drunk for an average of 103 hours, S.D.: 94. The non-SHS group (27 females, 7 males; mean age = 19.4 years, S.D.: 0.86) reported that they had never been directly exposed to SHS either at home, at work, at university, or within a social situation; they reported that they drank on average 8.47 units of alcohol per week, S.D.: 6.08, had been drinking for an average of 3.88 years, S.D.: 1.98, and had not drank for an average of 117 hours, S.D.: 108. As stated previously all 68 participants reported they did not use any illegal substance in addition to alcohol.

3. Measures and Procedure

Participants completed a series of brief questionnaires. A drug-use questionnaire was completed in which smoking and other drug use were assessed using a modified version of a Recreational Drug Use Questionnaire (RDUQ) used in previous research [24, 25]. This measured their smoking status; the number of hours exposed per week to SHS, the situation in which they were exposed and the number of years exposed to SHS (relating to the SHS group); the number of alcohol units consumed per week, length of alcohol use in years and when they last drank alcohol in hours. Similar questions were asked in relation to other drug use (e.g., cannabis, ecstasy). There were also "nonuse" options for all these drugs. Demographics (age, gender), whether they had previously suffered from/or were currently suffering from a substance dependence disorder, clinical amnesia, or some other psychiatric condition, were also measured on the questionnaire.

As previous research has indicated that there may be an association between depression and cognitive failures [26, 27], all participants completed the Hospital Anxiety and Depression Scale (HADS) [28] which is a 14-item standardised self-report questionnaire. Seven items measured generalised anxiety symptoms and 7 measured generalised depressive symptoms. Separate overall scores were obtained for the anxiety and depression constructs, each ranging from between 0 to 21, with a higher score indicating more severe symptoms. The HADS has been shown to be a valid and reliable measure of mood in nonclinical samples [29].

Prospective memory was assessed using the PM scale from the Prospective and Retrospective Memory Questionnaire (PRMQ) which is a self-report measure developed by previous authors [30]. The retrospective memory (RM) subscale of the PRMQ was also calculated since RM is related to both PM and EF. The PRMQ shows high internal consistency, with the reliability on Cronbach's alpha being 0.89. The PRMQ assesses self-reported prospective and retrospective memory slips in everyday life. Table 1 contains the full list of PM and RM questions contained in the PRMQ. The participant rated how often they experienced such failures on a 5-point scale from "very often" (5) to "never" (1) by circling the response that best reflects their memory ability. A mean score for PM slips/failures was calculated, along with a mean score for RM slips/failures, in both cases with a higher score indicating more memory slips/failures.

Executive function was measured using an Executive Function Questionnaire (EFQ) devised and validated by previous research [31]. The questionnaire is comprised of a series of questions designed to estimate deficits in the main components of executive function—including attentional difficulties, problems in concentration, one's ability of multitask, perseverance on a task, and impulse control. The EFQ shows high internal consistency, with the reliability on Cronbach's alpha being 0.78. For each item, participants responded by circling one response from a four-point scale (1) no problems experienced; (2) a few problems experienced; (3) more than a few problems experienced; (4) a great many problems experienced. Table 2 contains the full list of executive questions contained in the EFQ. The total scale score was computed by summing the responses to the six items and this total score was intended to reflect the participant's overall experience of executive problems rather than any specific aspect thereof, with a higher score indicating more executive deficits experienced.

The research received ethical approval from the School of Life Sciences Ethics Committee at Northumbria University. Participants were recruited on a voluntary basis and tested individually in a controlled laboratory situation. The PRMQ was administered first, followed by the EFQ, HADS, and then the personal characteristics/drug-use questionnaire. After completing the study participants were thanked for their cooperation and fully debriefed.

4. Results and Discussion

Chi-square analysis revealed no significant difference in the number of males and females between the SHS and non-SHS groups ($\chi^2(1) = 0.40, P = 0.52$). In order to observe what independent impact each of the covariates had upon prospective memory (PM) and executive function (EF), as well as what impact exposure to SHS has upon PM and EF after controlling for these covariates, two univariate ANCOVAS were applied to the PM and EF data (controlling for age, weekly alcohol use, anxiety and depression scores, and self-reported retrospective memory (RM) scores). The first ANCOVA revealed no significant independent impact of age upon PM $F (1, 62) = 0.79, P = .37$, no significant independent impact of weekly alcohol use upon PM $F (1, 62) = 2.17, P = .14$, no significant independent impact of HADS anxiety upon PM $F (1, 62) = 0.29, P = .59$, no significant independent impact of HADS depression upon PM $F (1, 62) = 0.24, P = .95$, but RM did have a significant impact upon PM $F (1, 62) = 73.8, P < .001$. After controlling for variations in these covariates a significant impact of SHS upon PM remained $F (1, 62) = 4.33, P < .05$. Inspection of the means showed that the SHS group reported more PM errors than the non-SHS group (see Table 3). The second ANCOVA revealed no significant independent impact of age upon EF $F (1, 62) = 0.00, P = .98$, no significant independent impact of weekly alcohol use upon EF $F (1, 62) = 1.59, P = .21$; however, there was a significant independent impact of HADS anxiety upon EF $F (1, 62) = 8.80, P < .01$, and a significant independent impact of HADS depression upon EF $F (1, 62) = 7.66, P < .01$, as well as a significant independent impact of RM upon EF $F (1, 62) = 4.33, P < .05$. After controlling for variations in these covariates a significant impact of SHS upon EF remained $F (1, 62) = 4.32, P < .05$. Inspection of the means showed that the SHS group reported more EF deficits than the non-SHS group (see Table 3). A Pearson Product Moment correlation revealed a significant positive correlation between scores on the EF and PM measures $r (68) = .215, P < .05$, indicating more failures reported on the EF measures corresponded with greater memory lapses on the PM measure.

The main finding from this study was that both increased frequency of self-reported PM lapses and self-reported deficits in EF were associated with exposure to second-hand smoking in the SHS group when compared with the non-SHS group. Thus, those participants who had never smoked but who reported being regularly exposed to SHS in confined spaces for prolonged periods of time on several occasions per week and over several years showed significantly more forgetting on everyday PM tasks (such as forgetting future activities one had planned to do) as well as greater deficits in EF (such failures in attention, planning, and multitasking), when compared with a group of never smokers who had not been exposed to SHS. To our knowledge this is the first analysis to observe a relationship between SHS exposure in a never-smoked group and both PM and EF deficits within the same cohort of participants. We controlled for a wide range of covariables that are potential confounders in cognitive research. Having reduced PM capabilities can result in poorer performance on everyday tasks, such as

TABLE 1: Self-reported memory slips for prospective memory items (questions: 1, 3, 5, 7, 10, 12, 14, 16) and retrospective memory items (questions: 2, 4, 6, 8, 9, 11, 13, 15).

(1) Do you decide to do something in a few minutes' time and then forget to do it?				
Very often	Quite often	Sometimes	Rarely	Never
(2) Do you fail to recognize a place you have visited before?				
Very often	Quite often	Sometimes	Rarely	Never
(3) Do you fail to do something you were supposed to do a few minutes later even though it is there in front of you, like taking a pill or turning off the kettle?				
Very often	Quite often	Sometimes	Rarely	Never
(4) Do you forget something that you were told a few minutes before?				
Very often	Quite often	Sometimes	Rarely	Never
(5) Do you forget appointments if you are not prompted by someone else or by a reminder such as a calendar or diary?				
Very often	Quite often	Sometimes	Rarely	Never
(6) Do you fail to recognize a character in a radio or television show from scene to scene?				
Very often	Quite often	Sometimes	Rarely	Never
(7) Do you forget to buy something you planned to buy, like a birthday card, even when you see the shop?				
Very often	Quite often	Sometimes	Rarely	Never
(8) Do you fail to recall things that have happened to you in the last few days?				
Very often	Quite often	Sometimes	Rarely	Never
(9) Do you repeat the same story to the same person on different occasions?				
Very often	Quite often	Sometimes	Rarely	Never
(10) Do you intend to take something with you, before leaving a room or going out, but minutes later leave it behind, even though it is there in front of you?				
Very often	Quite often	Sometimes	Rarely	Never
(11) Do you mislay something that you have just put down, like a magazine or glasses?				
Very often	Quite often	Sometimes	Rarely	Never
(12) Do you fail to mention or give something to a visitor that you were asked to pass on?				
Very often	Quite often	Sometimes	Rarely	Never
(13) Do you look at something without realising you have seen it moments before?				
Very often	Quite often	Sometimes	Rarely	Never
(14) If you tried to contact a friend or relative who was out, would you forget to try again later?				
Very often	Quite often	Sometimes	Rarely	Never
(15) Do you forget what you watched on television the previous day?				
Very often	Quite often	Sometimes	Rarely	Never
(16) Do you forget to tell someone something you had meant to mention a few minutes ago?				
Very often	Quite often	Sometimes	Rarely	Never

remembering meetings, chores one has to perform, and so forth, and having a compromised EF can only add to these problems. It is important therefore to observe whether the findings here are replicable under a variety of tasks that tap into PM and EF. Given that this was a relatively young cohort (with 97% of the SHS exposed group being under the age of 25 years (100% in the case of the non-SHS group)), the findings suggest that putative cognitive deficits as a result of prolonged exposure to SHS can start to occur after a relatively short period of time (the mean SHS exposure time in this study was just over 6 years) even in young people.

As suggested earlier, these may be important findings, since only a handful of studies to date have observed cognitive and intellectual deficits associated with prolonged exposure to SHS in children [3, 4], as well as observing an association between SHS exposure and deficits in the neurocognitive function of adolescent and adult populations [5–7], but none of these previous studies have assessed cognitive function directly, nor have they done so in relation to everyday remembering. Given that PM and EF are seen as essential to independent living [13, 19], exploring the relationship between exposure to SHS and deficits in these cognitive domains may be of paramount importance. A particular strength of this study was the number of "controls" adopted; that is, anyone who reported using an illegal drug (such as ecstasy or cannabis), who drank heavily or had drunk any alcohol within the past 48 hours, or reported suffering from a clinical psychiatric condition as excluded from the study. The findings were also observed after controlling for between-group variations on age, gender, weekly alcohol use, mood (anxiety and depression scores), and self-reported retrospective memory scores. Although the present study

TABLE 2: The executive items from the executive function questionnaire.

(1) Do you find it difficult to keep your attention on a particular task?
(2) Do you find yourself having problems concentrating on a task?
(3) Do you have difficulty carrying out more than one task at a time?
(4) Do you tend to "lose" your train of thoughts?
(5) Do you have difficulty seeing through something that you have started?
(6) Do you find yourself acting on "impulse"?

TABLE 3: Adjusted mean scores on the self-reported PM lapses and EF deficits.

	Self-reports	
	PM lapses	EF deficits
SHS group	2.84 (0.54)	14.0 (3.69)
Non-SHS group	2.36 (0.47)	11.3 (2.38)

Note. Standard errors are given in brackets.

found a relationship between exposure to SHS, reduced PM performance, and deficits in EF which were more profound in a never-smoked group who were exposed to SHS, the precise nature of this relationship needs further exploration in future research. Since there is evidence that preexisting deficits in EF are associated with more "risky" behaviour, including a greater risk of drug taking and more risky sexual activity, [32]. It is feasible that premorbid deficits in EF has resulted in greater exposure to SHS which, in turn, has led to the impairments in everyday PM found here. Those in the non-SHS exposure group may simply have had more proficient EF, opted not to engage in "risky behavior" (i.e. not expose themselves to SHS) and therefore have a more intact everyday PM as a result. This does not rule out the possibility that prolonged exposure to SHS results in decrements in both EF and PM. Future research should test these competing hypotheses by employing a longitudinal study comparing all neversmokers on EF scores before they became exposed to SHS and then comparing these with postexposure PM scores before any firm causality can be established.

The current study used self-report measures of both PM and EF. Whilst self-reports of both PM and EF have been useful in uncovering deficits in these domains in a range of drug users in the past, including excessive alcohol users [24] and ecstasy/cannabis polydrug users [25], it would be advantageous to confirm such findings using objective measures of PM and EF. Using objective measures alongside self-reports can provide convergent evidence of PM and EF deficits associated with exposure to SHS, which can only act to bolster the argument that prolonged exposure to tobacco smoke leads to cognitive impairments, for example, the CAMPROMPT which assesses time-and-event based PM [33] and the Reverse Digit Span as an objective measure of EF [11]. The reliance on self-reports of memory lapses in a group who may already have compromised memory problems

due to prolonged SHS exposure (the SHS group) raises the possibility of a "memory paradox," in which participants with faulty memories may inaccurately recall their memory failures. However, given that this is not a highly publicised area within the public domain (due to the scarcity of research in this field) it is unlikely that the SHS group would have a heightened awareness of the everyday memory problems associated with exposure to SHS. Indeed, several studies have shown that participants with a range of pathologies are more likely to underestimate their memory deficits [34, 35]. Further investigations, including the use of objective measures of PM and EF, as well as longitudinal studies that plot the decline in everyday memory associated with a greater length of time exposed to SHS, are also needed. One important area for further work would be to elucidate the relationship between biological mechanisms, SHS exposure, and cognitive deficits (such as the ones observed in this study). For example, exposure to SHS in neversmokers has been found to lead to a range of cardiovascular diseases similar to those observed in active smokers [1, 2], which may in turn lead to an increased risk of cognitive impairment in adults [7]. Future work should consider measuring health indices alongside PM and EF in never smokers exposed to SHS in order to test whether it is SHS-exposure-related cardiovascular disease that may account for the deficits in PM and EF found here. Given that some recent work from animal studies suggests that prolonged exposure to the toxic mixtures emitted in tobacco smoke, such as the tobacco-specific procarcinogen 4-methylnitrosamino-1-(3-pyridyl)-1-butanone (NNK), causes neuronal damage in the brain [36], this too could offer potential for further work in order to observe whether direct neuronal damage from SHS leads to compromised cognitive function. Further work in this area should also assess a range of other potential cohort differences, such as socioeconomic status and lifestyle variables—since these too might be linked with "risky behavior." Finally, research could also be extended to observe what impact exposure to SHS has upon the health and cognition of children, an area that is fast becoming a major public health concern, one that is highlighted by the recent World Health Organisation reports on the global epidemic of smoking, including exposure to SHS [23].

5. Conclusion

Not only do the findings of this study confirm previous research indicating a range of memory deficits associated with SHS exposure in a never-smoked group, but also they have demonstrated both PM and EF deficits within the same cohort of never smokers who have been exposed to SHS, which are not found in a group of never smokers not exposed to SHS. We hope that the findings uncovered here act to improve knowledge about the wider effects of SHS exposure, specifically in relation to the everyday cognitive consequences found here. It is a further hope that the results obtained here can be of help in campaigns that raise awareness of the dangers of SHS exposure beyond the already established health consequences.

Conflict of Interests

The authors declare that no financial support of any kind has been received in relation to this study. The authors also declare that there is no conflict of interests in relation to this submission.

References

[1] D. F. Dietrich, J. Schwartz, C. Schindler et al., "Effects of passive smoking on heart rate variability, heart rate and blood pressure: an observational study," *International Journal of Epidemiology*, vol. 36, no. 4, pp. 834–840, 2007.

[2] M. D. Eisner, Y. Wang, T. J. Haight, J. Balmes, S. K. Hammond, and I. B. Tager, "Secondhand smoke exposure, pulmonary function, and cardiovascular mortality," *Annals of Epidemiology*, vol. 17, no. 5, pp. 364–373, 2007.

[3] B. Eskenazi and J. J. Bergmann, "Passive and active maternal smoking during pregnancy, as measured by serum cotinine, and postnatal smoke exposure. I. Effects on physical growth at age 5 years," *American Journal of Epidemiology*, vol. 142, no. 9, supplement, pp. S10–S18, 1995.

[4] K. E. Bauman, R. L. Flewelling, and J. LaPrelle, "Parental cigarette smoking and cognitive performance of children," *Health Psychology*, vol. 10, no. 4, pp. 282–288, 1991.

[5] K. Yolton, K. Dietrich, P. Auinger, B. P. Lanphear, and R. Hornung, "Exposure to environmental tobacco smoke and cognitive abilities among U.S. children and adolescents," *Environmental Health Perspectives*, vol. 113, no. 1, pp. 98–103, 2005.

[6] M. J. Friedrich, "Researchers report new clues to dementia," *The Journal of the American Medical Association*, vol. 298, no. 2, pp. 161–163, 2007.

[7] D. J. Llewellyn, L. A. Lang, K. M. Langa, F. Naughton, and F. E. Matthews, "Exposure to secondhand smoke and cognitive impairment in non-smokers: national cross sectional study with cotinine measurement," *British Medical Journal*, vol. 338, no. 7695, pp. 1–6, 2009.

[8] K. K. Teo, S. Ounpuu, S. Hawken et al., "Tobacco use and risk of myocardial infarction in 52 countries in the INTERHEART study: a case-control study," *The Lancet*, vol. 368, no. 9536, pp. 647–658, 2006.

[9] A. Penn, L. C. Chen, and C. A. Snyder, "Inhalation of steady-state sidestream smoke from one cigarette promotes arteriosclerotic plaque development," *Circulation*, vol. 90, no. 3, pp. 1363–1367, 1994.

[10] M. Brandimonte, G. O. Einstein, and M. A. McDaniel, *Prospective Memory: Theory and Applications*, Lawrence Erlbaum Associates, New York, NY, USA, 1996.

[11] A. Baddeley, "Working memory: looking back and looking forward," *Nature Reviews Neuroscience*, vol. 4, no. 10, pp. 829–839, 2003.

[12] A. D. Baddeley and G. J. Hitch, "Developments in the concept of working memory," *Neuropsychology*, vol. 8, no. 4, pp. 485–493, 1994.

[13] M. A. McDaniel and G. O. Einstein, *Prospective Memory: An Overview and Synthesis of an Emerging Field*, Sage, London, UK, 2007.

[14] P. S. Bisiacchi, "The neuropsychological approach in the study of prospective memory," in *Prospective Memory: Theory and Applications*, M. Brandimonte, G. O. Einstein, and M. A. McDaniel, Eds., Lawrence Erlbaum Associates, New York, NY, USA, 1996.

[15] P. W. Burgess, E. Veitch, A. de Lacy Costello, and T. Shallice, "The cognitive and neuroanatomical correlates of multitasking," *Neuropsychologia*, vol. 38, no. 6, pp. 848–863, 2000.

[16] C. A. Johnson, L. Xiao, P. Palmer et al., "Affective decision-making deficits, linked to a dysfunctional ventromedial prefrontal cortex, revealed in 10th grade Chinese adolescent binge drinkers," *Neuropsychologia*, vol. 46, no. 2, pp. 714–726, 2008.

[17] M. A. McDaniel, E. L. Glisky, S. R. Rubin, M. J. Guynn, and B. C. Routhieaux, "Prospective memory: a neuropsychological study," *Neuropsychology*, vol. 13, no. 1, pp. 103–110, 1999.

[18] E. K. Miller and J. D. Wallis, "Executive function and higher-order cognition: definition and neural substrates," in *Encyclopaedia of Neuroscience*, L. J. Squire, Ed., vol. 4, pp. 99–104, Academic Press, Oxford, UK, 2009.

[19] M. Kliegel, T. Jager, M. Altgassen, and D. Shum, "Clinical neuropsychology of prospective memory," in *Prospective Memory: Cognitive, Neuroscience, Developmental and Applied Perspectives*, M. Kliegel, M. A. McDaniel, and G. O. Einstein, Eds., pp. 283–308, Lawrence Erlbaum Associates, Hillsdale, NJ, USA, 2008.

[20] M. Martin, M. Kliegel, and M. A. McDaniel, "The involvement of executive functions in prospective memory performance of adults," *International Journal of Psychology*, vol. 38, no. 4, pp. 195–206, 2003.

[21] A. P. Shimamura, J. S. Janowsky, and L. R. Squire, "What is the role of frontal lobe damage in memory disorders?" in *Frontal Lobe Function and Dysfunction*, H. S. Levin, E. M. Eisenberg, and A. L. Benton, Eds., pp. 173–195, Oxford University Press, New York, NY, USA, 1991.

[22] P. W. Burgess, A. Quayle, and C. D. Frith, "Brain regions involved in prospective memory as determined by positron emission tomography," *Neuropsychologia*, vol. 39, no. 6, pp. 545–555, 2001.

[23] World Health Organisation, *WHO Report on the Global Tobacco Epidemic, 2009*, World Health Organisation, Geneva, Switzerland, 2009.

[24] T. M. Heffernan, "The impact of excessive alcohol use on prospective memory: a brief review," *Current Drug Abuse Reviews*, vol. 1, no. 1, pp. 36–41, 2008.

[25] J. Rodgers, T. Buchanan, A. B. Scholey, T. M. Heffernan, J. Ling, and A. C. Parrott, "Prospective memory: the influence of ecstasy, cannabis and nicotine use and the WWW," *The Open Addiction Journal*, vol. 4, pp. 44–45, 2011.

[26] A. C. Parrott, A. Morinan, M. Moss, and A. Scholey, *Understanding Drugs and Behaviour*, John Wiley & Sons, Chichester, UK, 2004.

[27] R. Antikainen, T. Hänninen, K. Honkalampi et al., "Mood improvement reduces memory complaints in depressed patients," *European Archives of Psychiatry and Clinical Neuroscience*, vol. 251, no. 1, pp. 6–11, 2001.

[28] A. S. Zigmond and R. P. Snaith, "The hospital anxiety and depression scale," *Acta Psychiatrica Scandinavica*, vol. 67, no. 6, pp. 361–370, 1983.

[29] J. R. Crawford, J. D. Henry, C. Crombie, and E. P. Taylor, "Normative data for the HADS from a large non-clinical sample," *British Journal of Clinical Psychology*, vol. 40, no. 4, pp. 429–434, 2001.

[30] J. R. Crawford, G. Smith, E. A. Maylor, S. Della Sala, and R. H. Logie, "The prospective and retrospective memory questionnaire (PRMQ): normative data and latent structure in a large non-clinical sample," *Memory*, vol. 11, no. 3, pp. 261–275, 2003.

[31] T. Buchanan, T. M. Heffernan, A. C. Parrott, J. Ling, J. Rodgers, and A. B. Scholey, "A short self-report measure of problems with executive function suitable for administration via the internet," *Behavior Research Methods*, vol. 42, no. 3, pp. 709–714, 2010.

[32] T. M. Pronk, J. C. Karremans, and D. H. J. Wigboldus, "How can you resist? Executive control helps romantically involved individuals to stay faithful," *Journal of Personality and Social Psychology*, vol. 100, no. 5, pp. 827–837, 2011.

[33] B. A. Wilson, H. Emslie, J. Foley, A. Shiel, P. Watson, and K. Hawkins, *The Cambridge Prospective Memory Test*, Harcourt-Assessment, London, UK, 2005.

[34] F. Andelman, E. Zuckerman-Feldhay, D. Hoffien, I. Fried, and M. Y. Neufeld, "Lateralization of deficit in self-awareness of memory in patients with intractable epilepsy," *Epilepsia*, vol. 45, no. 7, pp. 826–833, 2004.

[35] S. Sevush and N. Leve, "Denial of memory deficit in Alzheimer's disease," *American Journal of Psychiatry*, vol. 150, no. 5, pp. 748–751, 1993.

[36] D. Ghosh, M. K. Mishra, S. Das, D. K. Kaushik, and A. Basu, "Tobacco carcinogen induces microglial activation and subsequent neuronal damage," *Journal of Neurochemistry*, vol. 110, no. 3, pp. 1070–1081, 2009.

17

Pattern and Trend of Substance Abuse in Eastern Rural Iran: A Household Survey in a Rural Community

Hasan Ziaaddini,[1] Tayebeh Ziaaddini,[2] and Nouzar Nakhaee[3]

[1] Research Center for Health Services Management, Institute of Futures Studies in Health, Kerman University of Medical Sciences, Kerman, Iran

[2] Research Center for Social Determinants of Health, Institute of Futures Studies in Health, Kerman University of Medical Sciences, Kerman, Iran

[3] Neuroscience Research Center, Institute of Neuropharmacology, Kerman University of Medical Sciences, P.O. Box 76175-113, Kerman, Iran

Correspondence should be addressed to Nouzar Nakhaee; nakhaeen@kmu.ac.ir

Academic Editor: Raymond Niaura

Introduction and Aim. Substance abuse imposes hazards on human health in all biopsychosocial aspects. Limited studies exist on epidemiology of substance abuse and its trend in rural areas. The present study aimed to compare substance abuse in one of the rural areas of southeast Iran, in a 12-year period (2000 and 2012). *Design and Methods.* In a household survey conducted in 2012, in Dashtkhak/Kerman, 1200 individuals above 12 years of age completed a questionnaire to determine their frequency of substance abuse. The questionnaire included the following three areas: demographic characteristics, frequency of substance abuse and ease of access to various drugs. *Results.* Among 900 completed questionnaires, majority of the participants (61.8%) were below 30 years of age and among them 54.4% were male. Cigarette (17.0%), opium (15.7%) and opium residue (9.0%) were the most frequent substances abused on a daily basis. Based on the participant's opinion, we conclude that the ease of access to cigarette, waterpipe and opium contributed to their increase in consumption compared with earlier years. *Discussion and Conclusion.* The steady rise in substance abuse in rural communities demands immediate attention and emergency preventive measures from policy makers.

1. Introduction

Substance abuse poses a major political, social and health challenge worldwide [1]. Besides being a personal risk, addiction is a social problem and imposes harmful and permanent effects on society. At present, 3.6%–6.9% of adults (15–64-years-old individuals) are under the influence of illicit substances [2]. According to the World Drug Report 2013, since 2008, the number of illicit drug users has shown 18% increase; rise in population and ease of availability appears to be the two common reasons [2].

Substance abuse in Iran, one of the Middle East countries, has a historical origin. During World War I, among 250,000 individuals of the Tehran municipality, 25,000 were reported to be addicted to opium [3]. In recent centuries, opium has

been prescribed for pain relief in Iran by traditional physicians. These traditions are stronger among rural populations owing to a lack of access to trained physicians. The usage of opium had been so common in rural areas that mothers often exposed babies to opium in an effort to calm them and sleep better [3]. The past two centuries have seen several changes with respect to handling illicit substances in Iran, from open access to death penalty for carrying illicit drugs. At present, Iran policy against illicit drugs is considered to be a combination of *war on drugs* and *harm reduction* strategies. With regards to opium use, Iran ranks among the top three countries in the world [4]. Therefore, epidemiological studies in Iran can provide better understanding for national policy makers as well as for other researchers in the world. Although several studies on the prevalence of substance abuse in Iran have been reported, the majority have been limited to urban areas [5, 6]; studies in rural areas were limited or often included small sample size [7]. Approximate one third of the Iran population lives in rural areas [8]; hence, it is critical to evaluate the substance abuse pattern in rural areas. In addition, the majority of epidemiological studies focussed on the trends of substance abuse because drug use behaviours are often dynamic, and with time are affected by various factors such as drug availability [9].

The present study aimed to investigate the trends of substance abuse among the rural communities of the Kerman province, the largest province in Iran, during a 12-year period by comparing data for the years 2000 and 2012. This region was selected for two reasons. First, Kerman as an eastern province, due to neighborhood with Afghanistan, the largest oipioid producing country in the world, is at higher risk of substance use, especially in youth group. A previous study reported that the usage of waterpipe, cigarette and alcohol, among high school boys, in this area was 51.5%, 34.6% and 7.27%, respectively [10]. Historically, Kerman had highest of opium usage in Iran [11]; second, accessibility of data from earlier years from this region [11] makes it easy to compare and analyse the changes with time. To the best of our knowledge, this is the first report describing the trend of drug abuse in rural Iran.

2. Methods

A household survey was conducted in 2012 in Dashtkhak, a northeastern village of Kerman province with a total population of 4416. The research was conducted under the approval of the Ethical Committee of Kerman University of Medical Sciences (Approval code: K/90/516). Following a brief meeting with the village council, details regarding the aim of the study, protocols and information regarding the questionnaire were explained to the participants. Confidentiality agreement and informed consent form were provided before the study. A researcher along with community health workers distributed the questionnaires to each house. One participant above 12 years of age per household was chosen to complete the questionnaire. Upon completion of the questionnaire, participants dropped them in a sealed ballot. The community health workers assisted the uneducated participants in the survey. Community health workers are employed by The Ministry of Health and provide primary health care in rural areas. Because of their acquaintance with the residents, their involvement in this research provided a great benefit to acquire data in a timely manner [12].

The validity and reliability of the questionnaire used in this study has been confirmed in previous studies [11]. It focussed primarily on three areas: The demographic features, details on substance abuse and the availability of substance. For details on substance abuse, substance abused throughout the lifetime, the last 30 days and every day were accounted [9]. Considering the pattern of substance abuse in Iran [5, 10], the questionnaire included the following substances: cigarette, waterpipe, opium, shireh (opium residues), heroin, cannabis, *shisheh*, alcohol and sedatives. Substance availability was

TABLE 1: Demographic characteristics of rural residents ($n = 900$).

Characteristic	Frequency	%
Age (yrs)		
12–19	140	15.6
20–29	221	24.6
30–39	194	21.6
40–49	147	16.3
50–59	98	10.9
≥60	100	11.1
Gender		
Male	490	54.4
Female	410	45.6
Education		
Illiterate	113	12.6
Primary school	207	23.0
Incomplete secondary	244	27.1
Complete secondary	219	24.3
College	117	13.0
Marital status		
Single	257	28.6
Married	643	71.4
Separated/divorced	0	0
Job		
Housewife	262	29.1
Employee	123	13.7
Worker	118	13.1
Student (school)	117	13.0
Student (college)	55	6.1
Farmer	50	5.6
Tradesman	24	2.7
Soldier	15	1.7
Jobless	68	7.6
Others	68	7.6

counted using a four-degree Likert scale [9]. *Shireh* comprises opium residue obtained after opium consumption that is boiled and concentrated; this is more potent than opium. The primary component of shisheh is methamphetamine [13].

Data analysis was performed by calculating percentage values. The chi-square test was used to compare the frequency of substances abused between the two time points. Two separate multivariate logistic regression models for tobacco and the other drugs were included to assess the association between baseline characteristics and substance abuse. Data were analysed through the SPSS 20 software package.

3. Results

Among the 1200 distributed questionnaires, 900 participants responded and completed the questionnaires (response rate = 75.0%). Lack of interest and time proved to be the primary reasons for incomplete response. The average age and sex of non-respondents did not differ from those of respondents.

TABLE 2: Frequency of substance use among rural residents ($n = 900$).

Substance	Lifetime use			Past 30 days			Near-daily		
	n	%	95% CI	n	%	95% CI	n	%	95% CI
Cigarette	286	31.8	28.8–34.9	171	19.0	16.5–21.8	153	17.0	14.6–19.6
Waterpipe	321	35.7	32.6–38.8	99	11.0	9.1–13.2	33	3.7	2.6–5.0
Cannabis	18	2.0	1.2–3.9	8	0.9	0.4–1.7	5	0.6	0.2–1.2
Opium	333	37.0	33.9–40.2	180	20.0	17.5–23.7	141	15.7	13.4–18.2
Shireh (opium residue)	185	20.6	18.0–23.3	114	12.7	10.6–15.0	81	9.0	7.2–11.0
Heroin	39	4.3	3.1–5.8	25	2.8	1.8–4.0	22	2.4	1.6–3.6
Shisheh (amphetamine)	7	0.8	0.3–1.5	5	0.6	0.2–1.2	2	0.2	0.04–0.7
Alcohol	69	7.7	6.1–9.5	16	1.8	1.1–2.8	5	0.6	0.2–1.2
Sedatives	177	19.7	17.2–22.4	87	9.7	7.9–11.7	41	4.6	3.3–6.1

TABLE 3: Percentage of daily substance use among rural residents based on sex and age group ($n = 900$).

Substance	Sex			Age group (yrs)		
	Male	Female	P value	<30	≥30	P value
Cigarette	144 (29.4)	9 (2.2)	<0.001	26 (7.2)	127 (23.6)	<0.001
Waterpipe	26 (5.3)	7 (1.7)	0.004	23 (6.4)	10 (1.9)	<0.001
Cannabis	4 (0.8)	1 (0.2)	0.383	1 (0.3)	4 (0.7)	0.358
Opium	107 (21.8)	34 (8.3)	<0.001	17 (4.7)	124 (23.0)	<0.001
Shireh (opium residue)	68 (13.9)	13 (3.2)	<0.001	12 (3.3)	69 (12.8)	<0.001
Heroin	19 (3.9)	3 (0.7)	0.002	5 (1.4)	17 (3.2)	0.092
Shisheh (amphetamine)	1 (0.2)	1 (0.2)	1.00	0 (0.0)	2 (0.4)	0.247
Alcohol	3 (0.6)	2 (0.5)	0.255	3 (0.8)	2 (0.4)	0.363
Sedatives	23 (4.7)	18 (4.4)	0.828	10 (2.8)	31 (5.8)	0.036

The majority of respondents (61.8%) were below 30 years of age, and 54.4% among them were male (Table 1). Other demographic characteristics are presented in Table 1.

Opium, waterpipe and cigarette showed highest prevalence among all the other substance tested. Cigarettes, opium and *shireh* were on the most common daily abused drugs. Majority of the substances were consumed high among men compared with women (Table 2). Cigarette, opium and sedative usage was higher among the participants above 30 years compared with younger groups, whereas waterpipe consumption revealed a reverse pattern (Table 3). From the participant point of view, cigarette, opium and waterpipe were easily accessible compared with other substances (Table 4). Moreover, cigarette, opiates, heroin and sedatives consumption increased significantly in 2012 (Table 5).

Tobacco smoking was prevalent among male (OR = 10.8, CI 95%: 6.2–18.6) and unemployed participants (OR = 2.4, CI 95%: 1.4–4.3). Other drugs such as opium, heroin, cannabis, sedatives, alcohol and amphetamines were common among males (OR = 2.7, CI 95%: 1.9–4.0) and married (OR = 4.5, CI 95%: 2.4–8.5) and unemployed (OR = 2.4, CI 95%: 1.3–4.3) participants.

4. Discussion

Detailed analysis on the trend and pattern of substance abuse is necessary to develop preventive measures. The present study illustrates a substantial increase in substance abuse in a rural area over a 12-year period. Our study evaluates two different time periods in the same area using similar method, with a gap of 12 years; this offers the additional advantage for comparing the effect of substance abuse over time. Household surveys are considered as the gold standard for estimating the number of substance abusers [14], provided the participants are ensured of privacy and that they trust those collecting their information. Such mutual trust between village inhabitants and community health workers governs the rural regions in Iran [12]. The primary drawback of this study was its limitation to a single rural area, which requires caution in generalizing results. In addition, although response rates less than 70% were considered acceptable [15], non-participation of 25% of subjects in our study may limit data interpretation.

Kerman province, because of its borders with Afghanistan, is in the transit path for opium and heroin from Eastern borders to other parts of the country [5]. Since the early 19th century, heavy opium use among the natives has been connected to its easy access [3].

The ratio of male and female participants was similar in both 2000 and 2012. The participant population in the year 2000 was younger compared with that in 2012 ($P <$ 0.05). This is probably because of an increase in average life span in Iran in recent years [8]. The lifetime substance abuse pattern showed a minor difference compared with that of the near-daily pattern. Opium, waterpipe and cigarette had highest prevalence of substance abuse throughout life

TABLE 4: Perceived difficulty in getting each of drugs*.

Substance	Very easy	Easy	Difficult	Very difficult
Cigarette	474 (52.7)	232 (25.8)	63 (7.0)	131 (14.6)
Waterpipe	389 (43.2)	277 (30.8)	94 (10.4)	140 (15.6)
Cannabis	45 (5.0)	74 (8.2)	244 (27.1)	537 (59.7)
Opium	227 (25.2)	241 (26.8)	142 (15.8)	290 (32.2)
Shireh (opium residue)	188 (20.9)	213 (23.7)	160 (17.8)	339 (37.7)
Heroin	40 (4.4)	82 (9.1)	227 (25.2)	551 (61.2)
Shisheh (amphetamine)	14 (1.2)	41 (3.7)	209 (23.2)	636 (71.9)
Alcohol	50 (5.6)	92 (10.2)	211 (23.4)	547 (60.8)
Sedatives	136 (15.1)	171 (19.0)	176 (19.6)	417 (46.3)

*Figures are in percentages.

TABLE 5: Prevalence (%) of daily substance use among rural residents in 2000 and 2012.

Substance	2000 study N = 1668	Current study N = 900	P value
Cigarette	122 (7.3)	153 (17.0)	<0.001
Waterpipe	NS	33 (3.7)	—
Cannabis	6 (0.3)	5 (0.6)	0.683
Opium	91 (5.0)	141 (15.7)	<0.001
Shireh (opium residue)	22 (1.3)	81 (9.0)	<0.001
Heroin	5 (0.3)	22 (2.4)	<0.001
Shishehn (amphetamine)	NS	2 (0.2)	—
Alcohol	2 (0.1)	5 (0.6)	0.105
Sedatives	14 (0.8)	41 (4.6)	<0.001

*NS: not studied.

and opium, *shireh* and cigarette among the daily abused substances (Table 2). This study reveals that opium abuse is endemic in this region [9] with lifetime prevalence higher than that of cigarette smoking (Table 2). In comparison with the data from 2000 showed that, in 2012, except for cannabis and alcohol, abuse of all other substances increased significantly. *Shireh* and heroin abuse enhanced 7-8 times. Based on anecdotal data, one of the reasons for this increase may be the rise in the cost of opium [16]. The consumption of substances, such as waterpipe and *shisheh*, was not investigated in 2000; these substance gained popularity during the last few years and are now considered as re-emerging drugs [11, 12, 17]. Although methamphetamine consumption was low compared with that of opiates, in urban areas, a gradual switch from traditional substances such as opium to synthetic substances such as methamphetamine is observed [17]. However, according to the current study, substance abuse patterns in rural areas differ from those in urban areas. Sedative consumption increased 6-fold, which is probably caused by easy availability of prescription drugs. An earlier study conducted in one of the rural regions of northern Iran reported that 13.5% of the participants abused opium almost daily and 28.1% smoked cigarette daily [7]. In another

study, which analysed urine samples through anonymous unlinked testing, 14.5% showed opioid consumption, that is, similar to the rate of daily abuse of opium in our study (15.7%). A comparison of substance abuse among urban and rural population showed that opioid abuse is higher among rural population, whereas other substances such as alcohol waterpipe and cannabis were prevalent among urban population [10]. Substance consumption, except waterpipe, was higher among participants above 30 years of age compared with the younger age groups, indicating that waterpipe is regaining popularity among youth. In United States, it has been reported that except ecstasy and amphetamines, drug usage in the past year is relatively similar among adolescents in rural and urban regions [18]. Although new studies are in favour of higher usage of tobacco, cannabis and alcohol in U.S. and Australian rural students compared with urban students [19].

The substance abuse was also much higher among men compared with that among women (Table 3); the most obvious difference was observed for cigarette, suggesting the social stigma associated with cigarette smoking in women in Iranian culture [20], while the stigma associated with waterpipe consumption is significantly less [21]. Sedative consumption was similar among both men and women probably because of similar and easy access to prescription drugs and the prevalence of anxiety and insomnia in general population.

Access to *shisheh* was more difficult than that to other drugs. Approximately three quarters of rural population had easy access to cigarette and water pipe, and half of them had easy access to opium. Despite the law against usage of tobacco, sale of cigarette and waterpipe tobacco in public places is common in Iran. Waterpipe usage is common among youth and has increased in recent years, which can be often observed in coffee shops, parks and college dormitories [21]. Because alcohol was prohibited by religion, it was expected that access to alcohol be most difficult.

The logistic regression analysis showed that higher the difficulty towards access to tobacco, the less the probability of tobacco smoking (Table 6). In Iran, there is no close monitoring on tobacco sales to youth and cigarette smoking is socially well accepted in metropolitan areas than rural areas [20]. rural areas, cultural barrier appears to play a role

TABLE 6: Logistic regression analysis to examine baseline characteristics associated with tobacco and other drugs use.

Characteristics	Tobacco use			Other drugs use		
	Adjusted odds ratio	95% CI	P value	Adjusted odds ratio	95% CI	P value
Age						
<30 years	1	—	—	1	—	—
≥30 years	1.42	0.84–2.40	0.188	2.13	1.30–3.50	0.003
Sex						
Female	1	—	—	1	—	—
Male	10.78	6.24–18.60	0.001	2.74	1.87–3.99	0.001
Education						
Illiterate	1	—	—	1	—	—
Primary	1.52	0.43–1.44	0.193	0.94	0.55–1.62	0.836
Secondary	1.19	0.65–2.73	0.620	1.29	0.72–2.34	0.394
Higher	0.78	0.33–2.02	0.340	0.61	0.35–1.08	0.090
Marital status						
Unmarried	1	—	—	1	—	—
Married	1.78	1.01–3.20	0.049	4.46	2.35–8.46	0.001
Job						
Employed	1	—	—	1	—	—
Unemployed	2.42	1.36–4.28	0.003	2.38	1.31–4.34	0.005
Access difficulty	0.76	0.59–0.99	0.042	0.64	0.50–0.82	0.001

than geographical barrier, and the difficulty in access may be related to factors such as family supervision and cultural taboo on smoking by youth and women [21]. The higher probability of tobacco smoking among men was in-line with the earlier results from both the urban [20, 21] and rural [12] areas of Iran. The differences among men and women regarding drug abuse (OR = 2.7) were less prominent than tobacco smoking (OR = 10.8) (Table 6). It may be because of the fact that except for tobacco all other substance abuse is illegal in Iran [20]; while drug abuse is considered a taboo among men and women, usage of tobacco is socially accepted among men, whereas it is stigmatized among women [20, 21]. In contrast to drug abuse, age had no effect on tobacco smoking, perhaps because of the higher age at onset of drug abuse comparing with that of tobacco abuse [10, 21]. Drug abuse was more common among unemployed; a finding that may not imply causation because of an ambiguous order of variables (i.e. unemployment and drug abuse). Difficulty in access played a major role and clearly reduced drug abuse.

5. Conclusions

In conclusion, the present study shows increased prevalence of substance abuse among rural population in Iran. Easy access to the substance appears to contribute significantly to this trend. The pattern of drug usage among rural population differs from urban areas. The results of the present study emphasize the necessity of immediate multi-dimensional preventive measures to regulate substance abuse among rural communities.

Conflict of Interests

The authors declare that there is no conflict of interests regarding the publication of this article.

References

[1] M. Singer, "Drugs and development: the global impact of drug use and trafficking on social and economic development," International Journal of Drug Policy, vol. 19, no. 6, pp. 467–478, 2008.

[2] UNODC, World Drug Report 2013, United Nations Office on Drugs and Crime, Vienna, Austria, 2013.

[3] A. A. Afkhami, "From punishment to harm reduction: resecularization of addiction in contemporary Iran," in Contemporary Iran: Economy, Society, Politics, A. Gheissari, Ed., pp. 194–210, Oxford University Press, New York, NY, USA, 2009.

[4] UNODC, World Drug Report 2010, United Nations Office on Drugs and Crime, Vienna, Austria, 2010.

[5] N. Nakhaee, K. Divsalar, M. S. Meimandi, and S. Dabiri, "Estimating the prevalence of opiates use by unlinked anonymous urine drug testing: a pilot study in Iran," Substance Use and Misuse, vol. 43, no. 3-4, pp. 513–520, 2008.

[6] A. Mokri, "Brief overview of the status of drug abuse in Iran," Archives of Iranian Medicine, vol. 5, no. 3, pp. 184–190, 2002.

[7] A. Meysamie, M. Sedaghat, M. Mahmoodi, S. M. Ghodsi, and B. Eftekhar, "Opium use in a rural area of the Islamic Republic of Iran," Eastern Mediterranean Health Journal, vol. 15, no. 2, pp. 425–431, 2009.

[8] UNFPA, "UNFPA Iran: Country Profile," 2012, http://iran.unfpa.org/Country%20Profile.asp.

[9] World Health Organization, Guide to Drug Abuse Epidemiology, WHO/MSD/MSB/00.3, World Health Organization, Geneva, Switzerland, 2000.

[10] H. Ziaaddini, A. Sharifi, and N. Nakhaee, "The prevalence of at least one-time substance abuse among Kerman pre-university male students," *Addiction & Health*, vol. 3-4, pp. 103–110, 2010.

[11] H. Ziaaddini and R. Ziaaddini, "The household survey of drug abuse in Kerman, Iran," *Journal of Applied Science*, vol. 5, no. 2, pp. 380–382, 2005.

[12] A. Mirahmadizadeh and N. Nakhaee, "Prevalence of waterpipe smoking among rural pregnant women in Southern Iran," *Medical Principles and Practice*, vol. 17, no. 6, pp. 435–439, 2008.

[13] Z. A. Mehrjerdi, "Crystal in Iran: methamphetamine or heroin kerack," *Daru*, vol. 21, no. 1, p. 22, 2013.

[14] M. Hickman, C. Taylor, A. Chatterjee et al., "Estimating the prevalence of problematic drug use: a review of methods and their application," *Bulletin on Narcotics*, vol. 54, no. 1-2, pp. 15–32, 2002.

[15] S. M. Morton, D. K. Bandara, E. M. Robinson, and P. E. Carr, "In the 21st century, what is an acceptable response rate?" *Australian and New Zealand Journal of Public Health*, vol. 36, no. 2, pp. 106–108, 2012.

[16] F. Raisdana and A. G. Nakhjavani, "The drug market in Iran," *Annals of the American Academy of Political and Social Science*, vol. 582, pp. 149–166, 2002.

[17] S. Shariatirad, M. Maarefvand, and H. Ekhtiari, "Emergence of a methamphetamine crisis in Iran," *Drug and Alcohol Review*, vol. 32, pp. 223–224, 2012.

[18] J. C. Gfroerer, S. L. Larson, and J. D. Colliver, "Drug use patterns and trends in rural communities," *Journal of Rural Health*, vol. 23, no. 1, pp. 10–15, 2007.

[19] K. Coomber, J. W. Toumbourou, P. Miller, P. K. Staiger, S. A. Hemphill, and R. F. Catalano, "Rural adolescent alcohol, tobacco, and illicit drug use: a comparison of students in Victoria, Australia, and Washington State, United States," *Journal of Rural Health*, vol. 27, no. 4, pp. 409–415, 2011.

[20] N. Sarraf-Zadegan, M. Boshtam, S. Shahrokhi et al., "Tobacco use among Iranian men, women and adolescents," *European Journal of Public Health*, vol. 14, no. 1, pp. 76–78, 2004.

[21] A.-R. Sabahy, K. Divsalar, S. Bahreinifar, M. Marzban, and N. Nakhaee, "Waterpipe tobacco use among Iranian university students: correlates and perceived reasons for use," *International Journal of Tuberculosis and Lung Disease*, vol. 15, no. 6, pp. 844–847, 2011.

18

Exploring Spatial Associations between On-Sale Alcohol Availability, Neighborhood Population Characteristics, and Violent Crime in a Geographically Isolated City

Daikwon Han and Dennis M. Gorman

Department of Epidemiology & Biostatistics, School of Rural Public Health, Texas A&M University, College Station, TX 77843, USA

Correspondence should be addressed to Daikwon Han; dhan@tamhsc.edu

Academic Editor: Otto M. Lesch

Objectives. Despite the increasing evidence of the associations between alcohol availability and violence, there are still inconsistent findings on the effects of on- and off-sale alcohol outlets on violent crime. The aim of this study was to examine spatial associations between on-sale alcohol availability, neighborhood characteristics, and violent crime in a geographically isolated city in Texas. *Methods*. Geographically weighted regression (GWR) and global regression models were employed to analyze the nature of the spatial relationship between violent crime, neighborhood sociocultural characteristics, and on-sale alcohol environment. *Results*. We found strong effects of neighborhood characteristics combined with on-sale alcohol availability on violence outcomes. Several neighborhood variables combined with alcohol availability explained about 63% of the variability in violence. An additional 7% was explained by the GWR model, while spatially nonstationary associations between violence and some predictor variables were observed. *Conclusions*. This study provided more credible evidence of the influence of on-sale alcohol outlets on violence in a unique setting. These findings have important policy implications in addressing the question of public health consequences of alcohol-related violence in local contexts.

1. Introduction

Two-decades of ecological research has demonstrated that alcohol-related violence is not simply an individual-level problem but rather must be understood within the community context, and that alcohol availability and the opportunity that this creates for drinking are an integral part of this problem [1]. Both cross-sectional and longitudinal studies have been used to assess the ecological relationship of various outlet density measures and place/population characteristics with violent crime across small geographic scales, including Census block groups [2], Census tracts [3], neighborhoods [4, 5], and zip codes [6, 7]. Although the specific relationship has varied by study setting, general findings show that neighborhoods with higher availability of alcohol are more likely to have higher rates of violent crime. There has also been some debate within the field of alcohol epidemiology as to whether alcohol outlet type, specifically on-sale versus off-sale premises, has differential effects on rates of violence.

A recent study by Toomey and colleagues [5] found that the association with violence was stronger and more consistent in the case of on-sale than off-sale outlets although they noted that half of the previous studies that assessed on-sale outlets separately found no effect on violence. Moreover, there are ecological theories about drinking environments that focus on the role of on-sale outlets in attracting specific types of people into specific geographic locations and the types of interactions that occur within these microenvironments [8, 9].

Because there are still inconsistent findings of the effects of on-sale alcohol outlets on violent crime, this study was conducted to examine the nature of the relationship, with appropriate spatial methods, between on-sale alcohol availability, neighborhood population characteristics, and violent crime in a unique study setting. Specifically, the present study takes advantage of two features that distinguish it from previous research, and both of which arise from the nature of the study site, Lubbock, Texas. First, since alcohol was almost exclusively sold for on-premise consumption in Lubbock until September of 2009, this study site allows us to examine the effects of such premises on violence uncontaminated by the effect of off-sale premises. Second, Lubbock is geographically isolated from other large population centers and is surrounded by sparsely populated counties in which alcohol is not readily available. Thus, one might reasonably consider the sale and consumption of alcohol in Lubbock to be a closed system in which the alcohol-related problems that occur are likely to be a function of the alcohol sold within the city.

In addition, since spatial data are often characterized by two fundamental properties, spatial dependence and nonstationarity, statistical methods that are appropriate in spatial analyses were also employed to examine the nature of the spatial relationship between violent crime, neighborhood sociocultural characteristics, and on-sale alcohol environment. Specifically, Geographically Weighted Regression (GWR), combined with global regression models, was utilized in exploring local associations while taking into consideration spatial dependence and nonstationarity of the spatial data and identifying important covariates in the spatial associations between neighborhood population/place characteristics and violence.

2. Methods

2.1. Study Population and Data. As noted above, the city of Lubbock provides a fairly unique setting to investigate the relationship between on-sale alcohol availability and violence, because of its geographically isolated location and (prior to August, 2009) its retail alcohol market being comprised almost exclusively of on-premise outlets (only a handful of off-sale outlets existed in an area south of the city known as "The Strip"). The estimated population of the city for 2009 was 226,000, making it the 11th largest city in the state of Texas. The city is also home to Texas Technical University which had a student population of 30,049 in the fall semester of 2009. The closest population center to the north of Lubbock is Amarillo, which is 124 miles away and about a two-hour journey by car. The nearest cities after this (Oklahoma city, Fort Worth, Albuquerque, and Las Cruces) are each 300 to 400 miles away. In addition, the eight counties that surround Lubbock have low population density and three are totally "dry" (i.e., the sale of alcohol beverage is illegal). None of the remaining five is totally "wet": about half of the precincts in four of these countries are dry, and the one county that has no dry precincts allows only off-premise sales of beer and wine.

As part of a larger study designed to examine the effects of the introduction of off-sale licenses in the city on September 23, 2009 [10], the present analysis focuses on the association between on-sale alcohol outlet density and violent crime prior to the introduction of off-sale outlets, hence the discontinuation of the dataset in August, 2009. Three archival data sets were employed in the study. First, data pertaining to reports of violent crime (murder, rape, robbery, and aggravated assault) during the time period January, 2005 and August, 2009 were obtained directly from the city of Lubbock Police Department. The dataset contained the date, time, and street address for each violent crime incident. There were a total of 7327 violent crimes for the 56-month time period, of which 49 (0.7%) were murders, 374 (5.1%) rapes, 1422 (19.4%) robberies, and 5482 (74.8%) assaults. Close to 99% of these violent crimes were geocoded by street address using Centrus Desktop. These data were then aggregated to the census block group level and the violent crime rate was calculated as crimes per 1,000 persons.

Second, a list of all alcohol outlets active during the same 56-month time period in the city of Lubbock was obtained from the Texas Alcoholic Beverage Commission (ABC) online database, which includes the name, geographic location, and type of permit or license of the outlet. There were a total of 197 on-sale licenses over the study time period, and outlet density per 1000 residents was used as a measure of alcohol availability. All outlets were geocoded and aggregated to the census block group level in the analysis.

Third, neighborhood population and sociostructural variables were extracted from the 2006–2010 American Community Survey 5-year estimate [11]. Consistent with previous ecological studies of alcohol availability and violence [3, 4], 12 neighborhood sociostructural variables were used as potential covariates in the analysis. These 12 neighborhood sociostructural variables fell into three major categories: (1) *concentrated disadvantage*: % families below poverty, % households receiving public assistance, % unemployed over age 16, % female-headed households with children, % Black, and % Hispanic; (2) *residential instability*: % of residents over age 1 who have lived in the same house 1 year ago, % homes that are owner occupied, % vacant housing units; (3) *sociodemographic measures of the resident population*: adult to child ratio, population density, and % population that is male and aged 15–24.

2.2. Statistical Analyses. Multivariate regression analysis was first conducted to examine the relationship between alcohol outlet densities, neighborhood sociostructural characteristics, and violent crime rate. Specifically, a stepwise ordinary least square (OLS) procedure was run to identify significant explanatory variables, with a 0.01 significance level for entry and a 0.05 level for removal. The candidate covariates in the study were the 12 factors pertaining to neighborhood characteristics described previously. Before performing the regression analysis, percent Black and outlet density variables were log transformed to adjust for skew. The dependent variable (violent crime per 1,000 population) was also log transformed, and a small constant was added to transform zero values. Plots of leverage values were used to identify outlying extreme values, and the variance inflation factors (VIF) were obtained for each of the explanatory variables to assess multicollinearity. Residual plots and partial regression plots were also checked for nonrandom pattern and model specification to ensure the inclusion of all the important explanatory variables in the final model. Regressions were also run with mean replacement for a small number of missing neighborhood variables, but results essentially remained unchanged and therefore are not reported.

To explore spatial association in the relationships between alcohol outlet densities, neighborhood sociostructural characteristics and the violent crime rate across the study area, the Geographically Weighted Regression (GWR) method was also employed [12]. The GWR produces a separate parameter estimate of regression coefficients, goodness-of-fit, and significance assessment for each observation. To minimize potential problems associated with multiple testing and multicollinearity among predictor variables, those statistically valid and significant predictors identified using OLS procedures were used in GWR model. For GWR modeling, we used adaptive kernels based on bisquare weighting function due to the irregular shape of the study area [13]. This method is often preferred in identifying the optimal number of nearest neighbors, considering the density and size of samples. To identify the optimal size of kernels, we used the Akaike Information Criteria (AIC) optimization method which identifies the bandwidth that minimizes the AIC score and that accounts for the local variation in the size of the data set [12, 14]. Estimates of spatial autocorrelation (Moran's I) were also obtained to ensure that residuals were not spatially correlated. Monte-Carlo significance tests were conducted to assess statistical significance of nonstationarity for alcohol availability and each of the covariates [15]. The calibration of local GWR models was performed using the GWR 3.0 [12].

3. Results

Descriptive summary statistics (mean and standard deviations) for six neighborhood variables included in the model (percent Hispanic, percent Black, percent families below poverty, percent owner occupied, percent residential stability, and population density), on-sale outlet density, and violent crime rates are shown in Table 1. Summary statistics for each individual crime type (assault, robbery, rape, and murder) are also included in the table.

Table 2 presents the summary of regression parameters (coefficients, standard errors, t values, and 95% confidence intervals) and diagnostics (adjusted R-squared and AIC) for the OLS model of violent crime that was constructed with six neighborhood variables and on-sale alcohol outlet density. These predictors explained about 63% of the variance in violent crime (adjusted R-squared = 0.628) and were all statistically significant at P values of <0.01. The table shows that a 1% increase in on-sale outlet density was associated with a 0.25% increase in violent crime. Variance inflation factors (VIF) included in the table indicate that multicollinearity among explanatory variables was removed in the model.

The local GWR model was also constructed with the above neighborhood variables and on-sale alcohol outlet density (Table 3 and Figure 1). Figure 1 presents a map of the violent crime rate modeled using the GWR. The map clearly shows spatial patterns of violent crime rates after taking into account local variations of the neighbourhood sociostructural characteristics and including alcohol availability. Specifically, a higher rate of violent crime was identified in the north-east of the city where combined outlet

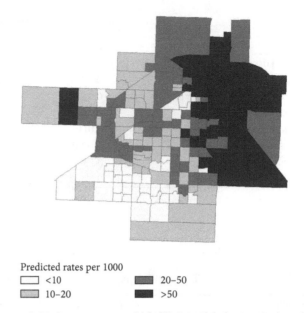

Predicted rates per 1000

☐ <10	▨ 20–50
▨ 10–20	■ >50

FIGURE 1: Violent crime rates (per 1000) modeled using Geographical Weighted Regression, Lubbock, Texas, 2005–2009.

TABLE 1: Descriptive summary statistics for violent crime, on-sale alcohol outlets, and neighborhood sociodemographic variables, 2005–2009, Lubbock, Texas ($n = 170$).

	Mean	Standard deviation
Neighborhood variables included in the model		
Percent Hispanic	30.9	24.5
Percent Black	8.6	15.2
Percent families below poverty	16.5	20.0
Percent owner occupied	55.6	27.7
Percent residential stability	73.0	17.7
Population density	4261	2764
Outlet density (per 1000)	1.3	3.9
Violent crime (per 1000)	44.1	75.0
Assault	31.7	42.9
Robbery	10.6	38.1
Rape	2.9	3.2
Murder	1.2	0.9

density and neighborhood characteristics have a relatively strong influence. Further, the parameters of each explanatory variable produced by the local GWR model (5-number summary values) differ across the study area with varying degrees of magnitude and sign of the statistical association (Table 3). We also identified block groups with positive and negative values of the t-statistic at the 95% level of significance, using standard values of ±1.96. Alcohol outlet density along with several covariates, including percent Black and percent Hispanic, indicated positively significant relationships in a majority of block groups (about 60%), while percent owner occupied and population density showed negatively significant relationships in most block groups within

TABLE 2: Ordinary least squares (OLS) model of violent crime (global model).

Variable	Estimate	Std. error	t value	95% CI	VIF[a]
Percent Hispanic	0.021	0.002	8.39	0.016, 0.026	1.169
Percent Black (log)	0.212	0.053	4.01	0.108, 0.317	1.207
Percent families below poverty	0.014	0.003	3.97	0.007, 0.021	1.533
Percent owner occupied	−0.014	0.004	−3.76	−0.021, −0.006	3.097
Percent residential stability	0.014	0.005	2.77	0.004, 0.023	2.384
Population density	−0.0001	0.000	−4.65	−0.000, −0.000	1.208
Outlet density (log)	0.250	0.066	3.78	0.119, 0.381	1.137
Intercept	2.109	0.340	6.19	1.437, 2.781	
Diagnostics					
Adjusted R^2			0.628		
AICc			388.46		

[a]Variance inflation factors.

TABLE 3: Geographically weighted regression (GWR) model of violent crime (local model).

Variable	Minimum	Lower quartile	Median	Upper quartile	Maximum
Percent Hispanic	0.018	0.021	0.022	0.023	0.024
Percent Black (log)	0.108	0.180	0.233	0.258	0.289
Percent families below poverty	0.001	0.007	0.011	0.015	0.022
Percent owner occupied	−0.025	−0.013	−0.012	−0.011	−0.008
Percent residential stability	−0.004	0.007	0.009	0.013	0.035
Population density	−0.0001	−0.0001	−0.0001	−0.0001	−0.0001
Outlet density (log)	0.071	0.147	0.246	0.346	0.399
Intercept	0.897	2.031	2.304	2.523	3.515
Diagnostics					
Adjusted R^2			0.704		
AICc			361.97		

the city (close to 90% of the block groups). Additionally, spatial nonstationarity of predictor variables was further assessed by the P values obtained from the Monte-Carlo tests. Two predictor variables (percent Black and percent Hispanic) exhibited statistically significant nonstationarity, while the rest of the variables, including alcohol outlet density, were not statistically significant. We further conducted sensitivity analyses in assessing statistical significance of spatial nonstationarity of predictor variables; results from the Monte-Carlo tests with all 12 sociostructural neighbourhood variables remained unchanged, indicating that errors due to model misspecification unlikely.

Finally, regression coefficients and diagnostic values were used to compare the performance between the two models. As indicated previously, the best OLS model explained slightly less than two-thirds of the variability in violence within the study area, while the GWR improved the model with an additional 7% in explained variance (mean adjusted R-squared value of 0.704). The AIC score for the GWR model (361.97) was much smaller than the AIC from the global OLS model (388.46), which suggests that the local GWR model provided a better fit to the data, and thus significant improvement over the global model.

The spatial distribution of local R-squared values produced by the GWR analysis is also presented in Figure 2.

Spatial variations in these local R-squared statistics demonstrate how the combined effects of neighborhood population and place characteristics (including outlet density) on violent crime vary across block groups within the city. This map also identifies geographic areas where the GWR produces an improvement in overall model fit with respect to the global model. More than 50% of census block groups showed an improvement over the R-squared of 0.63 from the global OLS model, especially in a majority of block groups east of the city.

4. Discussion

This study investigated whether violent crime is spatially and/or locally associated with neighborhood sociostructural characteristics, including the availability of alcohol through on-sale premises, in the city of Lubbock, Texas. Using the OLS procedure we identified several neighborhood sociostructural variables, including on-sale alcohol outlet density, that showed a statistically significant association with violent crime in the city, and which explained 63% of the variance in this outcome. An additional 7% was explained by the local GWR model, which explained more than two-thirds of the variability in violence within the study area. We also observed spatially varying population and neighborhood variables associated with violent crime within the study area, often not

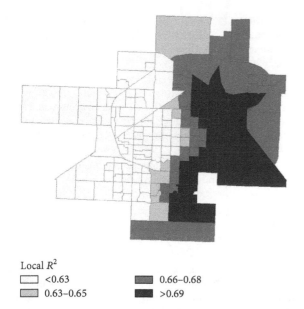

Local R^2
☐ <0.63   ▨ 0.66–0.68
▨ 0.63–0.65   ■ >0.69

FIGURE 2: Distribution of local R-squared values, Lubbock, Texas, 2005–2009.

captured by the global model. The findings provide evidence of the ecological association between on-sale alcohol outlets and violence overall and show that violence is spatially and locally associated with neighborhood and on-sale alcohol environment.

The findings concerning alcohol outlet density and violence add to a growing body of research that has examined the association between these two variables [1, 5]. As noted above, while a positive association between on-sale alcohol outlets and violence has been reported in a number of studies, overall the previous research in this area has produced mixed results with many studies reporting no association [5]. The current study may provide more credible evidence on the inconsistent associations reported previously as it allows assessment of the influence of on-sales outlets on violence in the almost total absence of off-sale outlets. We found that such outlets explained an additional 3% of the variance in violent crime in the OLS model. A number of mechanisms have been proposed as explanations of this relationship.

At the most basic level, alcohol consumption will increase as availability increases and this, in turn, will lead to a rise in both excessive drinking and alcohol-related harms [16]. Beyond availability, it has also been proposed that on-sale outlets can have a deleterious effect on local communities. For example, Livingston and colleagues argue that on-sale alcohol outlets can have an "amenity effect" which operates primarily in terms of the types of individuals that they attract into a neighborhood and the interactions that occur between them following the consumption of alcohol [8]. Along similar lines, Gruenewald's niche theory posits that alcohol outlets market their products to specific segments of the drinking population and that different types of drinkers are attracted to different types of drinking environments some of which are more conducive to the generation of violence than others [9].

The findings presented should be interpreted with caution given the limitations of the study. First, the question as

to whether neighborhood characteristics and outlet density are causally linked to the increased violence remains to be answered. Similarly, interpretations of our findings should consider limitations inherent due to the study design and measures used in the study; these include the use of population-based measures of violence and outlet density and potential aggregation problems of outlet density due to the cross-sectional study design. Study designs that take advantages of longitudinal changes in neighborhood characteristics and violence and that employ improved measures of violence (that consider population movement) and outlet density (that consider alcohol sales and duration of outlet operations) may help address this question [17].

Second, we cannot rule out the possibility that there may be other unmeasured neighborhood population and/or place characteristics that may be associated with violence. Other aspects of neighborhood social and built environments that may be directly or indirectly related to violence need to be further investigated, such as social capital, drug availability and other neighborhood institutions [18–20]. These too may require the use of methods other than those employed in our study [21]. Third, the results reported pertain to one isolated city in north-west Texas and may not be generalizable beyond this setting. Lastly, while GWR certainly provides the capability to explore and interpret the significance and sign of spatial and local associations, often undetected by conventional global models, it is not without limitations [22–24]. However, we additionally conducted sensitivity analyses to make sure that important predictor variables were not omitted in assessing statistical significance of spatial nonstationarity and to ensure that potential problems due to multiple testing and multicollinearity were not present by using statistically valid and significant predictors in the model.

Ethical Approval

The study protocol was approved by the Institutional Review Boards at Texas A&M University.

Conflict of Interests

The authors have declared that no conflict of interests exists.

Acknowledgments

The authors would like to thank Scott Horel for his assistance in geocoding. This work was supported by Grant no. 1R21AA020093-01A1 from the National Institute on Alcohol Abuse and Alcoholism.

References

[1] S. Popova, N. Giesbrecht, D. Bekmuradov, and J. Patra, "Hours and days of sale and density of alcohol outlets: impacts on alcohol consumption and damage: a systematic review," *Alcohol and Alcoholism*, vol. 44, no. 5, pp. 500–516, 2009.

[2] D. M. Gorman, P. W. Speer, P. J. Gruenewald, and E. W. Labouvie, "Spatial dynamics of alcohol availability, neighborhood

structure and violent crime," *Journal of Studies on Alcohol*, vol. 62, no. 5, pp. 628–636, 2001.

[3] L. Zhu, D. M. Gorman, and S. Horel, "Hierarchical Bayesian spatial models for alcohol availability, drug "hot spots" and violent crime," *International Journal of Health Geographics*, vol. 5, no. 54, 2006.

[4] H. Britt, B. P. Carlin, T. L. Toomey, and A. C. Wagenaar, "Neighborhood level spatial analysis of the relationship between alcohol outlet density and criminal violence," *Environmental and Ecological Statistics*, vol. 12, no. 4, pp. 411–426, 2005.

[5] T. L. Toomey, D. J. Erickson, B. P. Carlin et al., "The association between density of alcohol establishments and violent crime within urban neighbourhoods," *Alcoholism*, vol. 36, no. 8, pp. 1468–1473, 2012.

[6] P. G. Gruenewald, B. Freisthler, L. Remer, E. A. LaScala, and A. Treno, "Ecological models of alcohol outlets and violent assaults: crime potentials and geospatial analysis," *Addiction*, vol. 101, no. 5, pp. 666–677, 2006.

[7] R. Lipton and P. J. Gruenewald, "The spatial dynamics of violence and alcohol outlets," *Journal of Studies on Alcohol*, vol. 63, no. 2, pp. 187–195, 2002.

[8] M. Livingston, T. Chikritzhs, and R. Room, "Changing the density of alcohol outlets to reduce alcohol-related problems," *Drug and Alcohol Review*, vol. 26, no. 5, pp. 557–566, 2007.

[9] P. G. Gruenewald, "The spatial ecology of alcohol problems: Niche theory and assortative drinking," *Addiction*, vol. 102, no. 6, pp. 870–878, 2007.

[10] D. Han and D. M. Gorman, "Evaluating the effects of the introduction of off-sale alcohol outlets on violent crime," *Alcohol and Alcoholism*, vol. 48, no. 3, pp. 370–374, 2013.

[11] US Census Bureau, *American Community Survey (ACS): 2006–2010 5-Year Estimates*, U. S. Census Bureau, Suitland, Md, USA, 2012.

[12] A. S. Fotheringham, C. Brunsdon, and M. E. Charlton, *Geographically Weighted Regression: The Analysis of Spatially Varying Relationships*, Wiley, New York, NY, USA, 2002.

[13] C. Brunsdont, S. Fotheringham, and M. Charlton, "Geographically weighted regression-modelling spatial non-stationarity," *Journal of the Royal Statistical Society Series D*, vol. 47, no. 3, pp. 431–443, 1998.

[14] J. Mennis, "Mapping the results of geographically weighted regression," *Cartographic Journal*, vol. 43, no. 2, pp. 171–179, 2006.

[15] A. Hope, "A simplified Monte Carlo significance test procedure," *Journal of the Royal Statistical Society Series B*, vol. 30, pp. 582–598, 1968.

[16] E. W. Single, "The availability theory of alcohol-related problems," in *Theories on Alcoholism*, C. Chaudron and D. Wilkinson, Eds., Addiction Research Foundation, Toronto, Canada, 1998.

[17] M. Livingston, "A longitudinal analysis of alcohol outlet density and domestic violence," *Addiction*, vol. 106, no. 5, pp. 919–925, 2011.

[18] D. M. Gorman, L. Zhu, and S. Horel, "Drug 'hot-spots', alcohol availability and violence," *Drug and Alcohol Review*, vol. 24, no. 6, pp. 507–513, 2005.

[19] R. D. Peterson, L. J. Krivo, and M. A. Harris, "Disadvantage and neighborhood violent crime: do local institutions matter?" *Journal of Research in Crime and Delinquency*, vol. 37, no. 1, pp. 31–63, 2000.

[20] K. P. Theall, R. Scribner, D. Cohen, R. N. Bluthenthal, M. Schonlau, and T. A. Farley, "Social capital and the neighborhood alcohol environment," *Health and Place*, vol. 15, no. 1, pp. 323–332, 2009.

[21] C. Furr-Holden, K. Campbell, A. Milam, M. Smart, N. Ialongo, and P. Leaf, "Metric properties of the neighborhood inventory for environmental typology (NIfETy): an environmental assessment tool for measuring indicators of violence, alcohol, tobacco, and other drug exposures," *Evaluation Review*, vol. 34, no. 3, pp. 159–184, 2010.

[22] C. Graif and R. J. Sampson, "Spatial heterogeneity in the effects of immigration and diversity on neighborhood homicide rates," *Homicide Studies*, vol. 13, no. 3, pp. 242–260, 2009.

[23] A. Páez, S. Farber, and D. Wheeler, "A simulation-based study of geographically weighted regression as a method for investigating spatially varying relationships," *Environment and Planning A*, vol. 43, no. 12, pp. 2992–3010, 2011.

[24] L. A. Waller, L. Zhu, C. A. Gotway, D. M. Gorman, and P. J. Gruenewald, "Quantifying geographic variations in associations between alcohol distribution and violence: a comparison of geographically weighted regression and spatially varying coefficient models," *Stochastic Environmental Research and Risk Assessment*, vol. 21, no. 5, pp. 573–588, 2007.

Smoking and Other Drug Characteristics of Aboriginal and Non-Aboriginal Prisoners in Australia

Robyn L. Richmond,[1] Devon Indig,[1,2] Tony G. Butler,[3] Kay A. Wilhelm,[4] Vicki A. Archer,[2] and Alex D. Wodak[5]

[1] School of Public Health and Community Medicine, University of New South Wales, Kensington, Sydney, Australia
[2] Centre for Health Research in Criminal Justice, Justice Health, University of New South Wales, Suite 302, Level 2, 152 Bunnerong Road, Pagewood, NSW 2035, Australia
[3] National Centre in HIV Epidemiology and Clinical Research, University of New South Wales, Kensington, Sydney, Australia
[4] School of Psychiatry, Faculty of Medicine, University of New South Wales, Faces in the Street, St. Vincent's Health Urban Mental Health Research, St Vincent's Hospital, Level 4, O'Brien Centre, St Vincent's Hospital, 390 Victoria Street, Sydney, NSW 2010, Australia
[5] Alcohol and Drug Service, St. Vincent's Hospital, Darlinghurst, NSW 2010, Australia

Correspondence should be addressed to Robyn L. Richmond; r.richmond@unsw.edu.au

Academic Editor: Karen Cropsey

Introduction and Aim. Although tobacco and alcohol use have declined substantially in the Australian community, substance use among prisoners remains high. The aim was to compare the smoking, drug, and alcohol characteristics, sociodemographic profile, and general health of Aboriginal and non-Aboriginal male prisoners in a smoking cessation intervention. *Design and Methods.* This study was a descriptive cross-sectional analysis of data from 425 male prisoners who joined a quit smoking trial conducted at 18 correctional centres in NSW and Queensland using data collected by standardised self-report instruments. *Results.* Average age was 33 years with 15% from Aboriginal descent. Compared to non-Aboriginal prisoners, Aboriginal prisoners were significantly more likely to have left school with no qualifications, to have been institutionalised as a child, to be previously incarcerated, and commenced smoking at a younger age. The tobacco use profile of both groups was similar; most of them had a medium to high level of nicotine dependence, smoked roll your own tobacco, and were "serious" about quitting. *Discussion and Conclusion.* Despite differences in terms of sociodemographic characteristics and offending history, the smoking characteristics of Aboriginal and non-Aboriginal prisoners were similar. Incarceration offers an opportunity to encourage smoking cessation and reduction of drug use.

1. Introduction

Tobacco use causes a higher burden of disease than other behavioural risk factors, contributing 9.5% of the total burden in men and 6% in women and causes 16,000 deaths in Australia each year [1]. The 2010 National Drug Strategy Household Survey reported that the daily smoking prevalence in Australia has declined from 22% in 2001 to around 15% in 2010 [2]. However, specific groups such as Aboriginal people had higher rates than non-Aboriginal Australians (38% versus 17%) [2]. This higher rate of smoking contributes to the substantially increased burden of illness and disease experienced by Aboriginal people and contributes to reduced quality of life and premature death [3–5]. The prevalence of smoking among prisoners in 2009 was over five times higher (76% versus 15%) than the general community, and Aboriginal male prisoners were more likely to smoke (83% versus 71%) than non-Aboriginal male prisoners [6, 7]. Smoking tobacco is socially acceptable and regarded as an integral part of prison life where it is used as a de facto currency, to relieve boredom and stress, and as a social lubricant [8, 9]. Despite these high rates of smoking among prisoners, 70% of currently smoking prisoners had attempted to quit smoking [7, 10].

Excessive alcohol consumption is also a major risk factor for ill health and death, causing 3.8% of the burden of disease for males and 0.7% for females [1] while illicit drug use contributes 2.0% to the burden [1]. Prisoner populations have high levels of drug use and the Inmate Health Survey reports 44% of women and 42% of men had used illicit drugs while in prison with cannabis and heroin being the most common [6, 11]. Drug use is a significant and multifaceted problem contributing to injury, social and family disruption, workplace concerns, violence, crime and community safety issues, morbidity, and mortality [12].

Aboriginal people are disproportionately represented among the Australian prisoner population, reflecting approximately 2% of the Australian population but 26% of the Australian prison population, with an incarceration rate 14 times higher than for non-Aboriginal people [13]. Since 1990, the proportion of Aboriginal men in prison in full-time custody in NSW has increased from 9.9% to 22.1% [14].

This paper consists of a detailed analysis of the baseline data for a larger randomised controlled trial for smoking cessation among male prisoners in NSW and Queensland. The purpose of this paper is to compare the sociodemographics, offending history, drug and alcohol use, and smoking behaviours of male prisoners, identifying any differences between Aboriginal and non-Aboriginal inmates. Measuring these characteristics is critical to understanding how best to develop appropriate and targeted interventions. Incarceration offers an important, but underutilised, public health opportunity to improve the health of several key disadvantaged population groups who are overrepresented among prisoners.

2. Methods

From 2006 to 2010, we conducted a randomised controlled trial of a smoking cessation intervention among 425 male prisoners in 17 adult, men-only prisons in NSW and one prison in Queensland. Prisoners who were current smokers and who wanted to quit were invited to join the study through posters displayed in the prison clinics, flyers in the prisons, referrals from prison health clinic staff, and word of mouth between prison inmates. As a part of the study, we collected baseline data on demographic, smoking, and drug use characteristics.

2.1. Participants. Eligibility criteria for the intervention included male gender, current smoker, age over 18 years, no history of psychiatric illness (including current depression, as an antidepressant was used as an antismoking medication), no known allergy to nortriptyline or nicotine replacement therapy (NRT), no current treatment with another antidepressant or a major tranquiliser, and no history of cardiac disease (as determined by the medical records). Prisoners with current major depression were ineligible as they were likely to be taking antidepressant medication and there was potential for drug interactions, increased side effects and possibly increasing suicidality in a depressed prisoner. Female prisoners were not included as they only constitute

7% of the Australian prisoner population and tend to have much shorter sentences than men [13], thereby limiting availability for follow-up assessments at 6 and 12 months being conducted whilst in prison.

2.2. Measures Used. Three prison nurse interviewers collected information in face-to-face interviews covering sociodemographic characteristics, offending history, smoking behaviour, prior attempts to quit smoking, physical health status, mental health (Kessler Psychological Distress Scale, K-10) [15], alcohol use before entering prison, and drug use before and during incarceration. The 12-item Short-Form Survey (SF-12) was used to assess overall physical and mental well-being using the Physical Component Summary and Mental Component Summary scores [16]. Blood pressure was measured at baseline, with high blood pressure defined as systolic blood pressure of 140 or more and/or diastolic blood pressure of 90 or more. "Sufficient physical activity" was defined as at least 150 minutes of walking, moderate or vigorous activity per week over at least 5 occasions (at least 600 minutes over a four-week period), based on a definition from the NSW Centre for Physical Activity and Health [17]. Participants completed the Fagerström Test for Nicotine Dependence [18] with a score of 6+ regarded as moderate to high nicotine dependence. We used the stages of change model which measures smokers' readiness to quit and has been well validated in general samples [19].

Carbon monoxide (CO) was measured as the biomarker for tobacco consumption and exposure, which provides an immediate objective measure of use with good correlation between breath test and self-reported smoking [20]. CO allows detection of smoking over a 6–24-hour period and is recognised as an appropriate measure of tobacco use [21]. In our study CO was measured at several assessment points, including baseline, in expired breath using the Micro 4 Smokerlyzer breath analyzer (Bedfont Scientific Ltd., UK) using the recommended cut point for smoking of 10 ppm [21].

2.3. Ethics Approvals. Prisoners provided written informed consent to join the study. The study was independently approved by the University of New South Wales (UNSW) Human Resources Ethics Committee, NSW Department of Corrective Services Ethics Committee, Justice Health Human Research and Ethics Committee, Aboriginal Health and Medical Research Council Ethics Committee, and Queensland Corrective Services Research Committee.

2.4. Data Analysis. Data analysis was conducted using SAS version 9.2 [22]. Descriptive statistics were used to compare the characteristics of Aboriginal and non-Aboriginal prisoners using chi-square and t-tests, with 0.05 level of significance.

3. Results

3.1. Demographics and Offending History. Of 1751 male inmates wishing to join our study, 1326 were ineligible. The main reasons for ineligibility were imminent release date (35%), history of psychiatric disease (40%), cardiac history

TABLE 1: Demographics and offending history by Aboriginality.

Characteristics	Smoking cessation RCT			2009 NSW Inmate Health Survey		
	Aboriginal men % ($N = 64$)	Non-Aboriginal men % ($N = 361$)	Total men % ($N = 425$)	Aboriginal men % ($N = 259$)	Non-Aboriginal men % ($N = 538$)	Total men % ($N = 797$)
Mean age (±SD)	32.0 (9.7)	33.8 (10.2)	33.5 (10.2)	34.1[†] (11.8)	36.1 (13.7)	35.5 (13.2)
Age group						
<25 years	28.1	22.2	23.1	37.1	33.5	34.6
25–29 years	23.4	19.4	20.0	8.9	10.6	10.0
30–39 years	21.9	29.9	28.7	18.5	17.0	17.5
40+ years	26.6	28.5	28.2	35.5	39.0	37.9
Aboriginal origin	—	—	15.1	—	—	32.5
Country of birth: Australia	100.0[†]	70.2	74.9	99.6[†]	72.7	81.4
Left school with no qualification	56.3[†]	41.3	43.5	72.5[†]	42.5	52.3
Mean age when left school (+SD)	14.5[†] (1.7)	15.3 (2.0)	15.1 (2.0)	14.6 (1.3)	14.6 (1.2)	14.6 (1.2)
Institutionalised as a child (juvenile detention and/or placed in care)	56.3[†]	34.6	37.9	61.0[*†] 45.9[^†]	32.9[*] 21.7[^]	42.0[*] 29.6[^]
Being homeless prior to prison	9.4	6.7	7.1	13.9	10.1	11.3
Employed while in prison	67.2	72.9	72.0	55.6	61.5	59.6
Offending history						
Previously incarcerated	76.6[†]	61.5	63.8	80.7[†]	55.9	64.0
Median number adult prison terms (+SD)	3.0[†] (3.4)	2.0 (2.8)	2.0 (2.9)	3.0[†] (3.8)	2.0 (3.0)	2.0 (3.3)
Incarcerated 5+ years at baseline	15.6	18.6	18.1	9.3	12.3	11.3
Sentence length 5+ years	35.9	33.8	34.1	29.8[†]	42.3	38.4
Health status						
SF-12: mean physical component score	51.8 (8.9)	52.4 (7.0)	52.3 (7.3)	51.7 (9.7)	52.0 (10.2)	51.9 (10.0)
SF-12: mean mental component score	43.2 (7.0)	44.2 (6.5)	44.1 (6.6)	44.6 (15.1)	44.3 (14.2)	44.4 (14.5)
Insufficient physical activity	23.4	22.7	22.8	20.7	23.9	22.8
High blood pressure (140+ sys or 90+ dias)	1.6	5.0	4.5	14.5	14.8	14.7
Fair/poor self-rated health	23.4	16.3	17.4	24.8	22.5	23.3

[†]Statistically significant $P < 0.05$ comparing Aboriginal and non-Aboriginal male inmates. N/A: not available. [*]Ever juvenile detention; [^]ever placed in care as a child.

(5%) and not yet sentenced (20%). The mean age of the 425 participants was 33 years (median 32.0, range 18 to 65 years), which was consistent with the median age of 33.6 of prisoners across Australia [13] and was similar among Aboriginal and non-Aboriginal prisoners (Table 1). In our sample, 15% were of Aboriginal descent (consistent with the 22% Aboriginal origin in NSW) [23] but lower than the 33% Aboriginal in the 2009 Inmate Health Survey that deliberately oversampled on Aboriginal people [6]. Demographic results from the participants in our study have been compared with the results from the Inmate Health Surveys to demonstrate the comparability of our population and thus the generalisability of our results.

All the following comparisons were made between Aboriginal and non-Aboriginal prisoners. Aboriginal prisoners were significantly more likely to have left school with no qualification (56% versus 41%, $P < 0.03$), a finding consistent with the 2009 Inmate Health Survey. Aboriginal prisoners also left school at a significantly younger age (14.5 years versus 15.3 years, $P < 0.01$). Significantly more Aboriginal prisoners

(56% versus 35%, $P < 0.01$) reported being institutionalised as a child (i.e., juvenile detention and/or placed in care), consistent with 2009 Inmate Health Survey. Around three-quarters of prisoners (72%) were employed whilst in prison with no significant difference by Aboriginal status.

A significantly higher proportion of Aboriginal prisoners had been previously incarcerated (77% versus 62%, $P < 0.02$) and had significantly more adult prison terms (a median of 3.0 versus 2.0, $P < 0.02$), both consistent with 2009 Inmate Health Survey. No other offending-related characteristics were significantly different by Aboriginality. Nearly a fifth (18%) of the sample had already been incarcerated for five or more years at the time of recruitment and over a third (34%) had a sentence length of five years or more.

Consistent with the 2009 Inmate Health Survey, there were no significant differences by Aboriginality for the SF-12 Physical or Mental Component Scores and the mean SF-12 Mental Component Score (44.1) was considerably lower than the community norm (standardised at 50.0) [16]. Also consistent with the 2009 Inmate Health Survey the level of physical activity was good with two thirds (68%) reporting sufficient exercise compared to one third (32%) of similarly aged males in the general population [24]. High blood pressure was rare for study participants (4.5%) and much lower than that found in the 2009 Inmate Health Survey (14.7%) [6].

3.2. Smoking and Cessation Behaviours. All participants were current smokers, a requirement for joining the study. By comparison, 75% of males from the 2009 Inmate Health Survey were current smokers, with significantly more Aboriginal men smoking than non-Aboriginal men (83% versus 71%, $P < 0.01$). Among smokers, the majority of smoking-related behaviours did not differ between Aboriginality, and non-Aboriginal prisoners, with the exception that Aboriginal prisoners started smoking at a significantly younger age (12.7 years versus 13.9 years, $P < 0.05$). In the 2009 Inmate Health Survey, Aboriginal men also started smoking at a younger age than non-Aboriginal men (13.6 years versus 14.0 years, $P < 0.07$), but this was not found to be statistically significant. Both Aboriginal and non-Aboriginal prisoners had smoked for an average of 20 years, having started daily smoking at 15.5 years (Table 2). The average number of cigarettes smoked daily was 23, with 70% of prisoners smoking 20 or more cigarettes per day. This was substantially higher than found in the 2009 Inmate Health Survey, where only 24% smoked 21 or more cigarettes per day and non-Aboriginal men were significantly more likely to smoke than Aboriginal men (27.5% versus 18.3%, $P < 0.02$) [6].

The most popular (97%) form of tobacco used was hand rolled cigarettes made from loose leaf "White Ox" tobacco. The majority (83%) of prisoners had medium to high levels of dependence (≥ 6 on Fagerstrom Test of Dependence) and the mean expired CO level was 14 ppm. Approximately one-third (34%) of the participants shared a cell with a smoker, a finding that was lower than found in the 2009 Inmate Health Survey. Significantly more Aboriginal prisoners indicated one of the main reasons they smoked was because their spouse or partner smoked or that it helped them to fit into groups (59% versus 37%, $P < 0.01$) compared with non-Aboriginal prisoners.

On average, prisoners reported trying to quit 2.6 times in the past, with 13% remaining abstinent for a month or more in the past year. Over half (54%) had successfully quit for one day in the past year. Significantly more Aboriginal prisoners had tried quitting in the past year by lowering tar or nicotine content of their tobacco (14% versus 5%, $P < 0.01$) than non-Aboriginal prisoners. The most popular methods for quitting while living in the community were going cold turkey, cutting down consumption, and using a nicotine patch.

Although all reported that they were serious about quitting and planned to stop smoking, only half (49%) were "very sure" they would be able to do so. There were no differences by Aboriginality regarding intention to quit smoking with most determined to quit and between 40%–50% very sure of their ability to do so.

3.3. Drug and Alcohol Characteristics. Nearly all participants (95%) had "ever" used drugs but significantly more Aboriginal men had used drugs on a regular basis prior to prison (92% versus 79%, $P < 0.02$), consistent with the 2009 Inmate Health Survey. However, it is notable that the participants (all smokers) used drugs regularly at nearly twice the prevalence (81% versus 42%) as the general prison population in the 2009 Inmate Health Survey. This finding of increased drug use among smokers was consistent across all drug types and drug-related behaviours such as injecting and using drugs in prison. By contrast, risky alcohol use before entering prison was lower among the participants in our study who were all smokers compared to the general prisoner population in the 2009 Inmate Health Survey. Across both studies, Aboriginal men were significantly more likely than non-Aboriginal men to drink alcohol at risky levels prior to incarceration, including showing signs of risky and dependent drinking.

Table 3 shows that, among Aboriginal men, regular use of cannabis was significantly higher (80% versus 57%, $P < 0.01$) than non-Aboriginal men and more than twice as high (61% versus 26%) as in the 2009 Inmate Health Survey. Regular use of all drugs was higher among participants in our study compared to the 2009 Inmate Health Survey participants, including heroin (37% versus 9%), other opiates (16% versus 4%), amphetamines (49% versus 14%), cocaine (36% versus 5%), and tranquilisers (17% versus 5%). There were no other significant differences in drug use characteristics by Aboriginality. Compared to non-Aboriginal men, in the 2009 Inmate Health Survey, Aboriginal men had significantly higher prevalence of regularly using heroin or other opiates and significantly higher prevalence of ever injecting heroin or amphetamines but lower prevalence (39% versus 48%, $P < 0.02$) of ever using cocaine [6].

4. Discussion

This is the first study that describes the sociodemographic and tobacco, drug, and alcohol use characteristics of a sample of male smoking prisoners by Aboriginality.

People with low socioeconomic status, measured by level of education, are greatly overrepresented in prison. We found 44% of prisoners had left high school at Year 9 or before, with no educational qualification, a finding significantly higher for Aboriginal men. A similar result of 53% was reported in the 2009 NSW Inmate Health Survey, also significantly higher for Aboriginal men [7]. Smoking is related to lower education and lower income, two key variables of socio economic status [25–27]. Prisoner backgrounds are characterised by greater socioeconomic disadvantage as evidenced in lower levels of education, higher rates of unemployment prior to incarceration, and multiple contacts with the criminal justice system, with Aboriginal inmates experiencing greater disadvantage. Well-being has been found to be related to a high level of education [28]. However, in our study we report 17% of prisoners and as high as one quarter of Aboriginal prisoners rated their health as "fair" or "poor" in the last month.

TABLE 2: Smoking and cessation behaviours by Aboriginality.

Characteristics	Smoking cessation RCT			2009 NSW inmate health survey		
	Aboriginal men % ($N = 64$)	Non-aboriginal men % ($N = 361$)	Total men % ($N = 425$)	Aboriginal men % ($N = 259$)	Non-aboriginal men % ($N = 538$)	Total men % ($N = 797$)
Smoking behaviours and history						
Current smoker	100.0	100.0	100.0	83.2[†]	71.1	
Mean age when first smoked tobacco (+SD)	12.7[†] (4.3)	13.9 (4.2)	13.7 (4.3)	13.6 (5.0)	14.0 (4.5)	13.9 (4.7)
Mean age when first smoked tobacco daily (+SD)	15.1 (4.7)	15.5 (4.1)	15.5 (4.2)	N/A	N/A	N/A
Mean years when smoked tobacco (+SD)	19.2 (9.9)	19.9 (10.3)	19.8 (10.2)	N/A	N/A	N/A
Mean carbon monoxide reading (+SD)	13.1 (7.8)	14.5 (7.7)	14.3 (7.8)	N/A	N/A	N/A
Mean cigarettes smoked per day (+SD)	22.7 (8.4)	23.2 (10.0)	23.2 (9.8)	N/A	N/A	N/A
Smoking 20+ cigarettes per day	67.2	70.6	70.1	18.3[†*]	27.5	24.2
High tobacco dependence (Fagerstrom 6+)	84.4	82.6	82.8	N/A	N/A	N/A
Sharing a cell with a smoker	42.2	31.9	33.5	62.9	51.9	55.1
Smoking White Ox (loose tobacco)	98.4	97.0	97.2	97.8	94.9	96.6
Reason for smoking: spouse smoked/helps fit into group	59.4[†]	36.6	40.0	N/A	N/A	N/A
Smoking cessation history						
Quitting behaviours in past year						
Giving up more than one month	12.5	13.0	12.9	17.2	22.1	20.4
Trying to give up unsuccessfully	65.6	59.3	60.2	43.7	52.4	49.3
Lower tar or nicotine content	14.1[†]	5.3	6.6	4.0	9.6	7.6
Reduced amount of tobacco smoked	50.0	47.4	47.8	56.3	57.2	56.9
Quitting on purpose for 24 hours	59.4	52.6	53.7	N/A	N/A	N/A
Any type of quitting behaviour	75.0	73.1	73.4	82.7	81.6	82.0
Mean times of trying to quit smoking (+SD)	2.8 (3.3)	2.6 (7.4)	2.6 (7.9)	N/A	N/A	N/A
Stages of readiness to quit smoking						
Seriously thinking of cutting down	98.4	94.7	95.3	N/A	N/A	N/A
Seriously thinking about quitting	100.0	99.7	99.8	N/A	N/A	N/A
Plannig to quit smoking	100.0	99.2	99.3	N/A	N/A	N/A
Very sure of wanting to cut down smoking	92.2	89.2	89.7	N/A	N/A	N/A
Very sure of being able to cut down smoking	43.8	48.2	47.5	N/A	N/A	N/A
Very determined to cut down	81.3	83.9	83.5	N/A	N/A	N/A
Very sure of being able to quit smoking	40.6	50.1	48.7	N/A	N/A	N/A
Very determined to quit smoking	90.6	86.7	87.3	N/A	N/A	N/A

[†]Statistically significant $P < 0.05$ comparing Aboriginal and non-Aboriginal male inmates. [*]Categories started at 21+ cigarettes per day.

Cardiovascular disease, diabetes, sexually transmitted infections, and ear and eye disorders and injury are in excess among Aboriginal people living in the community compared with the broad Australian population [5, 24]. Poor health among Aboriginal people is attributed to dispossession, forced separation of children from family and communities, and disadvantage [5]. Subjective well-being is positively related to education but negatively correlated to smoking, consistent with our findings of a generally low level of education and poor health among male smoking inmates. The finding that prisoners' health compares unfavourably with the general population has been reported in the surveys of prison inmates in NSW [14] and in other studies [29, 30]. We found that more than a third of our prisoner population

TABLE 3: Drug and alcohol characteristics by Aboriginality.

Drug and alcohol use	Smoking cessation RCT			2009 NSW inmate health survey		
	Aboriginal men % (N = 64)	Non-aboriginal men % (N = 361)	Total men % (N = 425)	Aboriginal men % (N = 259)	Non-aboriginal men % (N = 538)	Total men % (N = 797)
Ever use any drugs	96.9	95.0	95.3	88.3	84.2	85.5
Regularly* use any drugs in year before prison	92.2[†]	79.0	80.9	50.8[†]	38.0	42.1
Ever use any drugs in prison	78.1[†]	63.2	65.4	48.0[†]	39.3	42.1
Ever inject any drugs	60.9	56.0	56.7	46.1[†]	37.2	40.1
Mean age when first injected (+SD)	18.9 (7.7)	17.9 (4.6)	18.0 (5.2)	18.5 (4.2)	18.5 (4.2)	18.5 (4.2)
Last injection in prison	32.4	33.7	33.5	22.0	22.2	22.2
AUDIT score 8+ prior to prison (risky drinker)	68.8[†]	48.5	51.5	74.2[†]	57.0	62.6
AUDIT score 20+ prior to prison (dependent drinker)	31.3[†]	18.6	20.5	44.1[†]	29.9	34.5
Drank 10+ drinks on typical day prior to prison	39.1[†]	24.7	26.8	57.8[†]	41.2	46.6
Drank 6+ drinks daily/almost daily prior to prison	26.6	19.9	20.9	39.8[†]	27.1	31.2
Cannabis						
Ever use	93.8	92.5	92.7	87.9[†]	81.6	83.6
Regularly use in year before prison	79.7[†]	57.1	60.5	34.4[†]	22.6	26.4
Ever use in prison	75.0[†]	57.1	59.8	35.9	31.2	32.7
Heroin						
Ever use	57.8	56.0	56.2	43.4	36.3	38.6
Regularly use in year before prison	40.6	37.1	37.7	13.7[†]	6.0	8.5
Ever inject	46.9	41.8	42.6	34.0[†]	26.5	28.9
Ever use in prison	32.8	34.9	34.6	17.2	15.2	15.9
Other opiates						
Ever use	37.5	36.8	36.9	20.7	18.2	19.0
Regularly use in year before prison	18.8	15.5	16.0	7.0[†]	3.0	4.3
Ever inject	29.7	24.1	24.9	15.6	12.6	13.6
Ever use in prison	15.6	19.4	18.8	5.9	5.6	5.7
Amphetamines						
Ever use	76.6	77.0	76.9	60.2	56.2	57.5
Regularly use in year before prison	46.9	49.0	48.7	17.2	13.0	14.3
Ever inject	53.1	44.6	45.9	37.5[†]	26.1	29.8
Ever use in prison	26.6	28.8	28.5	10.2	9.8	9.9
Cocaine						
Ever use	56.3	58.7	58.4	38.7[†]	47.9	44.9
Regularly use in year before prison	39.1	35.7	36.2	5.1	5.5	5.3
Ever inject	35.9	29.9	30.8	21.1	15.8	17.5
Ever use in prison	20.3	18.6	18.8	5.1	6.4	6.0
Tranquilisers						
Ever use	32.8	40.4	39.3	22.7	24.6	24.0
Regularly use in year before prison	15.6	17.7	17.4	5.1	5.5	5.3
Ever inject	6.3	7.8	7.5	3.1	3.6	3.4
Ever use in prison	18.8	18.0	18.1	6.3	8.1	7.5

[†]Statistically significant P < 0.05 comparing aboriginal and non-aboriginal male inmates. *Daily/almost daily use drugs prior to prison.

had medical and mental health conditions, and most had cardiovascular risk factors [31]. Our findings are important as these health issues can be used to motivate smokers to quit their habit. These results lend credence to the view that the prisoner setting is an important context to deliver evidence based health promotion interventions to improve health outcomes and reduce morbidity and mortality.

The NSW Inmate Census of 2009 reports that tobacco use is over four times higher in the correctional system compared to the general population [2, 6]. This finding has also been reported in the US studies of prisoner populations [29, 30]. Smoking profiles were similar among Aboriginal and non-Aboriginal inmates except that Aboriginal inmates were found to have started smoking at a younger age. Previous research examining the physical and mental health of Aboriginal and non-Aboriginal inmates in NSW found little difference in health status between these two populations across a diverse range of health indicators [32, 33]. However, we report elsewhere that the cardiovascular health of prisoners is far worse than males of similar age from the most disadvantaged backgrounds in the general population [31]. In that study we also reported that Aboriginal prisoners had significantly more cardiovascular risk factors than non-Aboriginal prisoners [31].

We report that, among our sample of smokers, current regular drug use was high, particularly for Aboriginal men in prison. In our study we found that Aboriginal prisoners were significantly more likely than non-Aboriginal men to be regular cannabis users. Further, we found that regular cannabis use was more than twice as high as compared to the participants in the Inmate Health Survey (60% versus 26%) and six times higher than the 2010 National Drug Strategy Household Survey [2, 7]. From data gained from our focus group study [8] we found that drug use is common among inmates in prison, with many initiating drug use while incarcerated. The reason that the prevalence of tobacco, cannabis and drug use is higher in prison compared to the general population is that drug use in the correctional system is endemic with drugs including cannabis and tobacco used as currency by prisoners.

Prisoners have a higher prevalence of illicit drug use compared to the broad Australian population [2, 6, 11]. Other research has identified strong associations between cannabis and tobacco among Aboriginal people, including the finding that cannabis use can sometimes be a gateway to tobacco use [34, 35]. Aboriginal men were also found to be significantly more likely than non-Aboriginal men to drink alcohol at risky or dependent levels prior to incarceration in both studies [34, 35]. There are 70% to 90% of heavy drinkers who are cigarette smokers [36, 37]. We expected that those who use tobacco as well as other drugs might find it more difficult to stop smoking compared with those who only smoked tobacco.

4.1. Strengths and Limitations of This Study. The strength of this study is that data are based on volunteer prisoners recruited to a smoking cessation RCT (to be reported elsewhere) who were representative of the general NSW prisoner population. Relying on self-reports may be imprecise and it is possible some respondents may have either minimised their tobacco use for social desirability or conversely exaggerated reports in order to be admitted to the randomised controlled trial to receive a smoking cessation intervention. This source of bias was minimised by the use of prison nurses as research assistants who have considerable experience taking medical and risk behaviour histories and working with the prisoner population. Further, we took biochemical measures (carbon monoxide) of tobacco use which provided an objective measure of smoking over a 6–24-hour period [21].

5. Conclusions

Only relatively recently have correctional communities realised the full extent of the burden of ill health which has been illuminated in the Inmate Health Surveys [6, 38]. However, these Inmate Health Surveys have limited information on tobacco and quit attempts. This paper provides unique information on tobacco use, quitting attempts and describes drug use in the prison setting.

The correctional system offers public health opportunities to detect and treat diseases, educate on unsafe practices, promote health and behaviour change, and offer continuity of care. High rates of tobacco and other drug use among inmates, combined with an interest in quitting, are an ideal scenario to promote smoking cessation, reduced drug use and healthier lifestyles and to provide appropriate, evidence-based interventions. Proactive smoking cessation programs and drug modification interventions delivered in the corrections system to inmates who already have chronic health conditions and cardiovascular risk factors may have a direct health benefit on communities, when they are released, including significant cost savings and social benefits. We are encouraged by the large number of prisoners who were already engaged in physical activities to promote health and well-being and the number of those who want to stop smoking or cut down their consumption.

Conflict of Interests

The authors declare that they have no conflict of interests.

Acknowledgments

This work was supported by the National Health and Medical Research Council (Project Grant 350829), the NSW Department of Health, and the Queensland Department of Health. NRT was provided free-of-charge by GlaxoSmithKline. Tony Butler is supported by the Centre for Health Advancement, NSW Department of Health. This trial from which these findings were generated is registered with the Australian New Zealand Clinical Trials Registry 12606000229572. The authors are grateful to V. A. Archer, the Project Manager for the study who ensured all components of the smoking cessation intervention were implemented. They would also like to acknowledge the prison research nurses, Anne Cole and Phe Affleck, who administered the baseline questionnaires and tenaciously followed up the prisoners, and Drs. Andrew Zdenkowski, Laurie Varga, and Ken Kuen who conducted the medical assessment of all participants for the study. They would also like to acknowledge Dr Alun Richards, Executive Director-Offender Health Services Directorate, Queensland Health, for introducing the study into Borallon Correctional Centre in Queensland. Invaluable assistance was provided by the research nurses Elizabeth Baxter, Luke McCreddie, Anne Cole and Phe Affleck in NSW and Adair Behrends in Queensland, as well as the Justice Health Pharmacy Chief pharmacists Hana Abdalla and Steven Crago, A/Data Coordinator Robyn Hetherington and Megan Kent A/Services Manager. Quitline was provided to the inmates by Quitline staff: Bronwyn Crosby, David Lester, Leah McLeod, Jennifer Blundell, Jake Docker, Jillian MacDonald and Matthew Nelson in NSW and Kerryn Nicks in Queensland. They would also like to acknowledge Joanne Hunnisett who entered and cleaned the considerable data bank and Fran Hyslop who also worked on the ethics applications and the literature review.

References

[1] S. Begg, T. Vos, B. Barker, C. Stevenson, L. Stanley, and A. Lopez, "The burden of disease and injury in Australia 2003," Cat. No. PHE 82, AIHW, Canberra, Australia, 2007.

[2] Australian Institute of Health Welfare, "2010 national drug strategy household survey report," Drug Statistics Series No. 25. Cat. no. PHE 145, AIHW, Canberra, Australia, 2011.

[3] Australian Bureau of Statistics, "National aboriginal and torres strait islander health survey 2004-2005," ABS Cat No. 4715.0, ABS, Canberra, Australia, 2006.

[4] T. Vos, B. Barker, S. Begg, L. Stanley, and A. D. Lopez, "Burden of disease and injury in aboriginal and torres strait Islander peoples: the indigenous health gap," *International Journal of Epidemiology*, vol. 38, no. 2, pp. 470–477, 2009.

[5] Australian Bureau of Statistics, "The health and welfare of Australia's aboriginal and torres strait Islander peoples," ABS Cat. No 4704.0, ABS, Canberra, Australia, 2010.

[6] D. Indig, L. Topp, B. Ross et al., "2009 NSW inmate health survey," Key Findings Report, Justice Health, Sydney, Australia, 2010.

[7] D. Indig, E. McEntyre, J. Page, and B. Ross, "2009 NSW inmate health survey," Aboriginal Health Report, Justice Health, Sydney, Australia, 2010.

[8] R. Richmond, T. Butler, K. Wilhelm, A. Wodak, M. Cunningham, and I. Anderson, "Tobacco in prisons: a focus group study," *Tobacco Control*, vol. 18, no. 3, pp. 176–182, 2009.

[9] T. Butler, R. Richmond, J. Belcher, K. Wilhelm, and A. Wodak, "Should smoking be banned in prisons?" *Tobacco Control*, vol. 16, no. 5, pp. 291–293, 2007.

[10] J. M. Belcher, T. Butler, R. L. Richmond, A. D. Wodak, and K. Wilhelm, "Smoking and its correlates in an Australian prisoner population," *Drug and Alcohol Review*, vol. 25, no. 4, pp. 343–348, 2006.

[11] T. Butler, M. Levy, K. Dolan, and J. Kaldor, "Drug use and its correlates in an Australian prisoner population," *Addiction Research and Theory*, vol. 11, no. 2, pp. 89–101, 2003.

[12] MCDS (Ministerial Council on Drug Strategy), *The National Drug Strategy 2010-2015*, 2011.

[13] Australian Bureau of Statistics, "Prisoners in Australia," ABS Catalogue Number 4517. 0, ABS, Canberra, Australia, 2011.

[14] S. Corben, "NSW inmate census 2010: summary of characteristics," Corrective Services NSW Statistical Publication No 36, Corrective Services NSW, Sydney, Australia, 2010.

[15] G. Andrews and T. Slade, "Interpreting scores on the Kessler Psychological Distress Scale (K10)," *Australian and New Zealand Journal of Public Health*, vol. 25, no. 6, pp. 494–497, 2001.

[16] J. E. Ware, M. Kosinski, and S. D. Keller, "A 12-item short-form health survey: construction of scales and preliminary tests of reliability and validity," *Medical Care*, vol. 34, no. 3, pp. 220–233, 1996.

[17] J. Chau, B. Smith, T. Chey, D. Merom, and A. Bauman, "Trends in population levels of sufficient physical activity in NSW, 1998 to 2005: full report," Report no. CPAH06-001c, NSW Centre for Physical Activity and Health, Sydney, Australia, 2007.

[18] T. F. Heatherton, L. T. Kozlowski, R. C. Frecker, and K. O. Fagerstrom, "The Fagerstrom test for nicotine dependence: a revision of the Fagerstrom Tolerance Questionnaire," *British Journal of Addiction*, vol. 86, no. 9, pp. 1119–1127, 1991.

[19] J. O. Prochaska, W. F. Velicer, J. M. Prochaska, and J. L. Johnson, "Size, consistency, and stability of stage effects for smoking cessation," *Addictive Behaviors*, vol. 29, no. 1, pp. 207–213, 2004.

[20] K. L. Cropsey, G. D. Eldridge, M. F. Weaver, G. C. Villalobos, and M. L. Stitzer, "Expired carbon monoxide levels in self-reported smokers and nonsmokers in prison," *Nicotine and Tobacco Research*, vol. 8, no. 5, pp. 653–659, 2006.

[21] SRNT Subcommittee on Biochemical Verification, "Biochemical verification of tobacco use and cessation," *Nicotine and Tobacco Research*, vol. 4, no. 2, pp. 149–159, 2002.

[22] SAS Institute, *The SAS System for Windows Version 9. 2. Cary*, SAS Institute, North Carolina, NC, USA, 2007.

[23] D. Indig, E. McEntyre, J. Page, and B. Ross, "2009 NSW inmate health survey," Aboriginal Health Report Appendix of Results, Justice Health, Sydney, Australia, 2010.

[24] Australian Bureau of Statistics, "National health survey: summary of results 2007-2008 Australia," ABS Cat. No. 4364.0, ABS, Canberra, Australia, 2010.

[25] S. J. McCann, "Subjective well-being, personality, demographic variables, and American state differences in smoking prevalence," *Nicotine & Tobacco Research*, vol. 12, no. 9, pp. 895–904, 2010.

[26] E. S. Soteriades and J. R. DiFranza, "Parent's socioeconomic status, adolescents' disposable income, and adolescents' smoking status in Massachusetts," *American Journal of Public Health*, vol. 93, no. 7, pp. 1155–1160, 2003.

[27] K. Stronks, H. D. van de Mheen, C. W. N. Looman, and J. P. Mackenbach, "Cultural, material, and psychosocial correlates of the socioeconomic gradient in smoking behavior among adults," *Preventive Medicine*, vol. 26, no. 5, pp. 754–766, 1997.

[28] R. A. Witter, M. A. Okun, W. A. Stock, and M. J. Haring, "Education and subjective well-being: a meta analysis." *Educational Evaluation and Policy Analysis*, vol. 6, no. 2, pp. 165–173, 1984.

[29] K. L. Cropsey and J. L. Kristeller, "Motivational factors related to quitting smoking among prisoners during a smoking ban," *Addictive Behaviors*, vol. 28, no. 6, pp. 1081–1093, 2003.

[30] K. L. Cropsey and J. L. Kristeller, "The effects of a prison smoking ban on smoking behavior and withdrawal symptoms," *Addictive Behaviors*, vol. 30, no. 3, pp. 589–594, 2005.

[31] R. Richmond, K. Wilhelm, D. Indig, T. Butler, V. Archer, and A. Wodak, "Cardiovascular risk among aboriginal and non-aboriginal smoking male prisoners: inequalities compared to the wider community," *BMC Public Health*, vol. 11, article 783, 2011.

[32] T. Butler, S. Allnutt, A. Kariminia, and D. Cain, "Mental health status of aboriginal and non-aboriginal Australian prisoners," *Australian and New Zealand Journal of Psychiatry*, vol. 41, no. 5, pp. 429–435, 2007.

[33] A. Kariminia, T. Butler, and M. Levy, "Aboriginal and non-aboriginal health differentials in Australian prisoners," *Australian and New Zealand Journal of Public Health*, vol. 31, no. 4, pp. 366–371, 2007.

[34] G. L. Humfleet and A. L. Haas, "Is marijuana use becoming a 'gateway' to nicotine dependence?" *Addiction*, vol. 99, no. 1, pp. 5–6, 2004.

[35] A. R. Clough, P. D'Abbs, S. Cairney et al., "Emerging patterns of cannabis and other substance use in Aboriginal communities in Arnhem Land, Northern Territory: a study of two communities," *Drug and Alcohol Review*, vol. 23, no. 4, pp. 381–390, 2004.

[36] J. A. Bowman and R. A. Walsh, "Smoking intervention within alcohol and other drug treatment services: a selective review with suggestions for practical management," *Drug and Alcohol Review*, vol. 22, no. 1, pp. 73–82, 2003.

[37] C. A. Patten, J. E. Martin, and N. Owen, "Can psychiatric and chemical dependency treatment units be smoke free?" *Journal of Substance Abuse Treatment*, vol. 13, no. 2, pp. 107–118, 1996.

[38] T. Butler and L. Milner, "The 2001 inmate health survey," Tech. Rep., NSW Corrections Health Service, Sydney, Australia, Canberra, Commonwealth of Australia, 2003, http://www.nationaldrugstrategy.gov.au/internet/drugstrategy/publishing.nsf/Content/nds2015.

20

Early Adolescents and Substance Use

Raimondo Maria Pavarin,[1] **and Dario Consonni**[2]

[1] *Epidemiological Monitoring Center on Addiction, DSM-DP, ASL Bologna, Via S. Isaia 94/A, 40100 Bologna, Italy*
[2] *Unit of Epidemiology, Department of Preventive Medicine, Fondazione IRCCS Ca' Granda-Ospedale Maggiore Policlinico, Via San Barnaba, 8-20122 Milan, Italy*

Correspondence should be addressed to Raimondo Maria Pavarin; raimondo.pavarin@ausl.bologna.it

Academic Editor: Raymond Niaura

1300 students (54.3% girls) 13–16 years old were interviewed in the urban area of Bologna during 2010. Random effect multiple logistic regression models were used. Results show a reciprocal relationship between alcohol use, tobacco, and cannabis. Most users were offered cannabis, began using at 14 years of age, and do not believe using is very dangerous. They live with only one parent, have more than 50 euros of spending money per month, and abuse alcohol, abuse that increases relative to the intensity of cigarette smoking. Legal/illegal dichotomy seems to overturn, where alcohol becomes a "drug" and the use of tobacco, similar to other drugs, is motivated as a solution to reduce anxiety, combat boredom, relax, and to ease loneliness.

1. Introduction

In Italy among 15 year olds, in the last year 9% have used cannabis at least once, 69% have used alcohol, and 34% have used tobacco, and this data increases at 16 years of age (17% cannabis, 80% alcohol, and 44% tobacco), with a greater prevalence of tobacco use among girls and alcohol and cannabis among boys [1]. Many try and then quit, but higher rates of continued use are evident for alcohol and tobacco [2].

Substance use in adolescence is an important predictor of possible continued use of illegal substances in adulthood, together with other risk factors: specific lifestyles outside the home (bar, discos, avd private parties), early start of sexual activity, a greater amount of spending money, frequenting urban environments or areas with a high prevalence and availability of illegal substances, the use of substances at home, family composition, and the development of various forms of sociability [3–9].

There is additional evidence that the decision to consume various substances is not connected only to specific contexts or individual characteristics, but that beliefs and expectations predict consumption styles. More recent studies are aimed at the decision-making processes of the adolescent where the possible costs and the potential expected benefits of consumption are considered [10–12]. In fact, given a set combination of experiences, abilities, information, and initiation of use, the choice of whether to use a substance followed by which to use, seems driven both by the function that it serves, as by the specific significances attributed to them by the consumer [13–22].

While most prevention programs are aimed at helping young people stay abstinent and to resist peer group pressure, there are few studies that describe the processes which drive the choice of utilizing diverse substances, studies that could help to develop and inform innovative approaches, especially in the education field and dissuasion efforts [17].

This study is aimed at identifying what drives early adolescents (13–16 years) to use substances.

2. Methods

Study Design and Participants. A cross-sectional study design was used. The target was composed of subjects between the ages of 13 and 16 years, recruited middle schools (third year) and high schools (first two years) in the province of Bologna.

In each school, there is a teacher who serves as a health referent, to whom a copy of the study protocol was sent and to whom the methodology and goals were explained.

At the participating schools, the interviewers, by appointment, met with the various classes, and after having explained to the students the goals and objectives of the study, they individually interviewed the young people in private who had obtained written permission from their parents.

To the young people, in addition to the guarantee of anonymity and the confidentiality of the interview, they were guaranteed that the results would not be separated by age group, but considered as a total. The interviews, carried out from February to May 2010, lasted approximately 10 minutes on average. Four interviewers who were experts in interacting with early adolescent were utilized.

Seven middle schools and two high schools participated.

Variables. A semistructured interview was created to be utilized in this study. Twenty people were interviewed in succession by two interviewers. Kappa statistics [23] were used to verify the comprehensibility of the questions, the congruity of the answers, and the interviewer's effect. The variables used obtained a K value over 0.50.

Variables utilized included demographic data (gender, age, domicile, and birth country); socioeconomic data (who do you live with, what grade, and monthly allowance); information about parents (occupational status); risk attributed to using various substances (score from 1 = *low* to 5 = *high*); use of substances in the last year (for each substance: age at first and last use, prevalent modality of use, modality of acquisition, and number of episodes of use); number of episodes of alcohol intoxication in the last year, and the CAGE test [24].

For each substance used, an open question was posed regarding the motive for use, and the responses were then codified into seven dichotomous variables (yes/no) after an analysis by a multidisciplinary team of experts including psychologists, psychiatrists, sociologists, and epidemiologists: to have fun and be with others, to improve sociability, curiosity, for pleasure, self-treatment for various types of malaise (anesthetic, analgesic, performance anxiety, and to alleviate sadness and depression), emulation, and to relax.

Statistical Analyses. Continuous and categorical variables were analyzed with Student's t and chi-squared test, respectively. To take into account possible correlation between students at each school, random effect multiple logistic regression models [25] were used to calculate odds ratios (ORs) with 95% confidence intervals (95% CI). All analyses were performed with Stata 11 [26].

3. Results

Study Subjects. A total of 1300 subjects were interviewed: 15.9% were 13 years old, 46.5% were 14 years old, 28.6% were 15 years old, and 8.9% were 16 years old. Slightly more than half were girls (54.3%), 8.9% were non-Italians. Just under half (48.8%) did not regularly receive an allowance, 43.5% received 50 euros or less each month, and 7.7% more than 50 euros (Table 1). Just more than one-third (36%) believed smoking cigarettes is not very dangerous, and 20% believed drinking alcohol is not very dangerous, 7% thought that cannabis is not very dangerous.

Regarding home life, 81.8% lived with both parents, 14.5% with their mother only, 1.3% with their father only, 2.5% with their mother and new partner, and 0.3% with their father and new partner.

At least one parent of 18.2% of subjects did not work: 1.7% of fathers were retired, 0.6% unemployed; 14% of mothers were housewives, 1.6% unemployed, and 0.2% retired.

Substances. Over the course of the last year, one subject in three smoked cigarettes, one in four drank alcohol, 14% were inebriated, 7% used illegal substances, and 48% were completely abstinent (Table 2).

Regarding illegal substances, 75 subjects used marijuana, 33 hashish, 6 hallucinogenic mushrooms, 3 cocaine, 3 ketamine green (all girls) 2 LSD (both boys), 1 "speed," and 1 salvia divinorum.

Average monthly expenditure for alcohol was 39 euros (data from 91 subjects), 42 euros for tobacco (data from 171 subjects), and 44 euros for cannabis (data from 37 subjects).

Alcohol. Average age of first use was around 13 years (boys 12.9, girls 13.1) and lasted two years (boys 2.6, girls 2.4). Boys had a higher prevalence of use and a lower perception of risk.

184 subjects were inebriated at least once in the last year, 3.7% at least five times, data that does not change based on gender.

With regard to the CAGE test, where there were no gender differences, 4% thought they should reduce their drinking, 2.6% experienced discomfort or feelings of guilt due to drinking habits, 1.5% drank alcohol at least once upon waking, and 1.3% were criticized for their drinking habits. 2.3% responded positive to at least two items on the test, 0.8% (10 subjects) to at least three.

Tobacco. The average age of first use was 13.4 years and lasted 2.1 years, with slight differences between boys and girls.

Girls had a higher prevalence of use and a lower perception of risk.

8% smoked fewer than 5 cigarettes a day, 4% from 5 to 9 cigarettes a day, and 4% more than 9, with more intense use among girls (more than 5 cigarettes a day: girls 9%, boys 6%).

Cannabis. For both genders the average age of first use was 14.2 years and lasted 1.5 years, 5% consumed very few times, and 1% more than 15 times in the last year.

Males had a higher prevalence of use and a lower perception of risk.

Regarding the modality of acquisition, to 61% of users it was offered, 34% used the same seller regularly, 6% acquired sporadically, and 5% sought out specific environments.

Subjects who used cannabis were younger on average when they started using tobacco (12.99 years, 95% CI 12.70–13.27) than those who did not use cannabis (13.46 years 95% CI 13.35–13.58, $P = 0.0003$).

Risk Profiles. To construct a profile of users of various substances, a multivariate analysis was carried out using logistic regression (Table 3). To take into account possible correlations between students at each school, random effect multiple logistic regression models were used to calculate odds ratios (ORs) and 95% confidence intervals (95% CI). The variables used in the model were gender, age, housing situation, parental occupational status, economic availability, perception of risk, and substance used (number of obs 1300).

TABLE 1: Characteristics of interviewed subjects.

		Males (594)	Females (706)	Males %	Females %	P
Age (years)	13	97	110	16.3	15.6	0.48
	14	280	325	47.1	46.0	
	15	172	200	29.0	28.3	
	16	45	71	7.6	10.1	
Nationality	Italian	530	654	89.2	92.6	0.03
	Other	64	52	10.8	7.4	
Lives with	Both natural parents	501	556	84.3	78.8	0.04
	Only one parent	78	127	13.1	18.0	
	Stepfamily	15	22	2.5	3.1	
Do parents work?	Only one	110	127	18.5	18.0	0.81
	Both	484	579	81.5	82.0	
Monthly allowance	≤50 euros	266	300	44.8	42.5	0.68
	>50 euros	46	54	7.7	7.7	
	No allowance	282	352	49.9	47.5	

TABLE 2: Substances used in the last year.

		Males (594)	Females (706)	Total (1300)	Males %	Females %	Total %	P
Alcohol	Abstinent	424	544	968	74.4	77.1	74.5	0.05
	Alcohol, no inebriation	80	69	149	11.5	9.8	11.5	
	Inebriation	90	93	183	14.1	13.2	14.1	
	Low perception of risk	156	109	265	26.3	15.4	20.4	<0.001
Tobacco	Abstinent	419	478	897	70.5	67.7	69.0	0.25
	<5 cigarettes/day	137	166	303	23.1	23.5	23.3	
	≥5 cigarettes/day	38	62	100	6.4	8.8	7.7	
	Low perception of risk	230	235	465	38.7	33.3	35.8	0.12
Cannabis	Abstinent	547	668	1215	92.1	94.6	93.5	0.14
	<15 episodes	39	29	68	6.6	4.1	5.2	
	≥15 episodes	8	9	17	1.4	1.3	1.3	
	Low perception of risk	53	38	91	8.9	5.4	7.0	0.03

Regarding alcohol use, the following users were highlighted: males, with more than 50 euros a month to spend, had a low perception of the dangers of alcohol, who used tobacco (increases with intensity) and cannabis.

Regarding tobacco use, the following stands out: females, with both parents employed, who had a low perception of the dangers of tobacco, used alcohol and cannabis. Probability increased in subjects with recent episodes of inebriation.

Regarding cannabis the following were highlighted: males, who lived with only one parent, who had more than 50 euros a month to spend, and a low perception of the dangers of cannabis, used tobacco (increases with intensity) and had recent episodes of inebriation.

Those Who Abstain. The same analysis, repeated for those who abstain entirely, highlighted subjects who live with both

parents (OR 1.36, 95% CI 1.0–1.86), had less than 50 euros to spend per month (OR 2.93, 95% CI 1.84–4.66), with only one parent employed (OR 1.94, 95% CI 1.39–2.72), and had a high perception of the dangers of alcohol (OR 1.44, 95% CI 1.11–1.87), tobacco (OR 1.95, 95% CI 1.41–2.71), and cannabis (OR 1.95, 95% CI 1.48–2.55).

Motives of Use. Tobacco use was motivated by curiosity (37%), pleasure (17%), emulation (10%), relax (7%), and self-treatment (7%); alcohol is associated with entertainment (30%), sociability (26%), curiosity (19%), and pleasure (15%); cannabis is used out of curiosity (48%), sociability (25%), pleasure (14%), and entertainment (11%).

Seven variables were constructed, derived from adding the motives of use of any substance (40% used out of curiosity, 22% to improve social relations, 21% to have fun, 19% for

TABLE 3: Profile of subjects who used substances in the last year—random effect multiple logistic regression[*].

	Alcohol[**]		Tobacco[**]		Cannabis[**]	
	OR	95% CI	OR	95% CI	OR	95% CI
Male	1.44	1.06–1.96	0.72	0.54–0.95	2.81	1.48–5.34
Lives with only one parent	1.12	0.75–1.66	1.03	0.71–1.50	2.44	1.21–4.92
Both parents work	1.23	0.80–1.89	2.01	1.32–3.05	1.81	0.64–5.06
Monthly allowance > 50 €	1.78	1.08–2.95	1.58	0.96–2.59	2.35	1.10–5.02
Low alcohol risk	1.92	1.35–2.74	0.74	0.51–1.07	0.68	0.33–1.39
Low tobacco risk	1.05	0.77–1.44	1.89	1.41–2.53	1.17	0.61–2.23
Low cannabis risk	1.27	0.71–2.26	1.53	0.85–2.75	14.20	6.68–30.18
Tobacco abstinent	1.00	—	1.00	—	1	
<5 cigarettes/day	3.08	2.24–4.24			2.88	1.27–6.50
≥5 cigarettes/day	14.38	7.86–26.29			23.31	9.49–57.27
Alcohol abstinent	—	—	1.00		1.00	—
Alcohol no inebriation			2.26	1.53–3.33	1.26	0.46–3.41
Alcohol inebriation			7.66	5.09–11.53	4.33	2.07–9.04
Use of cannabis						
No	1.00	—	1.00	—	—	—
Yes	2.74	1.41–5.31	5.31	2.59–10.86		

[*]Adjusted by age, [**]Number of obs 1300.

TABLE 4: Motives substances use—random effect multiple logistic regression model[*].

	Tobacco			Alcohol			Cannabis		
	Yes/no	OR	95% CI	Yes/no	OR	95% CI	Yes/no	OR	95% CI
Entertainment	77/324	1.45	0.87–2.42	111/221	76.12	30.12–192.41	31/54	1.76	0.98–3.18
Sociability	77/324	1.54	0.94–2.53	99/233	15.93	9.10–27.87	32/53	2.0	1.12–3.57
Curiosity	177/224	13.69	9.17–20.43	116/216	1.99	1.36–2.89	45/40	1.75	1.02–3.01
Pleasure	87/314	8.08	4.52–14.46	72/260	3.21	1.95–5.31	34/51	2.55	1.44–5.23
Emulation	40/361	15.85	4.40–39.20	24/308	1.64	0.84–3.20	4/81	0.41	0.13–1.27
Relax	31/370	47.59	6.28–360.50	23/309	3.35	1.43–7.84	7/78	1.02	0.40–2.64
Self-treatment	31/370	18.59	5.38–64.28	18/314	0.96	0.42–2.16	10/75	2.14	0.87–5.26

[*]Adjusted for gender and age.

pleasure, 8% to emulate others, 6% to self-treat, and 6% for relaxation), and the probability of use was calculated of the various substances adjusting for gender and age.

Considering values that were statistically significant at 95%, the use of any substance to emulate others and self-treat was more probable for those who smoked cigarettes; consumption for entertainment reasons was more probable for those who use alcohol; relaxation was a motivation for those who use alcohol or tobacco; increasing sociability was probable for who use alcohol or cannabis; for pleasure and for curiosity instead seemed to motivate use of all three different substances (Table 4).

4. Discussion

The results, which show a high use of tobacco and widespread alcohol abuse, indicate a relationship between use of substances, parental absence, a lot of spending money and low perception of risk. This is confirmed by the profiles of

abstinent subjects, from families with one parent employed outside the house, with less than 50 euro available a month, and who had a high perception of the dangers of the various substances.

The probability of using alcohol was higher for males, who had more money available, and increased as cigarette smoking increased.

With regard to tobacco, the probability of recent use was higher among females, among subjects whose parents both work, and among those who used alcohol or cannabis.

Most cannabis users were offered the drug, began using at 14 and were more likely to not believe it as very dangerous, lived with only one parent, had more than 50 euros spending money per month, abused alcohol, and use increased as cigarette smoking increased. It is notable that these subjects began smoking cigarettes before others did.

With regard to motives of use, except for curiosity and pleasure-seeking, which seemed common to all substances, self-treatment and emulation appeared specific for tobacco users, and entertainment for users of alcohol, while use for relaxation affected both; improving social relations was more probable among those who used alcohol or cannabis.

With regard to available spending money and use of the various substances, previous studies have found a relationship to smoking even small amounts of tobacco [27–29], an increase in use of illegal substances in relation to increasing monetary availability [30], and an increase in alcohol use related to increases in available spending money for leisure time activities [31]. Contrary to expectation, some studies have reported that adolescents from higher social classes presented a significantly higher percentage of alcohol and tobacco consumption than their counterparts from lower social classes, while others have reported a greater risk to start smoking cigarettes, marijuana, and drinking alcohol related to situations of socioeconomic disadvantage [32, 33].

The reciprocal relationship between use of various legal and illegal substances has been reported by recent studies, where the importance of this aspect has been presented regarding the planning of prevention strategies [34, 35].

With regard to risk attributed to the use of various substances, we found confirmation of studies of tobacco and marijuana, where the subjective perception of dangerous behavior seemed to exercise a protective function [36, 37].

With regard to family, a protective effect was shown for intact families (both father and mother), where particular attention was reported regarding adolescents in transition into new family structures [38, 39]. Parental control seemed initially to prevent marijuana use, but the effects weakened throughout adolescence [40].

5. Conclusions

This study presents some objective limits that indicate prudence in generalizing the results: only subjects who obtained consent from their parents were interviewed and the information communicated in the interviews could have been influenced by various factors, including the situation and the location. Despite this, the results offer useful indications for future prevention projects specific to early adolescents.

Family composition, available spending money, and risk perception seem to influence nonconsumption more than consumption, suggesting that they should be considered as protective factors that work together, to use as indicators of a serene environment, communication, and parental presence. In fact, when only one parent works, there was a low availability of spending money and a high perception of risk connected to use of any substance; there was a higher probability of finding subjects who were completely abstinent.

A strong association was shown between the use of alcohol, tobacco, and cannabis, where we found that those who used a specific substance did not believe it to be very dangerous. Particularly, a relationship was reported between early use of tobacco and later use of cannabis, which seems to delineate a specific progression, warranting further study. With regard to money, greater availability seemed to play a role in the use of alcohol and cannabis, but not in the use of

tobacco. While various substances were consumed for similar reasons, providing plausible explanations to the succession of use and poly use, we found emulation and self-treatment to be specific motivations for tobacco use and entertainment to be specific for alcohol use.

Among early adolescents, the legal/illegal dichotomy seems to overturn, where alcohol loses its functions related to alimentation and social relationships to become a "drug" for all intents and purposes, and the use of tobacco, similar to other drugs, is motivated as a solution to reduce anxiety, combat boredom, relax, and to ease loneliness.

Conflict of Interests

The authors report no conflict of interests.

References

[1] http://www.epid.ifc.cnr.it/Espad/materiale.htm.

[2] EMCDDA, "Annual report on the state of the drugs problem in Europe 2010," Lisbon, Portugal, 2010, http://www.emcdda.europa.eu.

[3] W. Latimer and J. Zur, "Epidemiologic trends of adolescent use of alcohol, tobacco, and other drugs," *Child and Adolescent Psychiatric Clinics of North America*, vol. 19, no. 3, pp. 451–464, 2010.

[4] A. W. Tu, P. A. Ratner, and J. L. Johnson, "Gender differences in the correlates of adolescents' cannabis use," *Substance Use and Misuse*, vol. 43, no. 10, pp. 1438–1463, 2008.

[5] M. Guxens, M. Nebot, and C. Ariza, "Age and sex differences in factors associated with the onset of cannabis use: a cohort study," *Drug and Alcohol Dependence*, vol. 88, no. 2-3, pp. 234–243, 2007.

[6] M. R. Hayatbakhsh, J. M. Najman, W. Bor, M. J. O'Callaghan, and G. M. Williams, "Multiple risk factor model predicting cannabis use and use disorders: a longitudinal study," *American Journal of Drug and Alcohol Abuse*, vol. 35, no. 6, pp. 399–407, 2009.

[7] M. Nation and C. A. Heflinger, "Risk factors for serious alcohol and drug use: the role of psychosocial variables in predicting the frequency of substance use among adolescents," *American Journal of Drug and Alcohol Abuse*, vol. 32, no. 3, pp. 415–433, 2006.

[8] I. Sutherland and J. P. Shepherd, "Social dimensions of adolescent substance use," *Addiction*, vol. 96, no. 3, pp. 445–458, 2001.

[9] OEDT-Focus sulle droghe, "Misurare la prevalenza e l'incidenza del consumo di stupefacenti," 2002, http://www.emcdda.europa.eu/attachements.cfm/att_33481_IT_Dif03it.pdf.

[10] H. Parker, J. Aldridge, F. Measham, and P. Haynes, *Illegal Leisure: The Normalisation of Adolescent Recreational Drug Use*, Routledge, London, UK, 1998.

[11] H. Parker, L. Williams, and J. Aldridge, "The normalization of 'sensible' recreational drug use: further evidence from the North West England longitudinal study," *Sociology*, vol. 36, no. 4, pp. 941–964, 2002.

[12] F. Measham and M. Shiner, "The legacy of 'normalisation': the role of classical and contemporary criminological theory in understanding young people's drug use," *International Journal of Drug Policy*, vol. 20, no. 6, pp. 502–508, 2009.

[13] W. M. Cox and E. Klinger, "A motivational model of alcohol use," *Journal of Abnormal Psychology*, vol. 97, no. 2, pp. 168–180, 1988.

[14] E. Kuntsche, R. Knibbe, G. Gmel, and R. Engels, "Why do young people drink? A review of drinking motives," *Clinical Psychology Review*, vol. 25, no. 7, pp. 841–861, 2005.

[15] A. van der Poel, G. Rodenburg, M. Dijkstra, M. Stoele, and D. van de Mheen, "Trends, motivations and settings of recreational cocaine use by adolescents and young adults in the Netherlands," *International Journal of Drug Policy*, vol. 20, no. 2, pp. 143–151, 2009.

[16] T. M. Brunt, M. van Laar, R. J. M. Niesink, and W. van den Brink, "The relationship of quality and price of the psychostimulants cocaine and amphetamine with health care outcomes," *Drug and Alcohol Dependence*, vol. 111, no. 1-2, pp. 21–29, 2010.

[17] A. Boys, J. Marsden, and J. Strang, "Understanding reasons for drug use amongst young people: a functional perspective," *Health Education Research*, vol. 16, no. 4, pp. 457–469, 2001.

[18] A. Boys and J. Marsden, "Perceived functions predict intensity of use and problems in young polysubstance users," *Addiction*, vol. 98, no. 7, pp. 951–963, 2003.

[19] A. Boys, J. Marsden, P. Griffiths, and J. Strang, "Drug use functions predict cocaine-related problems in young people," *Drug and Alcohol Review*, vol. 19, no. 2, pp. 181–190, 2000.

[20] J. Ahmadi and A. Ghanizadeh, "Motivations for use of opiates among addicts seeking treatment in shiraz," *Psychological Reports*, vol. 87, no. 3, pp. 1158–1164, 2000.

[21] C. M. Lee, C. Neighbors, and B. A. Woods, "Marijuana motives: young adults' reasons for using marijuana," *Addictive Behaviors*, vol. 32, no. 7, pp. 1384–1394, 2007.

[22] M. J. Zvolensky, A. A. Vujanovic, A. Bernstein, M. O. Bonn-Miller, E. C. Marshall, and T. M. Leyro, "Marijuana use motives: a confirmatory test and evaluation among young adult marijuana users," *Addictive Behaviors*, vol. 32, no. 12, pp. 3122–3130, 2007.

[23] B. K. Armstrong, E. White, and R. Saracci, *Principles of Exposure Measurement in Epidemiology*, Oxford University Press, Oxford, 1992.

[24] M. W. Bernadt, J. Mumford, and C. Taylor, "Comparison of questionnaire and laboratory tests in the detection of excessive drinking and alcoholism," *Lancet*, vol. 1, no. 8267, pp. 325–328, 1982.

[25] N. J. Horton, "Review of multilevel and longitudinal modeling using Stata, second edition, by Sophia Rabe-Hesketh and Anders Skrondal," *Stata Journal*, vol. 8, no. 4, pp. 579–582, 2008.

[26] StataCorp, "Stata: release 11. statistical software," StataCorp LP, College Station, Tex, USA, 2009.

[27] J. Van Reek, R. Knibbe, and T. Van Iwaarden, "Policy elements as predictors of smoking and drinking behaviour: the Dutch cohort study of secondary schoolchildren," *Health Policy*, vol. 26, no. 1, pp. 5–18, 1993.

[28] C. Reddy-Jacobs, M. M. Téllez-Rojo, F. Meneses-González, J. Campuzano-Rincón, and M. Hernández-Ávila, "Poverty, youth and consumption of tobacco in Mexico," *Salud Publica de Mexico*, vol. 48, no. 3, supplement 1, pp. S83–S90, 2006.

[29] D. Kostova, H. Ross, E. Blecher, and S. Markowitz, "Is youth smoking responsive to cigarette prices? Evidence from low- and middle-income countries," *Tobacco Control*, vol. 20, no. 6, pp. 419–424, 2011.

[30] M. S. Burrone, S. M. Bueno, M. L. de Costa Jr., J. Enders, R. A. Fernández, and G. P. Vasters, "Análisis de la frecuencia de experimentación y consumo de drogas de alumnos de escuelas de nivel medio," *Revista Latino-Americana de Enfermagem*, vol. 18, pp. 648–654, 2010.

[31] O. Rahkonen and S. Ahlstrom, "Trends in drinking habits among Finnish youth from 1973 to 1987," *British Journal of Addiction*, vol. 84, no. 9, pp. 1075–1083, 1989.

[32] E. M. M. Pratta and M. A. Dos Santos, "Adolescence and the consumption of psychoactive substances: the impact of the socioeconomic status," *Revista Latino-Americana de Enfermagem*, vol. 15, pp. 806–811, 2007.

[33] M. Lemstra, N. R. Bennett, C. Neudorf et al., "A meta-analysis of marijuana and alcohol use by socio-economic status in adolescents aged 10—15 years," *Canadian Journal of Public Health*, vol. 99, no. 3, pp. 172–177, 2008.

[34] E. G. García, B. C. Blasco, R. J. López, and A. P. Pol, "Study of the factors associated with substance use in adolescence using association rules," *Adicciones*, vol. 22, no. 4, pp. 293–299, 2010.

[35] I. K. Wium-Andersen, M. K. Wium-Andersen, U. Becker, and S. F. Thomsen, "Predictors of age at onset of tobacco and cannabis use in Danish adolescents," *Clinical Respiratory Journal*, vol. 4, no. 3, pp. 162–167, 2010.

[36] N. Doran, P. E. Sanders, N. M. Bekman et al., "Mediating influences of negative affect and risk perception on the relationship between sensation seeking and adolescent cigarette smoking nicotine," *Nicotine & Tobacco Research*, vol. 13, no. 6, pp. 457–465, 2011.

[37] C. Lopez-Quintero and Y. Neumark, "Effects of risk perception of marijuana use on marijuana use and intentions to use among adolescents in Bogotá, Colombia," *Drug and Alcohol Dependence*, vol. 109, no. 1-3, pp. 65–72, 2010.

[38] R. J. Paxton, R. F. Valois, and J. W. Drane, "Is there a relationship between family structure and substance use among public middle school students?" *Journal of Child and Family Studies*, vol. 16, no. 5, pp. 593–605, 2007.

[39] V. Hemovich, A. Lac, and W. D. Crano, "Understanding early-onset drug and alcohol outcomes among youth: the role of family structure, social factors, and interpersonal perceptions of use," *Psychology, Health and Medicine*, vol. 16, no. 3, pp. 249–267, 2011.

[40] Z. Tang and R. G. Orwin, "Marijuana initiation among American youth and its risks as dynamic processes: prospective findings from a national longitudinal study," *Substance Use and Misuse*, vol. 44, no. 2, pp. 195–211, 2009.

21

Involvement in Specific HIV Risk Practices among Men Who Use the Internet to Find Male Partners for Unprotected Sex

Hugh Klein

Kensington Research Institute, 401 Schuyler Road, Silver Spring, MD 20910, USA

Correspondence should be addressed to Hugh Klein; hughk@aol.com

Academic Editor: Jennifer B. Unger

Purpose. Men who have sex with other men (MSM) account for more than one-half of all new HIV infections in the USA. This study reports on the prevalence of a variety of HIV risk behaviors in one specific subpopulation of risk-seeking MSM. *Methods.* The study was based on a national sample of 332 MSM who use the Internet to find partners for unprotected sex. Data collection was conducted via telephone interviews between January 2008 and May 2009. *Results.* Unprotected oral and anal sex was commonplace among study participants. Men engaged in a large number of other risky behaviors as well, including having had multiple recent sex partners (mean number = 11), simultaneous double-penile penetration of the anus (16%), eating semen out of another man's anus (17%), engaging in multiple-partner sexual encounters (47%), engaging in anonymous sex (51%), and having sex while "under the influence" (52%). *Conclusions.* HIV intervention and prevention programs need to address numerous behaviors that place MSM at risk for contracting/transmitting HIV. Merely focusing on unprotected anal sex does a disservice to members of this community, who typically engage in many types of behavioral risks, each of which requires addressing if HIV transmission rates are to be reduced.

1. Introduction

In recent years, evidence has been mounting to suggest that men who have sex with other men (MSM) increasingly are turning to the Internet to meet partners for sex. For example, in a sample of gay men who were recruited into a health promotion study via gay-oriented Internet websites, Bolding and colleagues' [1] multivariate analysis revealed that the amount of risky sex in which men engaged was a significant predictor of their use of Internet websites to locate sex partners. Bolding et al. also reported that 47% of the men in their sample said that, when they wanted to identify potential sex partners, they preferred using websites to frequenting bars or other "offline" venues. In another study [2], among men actively using the Internet as a means of locating potential sex partners, 97% reported actually having met someone online for sex, and 86% said that they used Internet MSM sex sites at least once a week to identify possible partners. Ogilvie and colleagues [3] found that MSM who used the Internet to initiate sexual relationships reported having had more sex partners during the previous year than their counterparts who did not use the Internet for this purpose. Berg [4] noted that, compared

with men who did not engage in bareback sex, barebacking men said that they met their sex partners online rather than offline more than twice as frequently. More recently, based on their study of gay and bisexual men traveling to a major Gay Pride celebration, Benotsch and colleagues [5] found that men who used the Internet to set up "dates" prior to their travel acknowledged having more sex partners and were more likely to report having sex with a new partner than men who did not use the Internet to identify potential sex partners prior to their vacation travel.

Not only are MSM using the Internet more frequently to meet potential sex partners, but they also appear to be using it specifically to find partners with whom they can engage in risky sexual acts. For example, based on their research on MSM in the Seattle area, Menza and colleagues [6] reported that the proportion of anal sex partners who had met online increased significantly from 2003 to 2006. Halkitis et al. [7] cited Internet websites and chat rooms as key sources that are partly responsible for the upsurge of unprotected sexual activities that they have observed among gay and bisexual men in the New York City area. In their study of rural versus urban MSM, Kakietek et al. [8] found that Internet use was associated with an increased risk for engaging in unprotected anal sex overall and, in particularly, an increased risk for engaging in unprotected insertive anal sex for the rural men in their sample. Rosser and colleagues's [9] study of men visiting one of the Internet's most-popular gay-oriented websites noted that reliance upon the Internet to identify sex partners was associated with approximately a doubling of the number of times engaging in unprotected anal intercourse with male partners.

It should be noted, however, that not all studies have found that using the Internet to meet sex partners is associated with increased risk. Examples include Chiasson et al. [10], Coleman et al. [11], Mustanski [12], and Mustanski and Newcomb [13]. Moreover, mixed results have been reported by other researchers (e.g., [14]), whose work found that barebacking MSM spent more time on the Internet looking for sex while simultaneously engaging in greater serosorting practices. Mixed findings were also reported by Jenness and colleagues [15], whose work showed that it was not meeting partners online per se that was associated with elevated HIV risk involvement among MSM, but rather, it is the combination of meeting some partners online and others offline that led to heightened risk for HIV. Although their findings were of borderline statistical significance, Berry et al. [16] concluded that using the Internet to identify sex partners is associated with an increased risk of engaging in unprotected anal intercourse among HIV-negative MSM, but not among HIV-positive MSM.

One argument that is made occasionally is that men using the Internet for the purported purpose of identifying sex partners may not, in actuality, be using it for that purpose. Instead, it has been suggested that the act of searching through profiles online may be an erotic act for some men, who have no realistic intention of meeting in person anyone with whom they have interacted online. For these persons, posting a sex-related profile online or responding to other people's online postings may be expressions of fantasy or manifestations of symbolic preferences rather than actual sexual desires. Published studies have shown that fantasizing about engaging in unprotected sex is related to lower intentions to use condoms during actual sexual situations [17] and, thus, is not a purely harmless behavior in and of itself. Moreover, research has also shown that MSM who use the Internet with the intention/hope of meeting partners face to face rather than limiting themselves exclusively to the online interaction are more likely to discuss unprotected sex and less likely to talk about sexual safety with those online-met partners [18]. Furthermore, based on a large-scale content analysis study of one of the largest bareback-focused websites on the Internet, Klein [19] concluded that "men who use the Internet to locate sexual partners are very likely to meet up with such individuals for sex (i.e., their ads/profiles are, far more often than not, not posted purely for fun, but rather with sexual hook-ups in mind) suggest[ing] that there may not be a great disconnect between ad/profile content and behavioral practices."

This leaves open the question of what risky behaviors are practiced "in real life" (as distinguished from fantasized sexual behaviors that are promised in online profiles or "cybersex" behaviors that are discussed online in chats/conversations that do not lead to in-person sexual encounters) by MSM who use the Internet to identify partners for sex. Although numerous authors (cited previously) have reported that identifying sex partners via the Internet is associated with involvement in risky behaviors vis-a-vis HIV, their research has provided very little information about the extent to which men seeking sex online engage in specific behaviors that place them or their sex partners at risk for contracting HIV. This is the subject of the present report.

This paper examines the extent to which one specific subpopulation of MSM (namely, those who use the Internet for the express purpose of finding partners with whom they can engage in unprotected sex) engages in various behaviors that place them and their sex partners at risk for contracting HIV. The research contributes to the scholarly literature by documenting the prevalence of specific risk practices undertaken when members of this population use the Internet to find sex partners. Moreover, this paper provides information about a variety of risk behaviors that have not been discussed much in the scholarly literature, but which are practiced with relative frequency by MSM. Included among these less-well-researched/discussed high-risk practices are ejaculating internally during sex, simultaneous double-penile penetration, oral-anal contact, sharing of previously used but uncleaned sex toys, multiple-partner sexual encounters, the number of drug-related problems experienced, and men's preferences for engaging in sexual relations while under the influence of alcohol and other drugs. Additionally, throughout the paper, comparisons of risk involvement are provided for men who are HIV-positive and those who are HIV-negative, as HIV serostatus has been found to be a strong predictor of risk behavior practices among MSM [20, 21]. The paper concludes by discussing the implications of these findings for prevention and intervention.

2. Methods

2.1. Procedures. The data reported in this paper come from *The Bareback Project*, a National Institute on Drug Abuse-funded study of men who use the Internet specifically to find other men with whom they can engage in unprotected sex. The data were collected between January 2008 and May 2009. A total of 332 men were recruited from 16 different websites. Some of the sites catered exclusively to unprotected sex (e.g., http://www.bareback .com/, http://www.barebackrt.com/) and some of them did not but made it possible for site users to identify which persons were looking for unprotected sex (e.g., http://www .men4sexnow.com/). In order to be eligible to participate in the study, men had to be aged 18 or older—a requirement that eliminated almost nobody because all of the sites used for this study required men to certify their age as that of an adult before they could become members or site users. In addition, participants had to be residents of the United States, so as to keep this a USA-focused study.

A nationwide sample of men was derived, with random selection being based on a combination of the first letter of the person's online username, his race/ethnicity (as listed in his profile), and the day of recruitment. Each day, members of the research staff working on recruitment had three letters or numerals assigned to them for their use that day. These letters and numerals were assigned randomly, using the software available at http://www.random.org/ (substituting the numbers 1 to 26 to represent, sequentially, the letters of the alphabet, and then using numbers after that to represent numerals). The first letter/numeral was restricted for use for recruiting Caucasian men only; the last two letters/numerals were to be used exclusively for recruiting men of color. (This oversampling technique for racial minority group men was adopted so as to compensate for the fact that men of color, especially African-American men, are more difficult to recruit into research studies than their Caucasian counterparts are.) In order for a particular person to be approached and asked to participate in the study, these letters/numerals had to correspond to the first letter/numeral of that individual's profile and that person's race/ethnicity, as stated in his profile, had to be a match for the Caucasian-versus-racial-minority-group-member designation on the daily randomization listing.

On recruitment sites where it was possible to know who was online at the time the recruiter was working, selection of potential study participants came from the pool of men who happened to be logged onto the site during the time block when the recruiter was working. All men who were online at the time the recruiter was working and whose profile name began with the appropriate letter/numeral were eligible to be approached. On recruitment sites where it was not possible to know who was online at the time the recruiter was working, ZIP codes were used to narrow down the pool of men who could be approached. To do this, in addition to the daily three letters/numerals that were assigned randomly to each recruiter throughout the study, each day, ten five-digit numbers were also assigned to each recruiter (five to be used for Caucasian men, five to be used for men of color). These five-digit numbers were random number combinations generated by the http://www.random.org/ software, and they were used in this study as proxies for ZIP codes. Recruiters entered the first five-digit number into the website's ZIP code search field (which site users typically utilized to identify potential sex partners who resided within a specified radius from their residence), selected a five-mile radius, and then viewed the profile names of all men meeting those criteria who had logged onto that site within the previous 24 hours. Those men were eligible to be invited to participate, and their profiles were reviewed for the letter/numeral match described previously for men who were online at the time that recruiters were working.

Recruitment efforts were undertaken seven days a week, during all hours of the day and nighttime, variable from week to week throughout the duration of the project. This was done to maximize the representativeness of the final research sample, in recognition of the fact that different people use the Internet at different times.

Depending upon the website involved, men were approached initially either via instant message or email (much more commonly via email). A brief overview of the study was provided as part of the initial approach and informed consent-related procedures, and all men were given the opportunity to ask questions about the study before deciding whether or not to participate.[1] A website link to the project's online home page was also made available, to provide men with additional information about the project and to help them feel secure in the legitimacy of the research endeavor. Interviews were conducted during all hours of the day and nighttime, seven days a week, based on interviewer availability and participants' preferences, to maximize convenience to the participants. Over the course of the 17-month study period, no person could be approached more than five times (once every 90 days) and asked to participate. Anyone who specifically indicated that he was not interested in taking part in the study was listed on the daily-updated contacts list as "no further contact—refused" and was not contacted again.

Participation in the study entailed the completion of a one-time, confidential telephone interview covering a wide array of topics. The decision to conduct the data collection via telephone interviews rather than via anonymous online surveys was made for a number of reasons. First, telephone interviews allowed the research team members to establish rapport with respondents, and this was deemed critical in light of the length of the questionnaire and the very personal nature of the questions being asked. Second, using telephone interviews enabled the research team to make sure that study participants understood all of the questions (something that cannot be achieved when online survey techniques are used) and helped people to "think through" some of the more complex questions asked during the interview. Third, *The Bareback Project* was a mixed-methods study, involving the collection of both quantitative and qualitative data. The latter would have been precluded had only an online survey been implemented.

The questionnaire was developed specifically for use in *The Bareback Project*, with many parts of the interview derived from standardized scales previously used and validated by other researchers. The interview covered such subjects as degree of "outness," perceived discrimination based on sexual orientation, general health practices, HIV testing history and serostatus, sexual practices (protected and unprotected) with partners met online and offline, risk-related preferences, risk-related hypotheticals, substance use, drug-related problems, Internet usage, psychological and psychosocial functioning, childhood maltreatment experiences, HIV/AIDS knowledge, and some basic demographic information. Interviews lasted an average of 69 minutes (median = 63, s.d. = 20.1, range = 30–210). Men who completed the interview were compensated $35 for their time. Prior to implementation in the field, the research protocol was approved by the institutional review boards at Morgan State University, where the principal investigator and one of the research assistants were affiliated, and George Mason University, where the other research assistant was located.

2.2. Measures Used. Men were asked separate questions about the number of different men with whom they had had *any* kind of sex during the past 30 days (continuous measure) and over the course of their lifetimes (continuous). Men who initially responded "don't know" were instructed "Please take a moment and think about it, and give me a number that you know is definitely safe—that is, the number of men with whom you have had any kind of sex that you know "It is definitely no less than |x| persons. For example, you definitely had sex with no fewer than 3 men, or no fewer than 30 men, or no fewer than 300 men, and so forth." In this manner, self-reports of the number of sex partners range from accurate to conservative estimates.

For insertive oral sex, receptive oral sex, insertive anal sex, and receptive anal sex, separate questions were asked about the number of times engaging in each behavior during the previous 30 days (continuous), the number of partners with whom men had engaged in each behavior during that time frame (continuous), the number of those times in which the insertive partner wore a condom (continuous), and the number of those times that the receptive partner received ejaculatory fluid directly inside of his mouth or anus (continuous). For these specific behaviors, men were also asked how many of the men in question were people who had met online, how many times they had each type of sex with those online-met partners, how many of those situations involved the use of a condom, and how many of those sex acts involved internal ejaculation.

Subsequently, participants were asked several questions (all using a past-30-days time frame of reference, all continuous measures) about their involvement in other sexual practices. The first questions asked about "the number of times that you and another man both put your penises into another man's anus at the same time" (i.e., double fucking), "the number of times that two men both put their penises into your anus at the same time" (i.e., being double fucked), and for both of these behaviors, the number of times that at least one of the insertive partners ejaculated directly inside of the receptive partner's anus. Men were also asked "How many times did you have sex where you put your mouth or tongue onto or inside of another man's anus?" (i.e., rimming) and then "How many of these times had you or someone else ejaculated into this man's anus beforehand?" (i.e., felching) and then "And how many of those times did you then feed the semen to one of your sex partners by a kiss or drooling it onto or into his mouth?" (i.e., snowballing). Information about sharing sex toys was obtained by asking men "How many times have you had sex where a sex toy like a dildo or a butt plug was used inside of you?" and then "How many of those times had that item been used by your partner beforehand, without being cleaned before you used it?" and then "How many times of those times did you give the sex toy to your partner to use, without cleaning it first?" Information about "pimping out" a sex partner or "being pimped out" by a sex partner was gathered by asking "How many times have you had sex where your partner brought several other men to have sex with you? Some people call this being passed around or being pimped out by your partner" and then "How many times have you had sex where you brought several men to have sex with your partner? Some people call this passing around the partner or pimping him out." Men's practices of multiple-partner sex were ascertained by asking "How many times have you had any kind of sex in a three-way arrangement, where you and your partner had one other man join you for sex?" and then "How many of those times were condom used [by anyone involved]?" and then "How many

times have you had any kind of sex involving more than a total of three people—what some people call group sex or orgies?" and then "How many of those times were condoms used [by anyone involved]?" To learn about men's anonymous sex practices, the questions read as follows: "Some people like to have anonymous sex—that is, sex with persons they know nothing about—and some people do not like to do this. Do you like having anonymous sex?" and then "How many times during the past 30 days have you had anonymous sex of any kind with someone?".

Drug use behaviors were inquired about in a separate section of the questionnaire. There, men were asked about lifetime usage (yes/no), age of first use (continuous), number of days of use during the preceding 30 days (continuous), number of times using on a "typical" day of use during the past 30 days (continuous), and the number of times using shortly before having sex with someone or while having sex with someone (continuous). These questions were asked separately for alcohol, marijuana, powdered cocaine, crack cocaine, heroin or other opiates, hallucinogens, ecstasy, club drugs other than ecstasy (e.g., ketamine/"Special K," GHB, etc.), methamphetamine, Viagra or its equivalent (excluded from the present paper's analysis of "illegal drug use"), and sedatives or depressant drugs that were not prescribed by a physician. The format for these questions was derived from the substance use section of the widely used, validated, and reliability-tested *Risk Behavior Assessment* [22]. Additionally, men were asked "Suppose for the moment that you could have access to any type of drugs you wanted—alcohol, cocaine, whatever. Which types of drugs, if any, would you yourself most like to use shortly before you had sex with someone or while you were having sex?" This question was constructed specifically for use in this study. Men were also asked about their lifetime and past-30-days experiences with 14 types of substance abuse problems (each asked in yes/no format), including needing more of a drug in order to get the same effect previously experienced, having problems with family members as a result of one's own substance use/abuse, being unsuccessful in one's efforts to quit or curtail one's own drug intake, and experiencing withdrawal symptoms when unable to get alcohol or another drug to use. These measures were derived from the *DSM-IV-TR* [23] for the diagnosis of substance abuse and substance dependency, but not all of the diagnostic criteria were included, nor were details about the clustering of substance abuse-related symptoms within the *DSM-IV-TR*'s specified 12-month period.

2.3. Statistical Analysis. Much of this work is based on the presentation of descriptive statistics, with the appropriate confidence intervals (CI_{95}) and/or standard deviations provided to accompany the percentages and means reported. Parts of the analysis, especially those whose results are summarized in Tables 3 and 5, entailed comparing men who were HIV-negative and those who were HIV-positive on the prevalence and/or extent of involvement in various risky practices. Whenever the dependent variable was continuous in nature (e.g., number of sex partners, number of times engaging in a particular type of sex), Student's t-tests were used. Whenever the dependent variable was dichotomous or categorical in nature (e.g., recent involvement in a particular type of risky sex, recent use of a particular illegal drug), chi-square tests were performed. Throughout Section 3, findings are reported as statistically significant whenever $P < .05$.

3. Results

3.1. Sample Characteristics. In total, 332 men participated in the study. They ranged in age from 18 to 72 (mean = 43.7, s.d. = 11.2, median = 43.2) (see Table 1). Racially, the sample is a fairly close approximation of the American population, with 74.1% being Caucasian, 9.0% each being African American and Latino, 5.1% self-identifying as biracial or multiracial, 2.4% being Asian, and 0.3% being Native American. The large majority of the men (89.5%) considered themselves to be gay and almost all of the rest (10.2%) said they were bisexual. On balance, men participating in *The Bareback Project* were fairly well educated. About 1 man in 7 (14.5%) had completed no more than high school, 34.3% had some college experience without earning a college degree, 28.9% had a bachelor's degree, and 22.3% were educated beyond the bachelor's level. Slightly more than one-half of the men (59.0%) reported being HIV-positive; most of the rest (38.6%) were HIV-negative.

Table 1 also shows that men in this study used the Internet to find sex partners with great regularity. More than two-thirds of the men (68.3%) reported looking online specifically for bareback sex partners at least three days a week, on average, and even more of them (84.0%) said that they used the Internet three or more days each week to find sex partners on sites that were not bareback focused. As a general rule, the more frequently men reported looking online for sex partners, the more time they tended to spend on each of the days that they were online engaged in this pursuit.

3.2. Sexual Activity. The large majority of the men (88.9%, CI_{95} = 86.5–92.2%) participating in *The Bareback Project* had been sexually active during the month prior to interview. Sexually active men reported an average of more than 11 sex partners (mean = 11.3, s.d. = 16.7, range = 1–151) during the past month. Over the course of their lifetime, the bottom quartile of men in the study reported having had anywhere from 1 to 79 sex partners, the next-higher quartile of men reported 80 to 275 sex partners, the next-higher quartile of men reported 276 to 975 sex partners, and the top quartile reported anywhere from 976 to 20,000 sex partners.[2]

Men who were HIV-negative and those who were HIV-positive were equally likely to report having been sexually active during the month prior to interview (88.2% versus 89.3%, χ^2_{1df} = 0.09, n.s.). Sexually active HIV-positive men reported significantly more sex partners during the month prior to interview than their HIV-negative counterparts (13.1 versus 8.7, t = 2.25, P = .025). HIV-positive men also reported more than three times as many lifetime sex partners than HIV-negative men did, on average (1648.5 versus 506.1, t = 4.20, $P < .001$).

Table 2 presents information pertaining to various sexual behaviors among men in the sample. Almost all of the sexually active men (94.2%, CI_{95} = 91.6–96.9%) reported having performed oral sex on another man during the month prior to interview. On average, they reported having done this with 7.6 different partners (s.d. = 13.1) a total of 12.2 times (i.e., usually once or twice with each man; s.d. = 17.6). Most of the time (54.7%, CI_{95} = 48.8–60.5%), the man accepted semen orally during these oral sex behaviors. Approximately one-half (55.4%) of men's partners for this type of sex were people they had met online.

Table 3 presents information comparing sexual risk behavior involvement of HIV-negative and HIV-positive men. This table shows that HIV-negative and HIV-positive men alike were highly likely to report having performed oral sex on another man during the month prior to interview (92.5% versus 95.4%, χ^2_{1df} = 1.12, n.s.). HIV-positive men engaged in this behavior with significantly more partners than their HIV-negative counterparts did (8.9 versus 5.7, t = 2.07, P = .040). Consistent with this, HIV-positive men performed oral sex on their partners significantly more times during the month prior to interview than their HIV-negative counterparts did (14.5 versus 8.8, t = 2.70, P = .007), with both groups engaging in this behavior an average of once or twice with each partner. As Table 3 shows, HIV-positive and HIV-negative men were about equally likely to have performed oral sex on men they had met online (80.8% versus 80.2%, χ^2_{1df} = 0.02, n.s.). Both groups were, from a statistical standpoint, equally likely to have performed oral sex on another man without the use of a condom (94.9% versus 90.8%, χ^2_{1df} = 1.82, n.s.). HIV-positive men, however, were significantly more likely than HIV-negative men to accept their partner's semen in their mouths when performing oral sex (59.9% versus 46.9%, χ^2_{1df} = 4.57, P = .033). In the interest of conserving space and reducing verbiage, throughout the remainder of Section 3, findings for HIV-negative and HIV-positive respondents will be highlighted only when statistically significant differences were observed.

As Table 2 shows, the large majority (90.5%, CI_{95} = 87.2–93.8%) of sexually active study participants said that another man had performed oral sex on them during the 30 days prior to interview. On average, they said that 6.4 men had done this (s.d. = 9.1) a total of 10.9 times (again, typically averaging once or twice per sex partner; s.d. = 14.0). Most of the time (55.3%, CI_{95} = 49.3–61.2%), men said that they did not ejaculate into their partner's mouth during oral sex. Approximately one-half (54.9%) of men's partners for this type of sex were people they had met online.

Most of the sexually active men participating in *The Bareback Project* (64.1%, CI_{95} = 58.6–69.5%) said that they had performed insertive anal sex on another man during the month prior to interview. They reported having done this with approximately four men on average (mean = 4.2, s.d. = 7.3), approximately two or three times per partner (mean = 10.5, s.d. = 12.7). Most of the time (69.3%, CI_{95} = 62.7–75.8%), men said that they ejaculated directly into their partner's anus during these activities. Men said that most (62.4%) of the people with whom they recently performed insertive anal sex were people they had met via the Internet. As Table 3 illustrates, although HIV-positive and HIV-negative men were comparably involved in most aspects of insertive anal

TABLE 1: Sample Characteristics.

Characteristic	N	%
Age		
18–29	44	13.3
30–39	69	20.8
40–49	109	32.9
50–59	81	24.5
60+	28	8.5
Race/ethnicity		
Caucasian	246	74.1
African American	30	9.0
Latino	30	9.0
Asian/Pacific Islander	8	2.4
Native American/Native Alaskan	1	0.3
Biracial/multiracial	17	5.1
Educational attainment		
High school graduate or less	48	14.5
Some college	114	34.3
College graduate	96	28.9
Postgraduate	74	22.3
Population density in area of residence		
Rural (<250 persons per square mile)	76	22.9
Urban (1,000+ persons per square mile)	198	59.6
Low density (1,000 to 2,500 persons)	(53)	(16.0)
Medium density (2,501 persons to 5,000 persons)	(67)	(33.8)
High density (5,001+ persons)	(88)	(44.4)
Relationship status		
Married or "involved"	87	26.2
Single	245	73.8
HIV serostatus		
Negative	128	38.6
Positive	196	59.0
Do not know	8	2.4
Sexual orientation		
Gay	297	89.5
Bisexual	34	10.2
Sexual role identity		
Total top	54	16.3
Versatile top	62	18.7
Versatile	60	18.1
Versatile bottom	92	27.7
Total bottom	64	19.3
Internet use—looking specifically for bareback partners		
Once or twice a week	105	31.7
<30 minutes each day	(74)	(70.5)
30 to 60 minutes each day	(24)	(22.9)
61 to 120 minutes each day	(5)	(4.8)
121+ minutes each day	(2)	(1.9)

TABLE 1: Continued.

Characteristic	N	%
Three to six times a week	121	36.6
<30 minutes each day	(74)	(61.2)
30 to 60 minutes each day	(33)	(27.3)
61 to 120 minutes each day	(8)	(6.6)
121+ minutes each day	(6)	(5.0)
Daily	105	31.7
<30 minutes each day	(47)	(44.8)
30 to 60 minutes each day	(29)	(27.6)
61 to 120 minutes each day	(12)	(11.4)
121+ minutes each day	(17)	(16.2)
Internet use—looking for sex partners, not bareback specific (in addition to looking for bareback partners)		
Once or twice a week	53	16.0
<30 minutes each day	(43)	(81.1)
30 to 60 minutes each day	(7)	(13.2)
61 to 120 minutes each day	(1)	(1.9)
121+ minutes each day	(2)	(3.8)
Three to six times a week	127	38.4
<30 minutes each day	(29)	(22.8)
30 to 60 minutes each day	(63)	(49.6)
61 to 120 minutes each day	(26)	(20.5)
121+ minutes each day	(9)	(7.1)
Daily	151	45.6
<30 minutes each day	(33)	(21.9)
30 to 60 minutes each day	(47)	(31.1)
61 to 120 minutes each day	(29)	(19.2)
121+ minutes each day	(41)	(27.3)

sex, the data did reveal that HIV-positive men were more likely than HIV-negative men to say that they had engaged in unprotected insertive anal sex during the preceding month (64.0% versus 50.8%, χ^2_{1df} = 5.09, P = .024).

A comparable percentage of the sexually active men (67.5%, CI_{95} = 62.1–72.8%) indicated that they had engaged in receptive anal sex during the preceding 30 days (see Table 2). On average, they had done this with four different sex partners (mean = 3.9, s.d. = 6.3) approximately two or three times each (mean = 9.3, s.d. = 11.4). The majority of the time (74.4%, CI_{95} = 68.3–80.4%), men said that their partners ejaculated directly inside of their anus. Most (58.6%) of the people with whom they reported recently having engaged in receptive anal sex were partners they had met online.

Table 3 shows that, when it came to receptive anal sex, HIV-negative and HIV-positive men often differed from one another. HIV-negative men were less likely to report this practice during the previous month (60.8% versus 72.0%, χ^2_{1df} = 4.04, P = .044). When they did engage in this behavior, HIV-negative men were less likely to engage in it without the use of condoms (51.7% versus 69.1%, χ^2_{1df} = 9.23, P = .002) and they were less likely to allow one of their

TABLE 2: Prevalence of selected sexual behaviors among sexually active men.

Sexual behavior	N	%
Oral sex—insertive		
No	17	5.8
Yes	277	94.2
With partners met online?		
No	53	19.1
Yes	224	80.9
Any of it unprotected?		
No	23	8.3
Yes	254	91.7
Any of it entailing internal ejaculation?		
No	125	45.1
Yes	152	54.9
Oral sex—receptive		
No	28	9.5
Yes	267	90.5
With partners met online?		
No	59	22.1
Yes	208	77.9
Any of it unprotected?		
No	16	6.0
Yes	251	94.0
Any of it entailing internal ejaculation?		
No	147	55.3
Yes	119	44.7
Anal sex—insertive		
No	106	35.9
Yes	189	64.1
With partners met online?		
No	32	16.9
Yes	157	83.1
Any of it unprotected?		
No	51	27.0
Yes	138	73.0
Any of it entailing internal ejaculation?		
No	58	30.7
Yes	131	69.3
Anal sex—receptive		
No	96	32.5
Yes	199	67.5
With partners met online?		
No	42	21.1
Yes	157	78.9
Any of it unprotected?		
No	64	32.3
Yes	134	67.7
Any of it entailing internal ejaculation?		
No	51	25.6
Yes	148	74.4

TABLE 2: Continued.

Sexual behavior	N	%
Sex partners in past 30 days		
1	38	12.9
2–5	109	36.9
6–10	52	17.6
11–20	61	20.7
21–30	16	5.4
31+	19	6.4
Double fucking—insertive		
No	265	89.8
Yes	30	10.2
Any of it unprotected?		
No	4	13.3
Yes	26	86.7
Any of it entailing internal ejaculation?		
No	10	33.3
Yes	20	66.7
Double fucking—receptive		
No	267	90.2
Yes	29	9.8
Any of it unprotected?		
No	5	17.2
Yes	24	82.8
Any of it entailing internal ejaculation?		
No	5	17.2
Yes	24	82.8
Oral-anal contact—insertive		
No	99	33.6
Yes	196	66.4
Any of it involving felching?		
No	147	75.0
Yes	49	25.0
Any of it involving snowballing?		
No	18	36.7
Yes	31	63.3
Oral-anal contact—receptive		
No	102	34.6
Yes	193	65.4
Sharing of used, uncleaned sex toys		
No	79	80.6
Yes	19	19.4
Any pimping out or being pimped out sexually?		
No	225	76.3
Yes	70	23.7
Multiple partner sexual encounters		
No	156	52.9
Yes	139	47.1

TABLE 2: Continued.

Sexual behavior	N	%
Any of it involving three ways?		
No	10	7.8
Yes	129	92.1
Any of it involving unprotected sex?		
No	24	18.6
Yes	105	81.4
Any of it involving larger-group encounters?		
No	60	43.2
Yes	79	56.8
Any of it involving unprotected sex?		
No	20	25.3
Yes	59	74.7
Anonymous sex encounters		
No	144	48.8
Yes	151	51.2

partners to ejaculate directly into their anus (65.8% versus 79.4%, $\chi^2_{1df} = 4.49$, $P = .034$).

3.3. Risky Sexual Practices.
Two-thirds of the sexually active men (66.7%, $CI_{95} = 61.3–72.1\%$) reported no condom whatsoever during the preceding month. HIV-positive men were significantly more likely than HIV-negative men to report no condom use whatsoever during the previous month (71.3% versus 60.0%, $\chi^2_{1df} = 4.06$, $P = .044$). The average overall rate of sexual protection was 8.1% (s.d. = 19.1) and more than one-third of all sex acts (mean = 37.3%, s.d. = 28.8) entailed internal ejaculation. HIV-positive men used condoms less frequently than HIV-negative men did (5.2% versus 12.2%, $t = 3.17$, $P = .002$). Both groups reported comparable rates of sex involving internal ejaculation (39.6% versus 33.9%, $t = 1.67$, n.s.).

The large majority of the men who had engaged in oral sex reported no condom use during this behavior (89.7%, $CI_{95} = 86.2–93.2\%$). The overall rate of engaging in protected oral sex was 4.1% (s.d. = 16.6). Approximately one-quarter of all oral sex acts resulted in the recipient partner accepting semen directly into the mouth or throat (mean = 27.7%, s.d. = 32.2). All of these figures were comparable for insertive and receptive oral sex, and no significant differences were found based on HIV serostatus.

Most of the men who had engaged in anal sex reported no condom use during this behavior (65.8%, $CI_{95} = 60.2–71.5\%$). Zero condom use during anal sex was more common among HIV-positive men than it was among HIV-negative men (71.4% versus 57.7%, $\chi^2_{1df} = 5.54$, $P = .019$). The overall rate of condom use during anal sex was 17.2% (s.d. = 31.9). This, too, differed for HIV-positive and HIV-negative men (10.5% versus 26.9%, $t = 4.31$, $P < .001$). More than one-half of all anal sex acts resulted in the recipient partner accepting semen directly into the anus (mean = 52.6%, s.d. = 37.8), with HIV-positive men being more likely than their HIV-negative

counterparts to engage in this behavior (57.8% versus 45.3%, $t = 2.72$, $P = .007$).

As Table 2 shows, double simultaneous penile-anal penetration (i.e., double fucking) was reported during the month prior to interview by approximately one-sixth of the men participating in The Bareback Project (15.9%, $CI_{95} = 11.8–20.1\%$). 10.2% of the men reported having engaged in this behavior insertively ($CI_{95} = 6.7–13.6\%$), with internal ejaculation occurring for one or both insertive partners 66.7% of the time ($CI_{95} = 49.8–83.5\%$). 9.5% of the men indicated that they had engaged in double fucking receptively during the month prior to interview ($CI_{95} = 6.1–12.8\%$), and the large majority of these instances (82.1%, $CI_{95} = 68.0–96.3\%$) involved one or both of the insertive partners ejaculating into the recipient man's anus. Analyses comparing HIV-positive and HIV-negative men (see Table 3) revealed that HIV-positive men were almost three times more likely to engage in insertive double fucking than HIV-negative men were (13.7% versus 5.0%, $\chi^2_{1df} = 5.92$, $P = .015$). HIV-positive men who engaged in receptive double fucking were considerably more likely than their HIV-negative counterparts to engage in this behavior when it entailed internal ejaculation (90.5% versus 57.1%, $\chi^2_{1df} = 3.98$, $P = .046$).

Oral-anal contact (i.e., rimming) was a common practice among men in this study (82.4%, $CI_{95} = 78.0–86.7\%$), with 66.4% of the men indicating that they had placed their mouth or tongue onto or into a sex partner's anus during the previous month ($CI_{95} = 61.0–71.8$) and 65.4% reporting that someone had done that to them ($CI_{95} = 60.0–70.8\%$). As Table 3 shows, HIV-positive men were more likely than HIV-negative men to report engaging in receptive oral-anal contact during the previous month (70.9% versus 57.5%, $\chi^2_{1df} = 5.65$, $P = .018$). Moreover, 16.6% of the sexually active men in the study (or 25.0% of those who acknowledged having been the insertive partner in oral-anal contact) said that they took this one

TABLE 3: Comparison of HIV-negative and HIV-positive men's involvement in selected sexual behaviors among sexually active men.

Sexual behavior	HIV-negative (% yes)	HIV-positive (% yes)	$P = \lvert x \rvert$
Oral sex—insertive			
Past 30 days	92.5	95.4	n.s.
With partners met online?	80.2	80.8	n.s.
Any of it unprotected?	90.8	94.9	n.s.
Any of it entailing internal ejaculation?	46.9	59.9	.033
Oral sex—receptive			
Past 30 days	94.2	88.0	n.s.
With partners met online?	78.8	77.3	n.s.
Any of it unprotected?	91.7	86.9	n.s.
Any of it entailing internal ejaculation?	43.8	45.5	n.s.
Anal sex—insertive			
Past 30 days	60.8	66.3	n.s.
With partners met online?	83.6	82.8	n.s.
Any of it unprotected?	50.8	64.0	.024
Any of it entailing internal ejaculation?	63.0	73.3	n.s.
Anal sex—receptive			
Past 30 days	60.8	72.0	.044
With partners met online?	80.8	77.8	n.s.
Any of it unprotected?	51.7	69.1	.002
Any of it entailing internal ejaculation?	65.8	79.4	.034
Sex partners in past 30 days			.002
1	14.2	12.0	
2–5	49.2	28.6	
6–10	15.0	19.4	
11–20	14.2	25.1	
21+	7.5	14.9	
Double Fucking—Insertive			
Past 30 days	5.0	13.7	.015
Any of it unprotected?	98.3	98.9	n.s.
Any of it entailing internal ejaculation?	66.7	66.7	n.s.
Double fucking—receptive			
Past 30 days	5.8	12.0	n.s.
Any of it unprotected?	97.5	99.4	n.s.
Any of it entailing internal ejaculation?	57.1	90.5	.046
Oral-anal contact—insertive			
Past 30 days	60.8	70.3	n.s.
Any of it involving felching?	24.7	25.2	n.s.
Any felching involving snowballing?	55.6	67.7	n.s.
Oral-anal contact—receptive	57.5	70.9	.018
Sharing of used, uncleaned sex toys	22.6	17.9	n.s.
Pimping out or being pimped out sexually	17.5	28.0	.037
Multiple-partner sexual encounters			
Past 30 days	33.3	56.6	<.001
Any of it involving three ways?	30.8	52.6	<.001
Any three ways involving unprotected sex?	24.2	49.1	<.001
Any of it involving larger-group encounters?	15.0	34.9	<.001
Any larger group encounters involving unprotected sex?	11.7	30.3	<.001
Anonymous sex encounters	41.7	57.7	.007

TABLE 4: Substance use behaviors.

Substance use behavior	N	%
Any illegal drug use in past 30 days?		
No	132	39.9
Yes	199	60.1
Which drug(s)?		
Marijuana	108	54.3
Cocaine	15	7.5
Crack	8	4.0
Heroin or other opiates	3	1.5
Hallucinogens	0	0.0
Ecstasy	8	4.0
Club drugs other than ecstasy	10	5.0
Methamphetamine	53	26.6
Sedatives or depressants	11	5.5
Any drug-related problems in past 30 days?		
No	239	72.2
Yes	92	27.8
How many? (out of 13 listed)		
1	40	43.5
2	22	23.9
3	11	12.0
4 or more	19	20.7
Any sex while "under the influence" in past 30 days?		
No	175	52.9
Yes	156	47.1
Which drug(s)? (top 3 listed; all others less common)		
Alcohol	89	57.1
Marijuana	78	50.0
Methamphetamine	51	32.7
Prefer to have sex while "under the influence"?		
No	148	44.6
Yes	184	55.4
Which drug(s)? (top 4 listed; all others less common)		
Alcohol	60	32.6
Marijuana	96	52.2
Ecstasy	37	20.1
Methamphetamine	60	32.6
Ever been in drug treatment?		
No	271	81.6
Yes	60	18.4
More than once?		
No	35	58.3
Yes	25	41.7

step further by eating semen out of the anus that they were rimming—a practice referred to as felching. Most of these men (63.3% of them or 10.5% of the sexually active sample)

reported taking this activity one step further still by then sharing that semen with a sex partner by kissing or drooling the semen into another man's mouth—a practice referred to as snowballing. These practices were fairly comparable among HIV-negative and HIV-positive men alike.

Less commonly reported was sharing of sex toys, such as dildos or butt plugs. Although approximately one-third (33.2%, $CI_{95} = 27.8–38.6\%$) of the sexually active men said that they had used sex toys during the month prior to interview, relatively few of these men (19.4% of them, $CI_{95} = 11.6–27.2\%$, or 6.4% of the men in the study) said that they recently shared a used, uncleaned sex toy with a sex partner. Taking a sex toy from a sex partner who had just used it, and then using it on oneself without cleaning it first, was reported by 3.7% of the men in the study ($CI_{95} = 1.6–5.9\%$) (i.e., 11.2% of those who reported any recent sex toy use). Using a sex toy and then giving it to a sex partner to use without cleaning it first was reported by 5.1% of the respondents ($CI_{95} = 2.6–7.6\%$) (i.e., 15.3% of those who reported any recent sex toy use).

Approximately one-quarter of the sexually active men (23.7%, $CI_{95} = 18.9–28.6\%$) in *The Bareback Project* said that, during the month prior to interview, they had invited several other men to a sexual encounter with the express purpose being to use one of their sex partners or in the alternative, that they had allowed a sex partner to invite other people to a sexual encounter with the express purpose to use them sexually. These behaviors are known as "pimping out" or "being pimped out by" a sex partner, and ordinarily they entail situations in which the inviting partner and the persons he has invited take turns using the "pimped out" partner for their sexual gratification without the "pimped out" partner having much, if any, say in what is done to him sexually. These practices were more common among HIV-positive men than among HIV-negative men (28.0% versus 17.5%, $\chi^2_{1df} = 4.34$, $P = .037$). Nearly one-fifth of the men in the study (19.3%, $CI_{95} = 14.8–23.8\%$) said that, in the previous month, at least one of their sex partners had done this to them, and about one-half as many (10.5%, $CI_{95} = 7.0–14.0\%$) said that they had done this to someone with whom they had sex.

Nearly one-half of the men participating in the study (47.1%, $CI_{95} = 41.4–52.8\%$) said that, during the month prior to interview, they had engaged in multiple-partner sex (i.e., three or more partners having sex together). The large majority of these men (92.8% of them or 43.7% of the total sample, $CI_{95} = 38.1–49.4\%$) said that this took the form of three-way sexual encounters, and about one-half (56.8% of the men reporting multiple-partner sex or 26.8% of the sexually active men in the study, $CI_{95} = 21.7–31.8\%$) said that this took the form of larger group sexual encounters or orgies. Condom use during multiple-partner sexual encounters tended to be slightly greater than it was overall for other types of sexual behaviors/scenarios, but was still very low: 13.0% of the three-way sexual encounters and 19.1% of the larger-group sexual encounters (accounting for 15.4% of all multiple-partner sexual encounters) involved the use of condoms by one or more of the participants.

These various multiple-partner sex measures all differed greatly based on men's HIV serostatus. Compared to their

TABLE 5: Differences between HIV-positive and HIV-negative men in substance use behaviors.

Substance use behavior	HIV-negative (% yes)	HIV-positive (% yes)	$P = \lvert x \rvert$
Any illegal drug use in past 30 days?	57.8	61.7	n.s.
Among recent users of any illegal drugs, which drug(s)?			
Marijuana	52.6	50.0	n.s.
Cocaine	3.0	5.6	n.s.
Crack	1.5	3.1	n.s.
Heroin or other opiates	0.7	1.0	n.s.
Hallucinogens	0.0	0.0	n.s.
Ecstasy	1.5	3.1	n.s.
Club drugs other than ecstasy	0.7	4.6	.044
Methamphetamine	8.2	21.4	.001
Sedatives or depressants	3.0	3.6	n.s.
Any drug problems in past 30 days?	25.9	29.1	n.s.
Among people with any recent drug problems, how many? (out of 13 listed)			n.s.
1	45.7	42.1	
2	22.9	24.6	
3	11.4	12.3	
4 or more	20.0	21.1	
Any sex while "under the influence" in past 30 days?	44.5	57.7	.026
Among people with any recent sex while "under the influence," which drug(s)? (top 3 listed; all others less common)			
Alcohol	29.1	31.4	n.s.
Marijuana	17.7	32.6	.004
Methamphetamine	25.7	43.8	n.s.
Prefer to have sex while "under the influence"?	42.7	64.3	<.001
Among those preferring to have sex while "under the influence," which drug(s)? (top 4 listed; all others less common)			
Alcohol	17.7	17.4	n.s.
Marijuana	19.9	35.2	.002
Ecstasy	11.0	11.2	n.s.
Methamphetamine	9.6	24.0	<.001
Ever been in drug treatment?	15.6	19.9	n.s.
Among those who have been in treatment before, been in treatment more than once?	57.1	33.3	n.s.

HIV-negative counterparts, HIV-positive men were more likely to engage in any type of multiple-partner sexual encounter (56.6% versus 33.3%, $\chi^2_{1df} = 5.43$, $P < .001$), a three-way sexual encounter (52.6% versus 30.8%, $\chi^2_{1df} = 13.67$, $P < .001$), a three-way sexual encounter involving unprotected sex (49.1% versus 24.2%, $\chi^2_{1df} = 18.67$, $P < .001$), a larger-group sexual encounter (34.9% versus 15.0%, $\chi^2_{1df} = 14.32$, $P < .001$), and a larger-group sexual encounter involving unprotected sex (30.3% versus 11.7%, $\chi^2_{1df} = 14.06$, $P < .001$). Moreover, rates of condom use during these multiple-partner sexual encounters differed for HIV-positive and HIV-negative men. Overall rates of condom use were significantly lower among the former than among the latter (11.3% versus 25.7%, $t = 2.49$, $P = .014$), in large part due to the intergroup differences in protection rates during three-way sexual encounters (8.2% versus 25.0%, $t = 2.81$, $P = .006$).

Approximately one-half (51.2%, $CI_{95} = 46.5–56.9\%$) of the sexually active men said that they had engaged in anonymous sex during the month prior to interview, with this practice being more common among HIV-positive men than it was among HIV-negative men (57.7% versus 41.7%, $\chi^2_{1df} = 7.34$, $P = .007$). Men who had engaged in recent anonymous sex did so an average of 7.8 times (s.d. = 12.5), and this figure was comparable for HIV-positive and HIV-negative men (7.7 versus 8.0, $t = 0.16$, n.s.).

3.4. *Drug Use Behaviors*. Table 4 summarizes findings for substance use and abuse among men in the sample, and Table 5 provides similar information with comparisons for HIV-negative and HIV-positive men. Most of the men participating in *The Bareback Project* (60.1%, $CI_{95} = 54.8$–65.4%) reported having used at least one illegal drug during the month prior to interview, and more than one-third of *these* men (38.3% of them or 23.0% of the total sample, $CI_{95} = 18.4$–27.5%) said that their use entailed the consumption of a drug that was "harder" than marijuana. These figures were similar for HIV-negative and HIV-positive men. The most common drugs of recent use were marijuana (51.1%, $CI_{95} = 46.7$–56.4%), methamphetamine (16.0%, $CI_{95} = 12.1$–20.0%), and powdered cocaine (4.5%, $CI_{95} = 2.3$–6.8%). Comparisons based on HIV serostatus revealed that HIV-positive men were more likely than their HIV-negative counterparts to report recent methamphetamine use (21.4% versus 8.2%, $\chi^2_{1df} = 10.48$, $P = .001$) and recent use of a club drug other than ecstasy (4.6% versus 0.7%, $\chi^2_{1df} = 4.05$, $P = .044$). Approximately one man in sixteen (6.0%, $CI_{95} = 3.5$–8.6%) said that he had injected a drug during the previous 30 days, and this behavior was more common among HIV-positive men than it was among HIV-negative men (10.2% versus 0%).

More than one-quarter of the men taking part in the study (27.8%, $CI_{95} = 23.0$–32.6%) said that their recent substance use had caused them to experience at least one drug-related problem and/or symptom of drug dependence, and the large majority of *these* men (92.9% of them or 26.0% of the total sample) reported experiencing two or more such problems/symptoms during the preceding month. The most-commonly-reported substance abuse problems and dependency symptoms were trying to make rules to control when or where one's own drug use would be permitted (16.9%, $CI_{95} = 12.9$–21.0%), continued substance use despite experiencing drug-related depression (9.4%, $CI_{95} = 6.2$–12.5%), losing interest in friends or activities as a result of drug (ab)use (8.5%, $CI_{95} = 5.5$–11.5%), needing to use more of a substance in order to get the same high as previously obtained (7.0%, $CI_{95} = 4.2$–9.7%), and an inability to quit or cut down on one's drug use (6.3%, $CI_{95} = 3.8$–9.0%).

When asked about their preferences for having sex while high or sober, most study participants (55.4%, $CI_{95} = 50.1$–60.8%) said that they would prefer to have sex while under the influence of alcohol and/or an illegal drug. This preference was even more pronounced among men who were infected with HIV than among those who were not (64.3% versus 42.7%, $\chi^2_{1df} = 15.22$, $P < .001$). The large majority of the persons preferring to have sex while "under the influence" (85.9% of them or 47.6% of the total sample, $CI_{95} = 42.2$–53.0%) said that they would prefer to have sex under the influence of at least one illegal drug, and most of *these* persons

(64.5% of them or 30.7% of the total sample, $CI_{95} = 25.8$–35.7%) said that they would prefer this drug to be something "harder" than marijuana. Moreover, 41.0% of respondents indicated a preference for both they themselves and their sex partners to be "under the influence" during sex ($CI_{95} = 35.7$–46.2%). This preference was more common among HIV-infected men than it was among HIV-uninfected men (49.5% versus 28.7%, $\chi^2_{1df} = 14.38$, $P < .001$). Most of the men who preferred to have sexual relations while both they themselves and their sex partner(s) were "under the influence" (72.8% of them or 29.8% of the sample, $CI_{95} = 24.9$–34.7%) preferred both they themselves and their sex partners to be high on an illegal drug during sex, with one-half of these individuals (14.5% of the total sample, $CI_{95} = 10.7$–18.2%) expressing a desire for both partners to be high on a "harder" drug than marijuana.

To a great extent, men's preferences for having sex while "under the influence" were consistent with their practices. More than one-half of the sexually active study participants (52.4%, $CI_{95} = 46.7$–58.1%) said that they had engaged in sex while high on alcohol *and/or* an illegal drug during the 30 days prior to interview. This practice was more common among HIV-positive men than it was among HIV-negative men (57.7% versus 44.5%, $\chi^2_{1df} = 4.93$, $P = .026$). More than one-third of the men in the study (39.1%, $CI_{95} = 33.5$–44.7%) reported having engaged in sex while high on an illegal drug, and about one-half of *these* men (58.1% of them, $CI_{95} = 48.7$–67.5%, or 20.7% of the total sample) said that that involved the use of a drug that was "harder" than marijuana.

4. Discussion

A number of interesting findings were revealed by this research. First, far from merely using the Internet for pure fantasy or cybersex purposes, during the year prior to interview, the large majority of the sexually active men participating in this study (98.0%, $CI_{95} = 96.3$–99.6%) actually met in person at least one sex partner originally identified via the Internet (mean = 35.6, SD = 57.6). Moreover, the large majority of the sexually active men participating in *The Bareback Project* reported having had multiple sex partners during the month prior to interview, with the "average" man reporting having had 11 recent sex partners. Other researchers have found a relationship between having multiple sex partners and elevated risk for HIV [24–26]. The present study is consistent with those findings. Compounding this problem, participants in *The Bareback Project* met a substantial proportion of their recent sex partners online, typically after having had relatively brief discussions with them. Most of their sex partners were, therefore, either strangers to them or persons about whom they knew little and with whom they typically engaged in minimal amounts of dialog prior to agreeing to meet for sex. Indeed, qualitative data from the study (not previously discussed) indicated that, in many instances, men in this study did little more than reading someone's profile, checking that person's online photograph(s) to determine their level of sexual interest in that person and then contacting the person with a sexual invitation to "hook up." Research has shown that partner communication is related inversely to

HIV risk involvement [27, 28]. Additional research has shown that sexual risk taking tends to be greater among MSM who meet their sex partners online [1, 7], with this elevated risk oftentimes being attributed, at least in part, to trusting information provided in online profiles and men's tendency not to engage in safer sex discussions with the men they meet online.

Intervention programs targeting risk-seeking MSM such as those who participated in the present study might use several different approaches to trying to reduce risk in this population. For example, they might work with men to reduce their number of sex partners, perhaps suggesting that they develop longer-term "friends with benefits" or "fuck buddies" arrangements with a smaller number of sex partners whom they can get to know better in terms of their sexual health rather than always looking for new partners about whom they know comparatively little with regard to their sexual health. This is purely a harm reduction approach rather than a risk-elimination approach to HIV risk reduction, but the former is likely to be more realistic than the latter. Another strategy might be to work with MSM who meet many of their sex partners online to teach them strategies that they can use to reduce their risk for acquiring or transmitting HIV with partners met this way. For example, interventionists could do more to educate men about the truthfulness (or lack thereof) of men's online profiles. Although many men realize that others are not always truthful about what they say about themselves online, data from The Bareback Project indicate that 24.2% of the men believed that online profiles are "very accurate" or "fairly accurate" with regard to the information they contain about a person's HIV serostatus. More education and skills building about how to overcome the occasional lack of truthfulness that pervades many men's online profiles and sexual advertisements might be an effective way of enabling some men to reduce their risk for HIV. This could include intervention components teaching improved partner communication skills.

Also worth considering would be the development and implementation of Internet-based educational and intervention efforts targeting men such as those who participated in The Bareback Project. In order to have an honest chance at succeeding, such endeavors would have to be engaging and consist of messages that risk-seeking MSM perceive to be helpful and practical in their lives. Utilizing sexually appealing men as "eye catchers," particularly on the first web page that men would encounter when visiting these educational/intervention programs' websites, is likely to be an effective technique at garnering their interest and willingness to visit other areas of the website. The community-based HIV prevention group DCFukit (see http://www.dcfukit.org) has utilized this strategy quite effectively in promoting its safer-sex kits and providing MSM with detailed, useful HIV information online. This organization's website is sleek, has a contemporary feeling to it, and is visually appealing (with plenty of photos of shirtless and partly- to mostly-naked men of various ages and races) and has even involved members of the gay pornography industry (in various stages of undress) in providing some of its website's online HIV prevention messages. Any Internet-based HIV prevention/intervention campaign designed to reach risk-seeking MSM should take into account what it takes to capture and then maintain the attention of members of this population, as this will be key if the endeavor is to have a chance at being effective. Recent research has shown that including HIV-positive persons' opinions and perspectives on website appeal and utility can be an effective strategy to maximize the potential usefulness of such an approach to providing HIV information [29]. Undoubtedly, this will apply to risk-seeking MSM as well.

Along these same lines, HIV education/intervention projects targeting risk-seeking MSM also might consider availing themselves of emergent technology when providing their messages for MSM. For example, recent evidence has been provided to suggest that men, especially young men, may be amenable to health messages provided via podcasts [30, 31]. As another example, only recently have researchers begun to explore the usefulness of providing health information and prevention content via text messaging, mobile phones, and the so-called smart phones [32]. Early results from these projects are promising particularly for the provision of sexual health and HIV-related information to young adults [33]. How effective these approaches can be at reaching risk-involved MSM remains to be seen, but initial study findings suggest that they are well worth exploring. Research will need to be conducted with regard to whether the use of emergent technologies such as these can be effective at reaching MSM of all ages, all races, and so forth or whether certain subgroups respond better than others to this type of HIV education/intervention approach. This would be a fruitful avenue for future research to pursue.

Another important finding coming from the present study is that a sizable proportion of oral and anal sex acts reported by the men in this study entailed internal ejaculation. The large majority of oral sex acts did not involve the use of a condom, and approximately one-quarter of the unprotected oral sex involved ejaculation into the mouth or throat. Nearly two-thirds of all anal sex acts involved no condom use, and more than one-half of these acts entailed ejaculation directly inside of the anus. Although it is a misconception that sex among MSM almost always involves internal ejaculation, it is nonetheless true that a sizable proportion of these men's sex acts do entail the sharing of semen between partners. The main implication of this finding is straightforward: interventionists working with unprotected sex-seeking MSM, such as those who took part in the present study, must find ways to increase condom usage among members of this population or decrease the frequency with which they engage in sexual relations involving internal ejaculation, or both.

Regarding the latter, it is likely that little can be done. Interventionists could work with MSM to encourage them to withdraw the penis (or to have their partners do so) prior to internal ejaculation. This is a practice that has been shown to reduce men's risk for HIV [34]. Another potential approach would be to encourage men to allow their partners to ejaculate on them rather than inside of them or to ejaculate onto their partners externally rather than internally. Although this would be unpalatable to many of the men who self-identify as "cum lovers" who specifically enjoy the taste or feel of semen (which was true for 60.7% of the men in this study), some might find it to be an acceptable compromise at least some of the time. It is a textbook example of the value of advocating a harm reduction approach, particularly when extinction of a particular behavior (in this instance, the risky practice of having sex involving internal ejaculation) is not a feasible or realistic goal.

Regarding the former, intervention strategies must consider the question of how to make condoms more appealing and less unpleasant to men who prefer intentional condomless sex. Previous research suggests that highlighting the sexual/sensory aspects of condom use and eroticizing safer sex might help increase condom use among MSM [35]. A number of community-based HIV prevention, education, and intervention programs around the United States have offered workshops about eroticizing safer sex, in an effort to teach members of the MSM community about specific strategies that can be undertaken to make condom use and other safer sex strategies more palatable. Programs such as those offered by Gay Men's Health Crisis in New York City [36], the Howard Brown Health Center in Chicago, and Project AIDS Resources and Knowledge (Project ARK) in St. Louis are to be applauded, as are population-specific approaches such as AIDS Project Los Angeles' Red Circle Project (targeting safer sex among Native Americans) and Bockting et al.'s [37] program targeting safer sex among transgendered persons. Likewise, in recent years, websites dedicated to promoting erotic safer sex have begun to appear on the Internet, and the present author believes that they offer great promise in combating HIV risk taking among MSM. Excellent examples of this may be found in the Washington, DC-based group's DCFukit website, at http://www.dcfukit.org. Finding innovative ways to eroticize safer sex may be an important approach to changing how MSM think about condom use, and that, in turn, is likely to be an effective way of reducing their involvement in risky sexual practices.

Another finding obtained in the present study that is well worth highlighting is that unprotected oral sex and unprotected anal sex were by no means the only HIV risk behaviors in which study participants had been engaging. Men fairly commonly reported recently having engaged in such risky practices as simultaneous double-penile penetration (a.k.a. "double fucking," 15.9%), eating semen out of a man's anus (a.k.a. "felching," 16.6%), having sex while under the influence of alcohol and/or other drugs (52.2%), "pimping out" a sex partner or "being pimped out" by a sex partner (23.7%), having multiple-partner sex (47.1%), and engaging in anonymous sex (51.2%). Other studies as well have reported these practices to be commonplace among MSM, including published reports focusing on the prevalence of felching (which was remarkably similar to that found in the present study; see [38]), the prevalence of engaging in multiple-partner sex (which was quite similar to that found in the present study; see [39]) and high-risk sex during multiple-partner sexual encounters [40, 41], the prevalence of engaging in anonymous sex (which again was similar to that found in the present study; see [42]), and the common cooccurrence of having sex and using alcohol and/or other drugs [43–45]. In order to be effective in their efforts to combat HIV among MSM such as those who participated in *The Bareback Project*, interventionists will have to develop specific

strategies to address the psychosexual needs attendant to each of these particular behaviors. The strategies that prove to be effective at reducing men's involvement in sharing sex toys, for example, are not likely to be equally effective at reducing multiple-partner sexual encounters because the behaviors themselves are very different and the arousal elements that these behaviors satisfy are also very different. Kalichman and Grebler [25] have written about the need to address having multiple concurrent sex partners. Klein [46] has spoken about strategies that might be employed to reduce the risks associated with felching practices among MSM. Fernández and colleagues [47] and Schönnesson and colleagues [48] discussed how interventions might target substance abuse-related risk practices among MSM. These authors' works demonstrate quite clearly how different the HIV intervention needs are likely to be for MSM-targeted endeavors, based on the specific behavior(s) that these interventions wish to affect. Reviewing writings such as these, and considering them in light of the present study's findings regarding the variety of risky practices in which men engaged, makes one thing abundantly clear: reducing HIV risk among MSM such as those who participated in *The Bareback Project* is going to be a complex process.

Another noteworthy finding documented in the present study was the fact that, on many dimensions of HIV risk, HIV-positive and HIV-negative men differed from one another. Although by no means did the two groups differ from one another in terms of their involvement in all of the risk behaviors examined in this paper, in all instances (without exception) in which a difference was found between the two groups, it was always in the direction of HIV-positive men being more likely to engage in the risk practice than their HIV-negative counterparts. To some extent, this is probably due to a false belief on the part of many HIV-infected men that having HIV means that they no longer need to concern themselves as much about their sexual health practices and their drug use behaviors. From their perspective, they already have HIV, so how much worse can it be/get if they engage in high-risk behaviors? Overlooked by adhering to this perspective, of course, is consideration of becoming infected with a new strain of HIV that is resistant to their current medications, becoming infected with a sexually transmitted infection other than HIV, or the enhanced possibility of infecting one's sex partners with HIV by virtue of practicing these high-risk behaviors.

In recent years, numerous public health efforts focusing on HIV-infected MSM have devoted considerable attention to developing effective strategies that can reduce HIV risk behavior involvement in this population. These initiatives have come to be known as "prevention with positives" programs, in which HIV-positive men (and sometimes their sex partners as well, especially if they are involved in ongoing sexual relationships with these partners) are targeted for enhanced, intensive educational, prevention, and/or intervention messages. Important recent research addressing the importance of these programs has included the works published by Wei and colleagues [49], Hatfield and colleagues [50], Crepaz and colleagues [51], Rutledge [52], and Stall and Van Griensven [53] (among many others), with most of these authors having devoted considerable time and attention to discussing strategies for implementing more effective "prevention with positives" programs and the challenges faced by such programs. The findings obtained in the present study support the need for these types of programs in the ongoing effort to curtail the spread of HIV.

Two additional discussion-worthy findings obtained in the present research both pertain to substance use/abuse. The use of illegal drugs was widespread in this research population, and recent use was much more prevalent among study participants (60.1%) than would be expected among men in the US general population (9.9%) [54]. Moreover, most of the study participants (56.4%) said that they prefer to have sex while under the influence of alcohol and/or illegal drugs rather than while sober, with the large majority of these men (85.9% of them) indicating a preference for having sex while high on an illegal drug. Indeed, more than one-half of the men who took part in this study (52.2%) reported recently having engaged in sexual relations at a time when they were not sober. These findings are of great concern, because there is a well-established association between substance use/abuse and involvement in risky sex [55–57]. Clearly, there is a need for substance abuse prevention education, drug abuse intervention services, and substance abuse treatment among men who use the Internet to find partners for unprotected sex. Other scholars as well have spoken of the need for these types of services among MSM [58–60]; the present study supports their contention. Completing drug treatment has been shown to be effective at helping to reduce HIV risk practices in a variety of population groups [61, 62], including MSM [63, 64]. The key to implementing effective drug abuse prevention and treatment services will be making sure that these programs are sensitive to the needs of gay and bisexual men and that they are designed in a culturally appropriate manner. In recent years, several such programs have evolved around the United States, offering treatment services specifically for gay men due to their unique needs for substance abuse recovery. Examples include Freedom Rings (Jacksonville, FL,), Michael's House (Palm Springs, CA, MSA), Out Interventions (Venice, CA, MSA), Pride Institute (Dallas, TX), and Rainbow Recovery (Laguna Beach, CA, MSA).

4.1. Potential Limitations. Before concluding, the author wishes to acknowledge two potential limitations of this research. First, the data in this study are based on uncorroborated self-reports. Therefore, it is unknown whether participants underreported or overreported their involvement in risky behaviors. The self-reported data probably can be trusted, however, as noted by other authors of previous studies with similar populations [65]. This is particularly relevant for self-reported measures that involve relatively small occurrences (e.g., number of times having a particular kind of sex during the previous 30 days), which characterize the substantial majority of the data collected in this study [66]. Other researchers have also commented favorably on the reliability of self-reported information in their studies regarding topics such as condom use [67].

A second potential limitation is the possibility of recall bias. For most of the measures used, respondents were asked about their beliefs, attitudes, and behaviors during the past 7 or 30 days. These time frames were chosen specifically: (1) to incorporate a large enough time frame in order to facilitate meaningful variability from person to person, and (2) to minimize recall bias. Although the authors cannot determine the exact extent to which recall bias affected the data, other researchers who have used similar measures have reported that recall bias is sufficiently minimal that its impact upon study findings is likely to be negligible [68, 69]. This seems to be especially true when the recall period is small [70, 71], as was the case for most of the main measures used in the present study.

A third limitation of this research is the unknown extent to which findings may be generalized. As with many published studies focusing on risk practices among MSM, the present study had a larger-than-expected proportion of well-educated men. HIV-positive men were overrepresented as well, which is not surprising when one considers that the study population was comprised by men seeking unprotected sex online. Although study participants were selected at random from the various websites used for recruitment purposes, there is no way to know how well these individuals represent unprotected sex-seeking MSM more broadly. What the present study population does represent, however, is a sample of risk-seeking MSM who actively use the Internet to identify potential sex partners.

5. Conclusion

In conclusion, all of the preceding findings—men's large numbers of recent sex partners, their propensity for initially identifying sex partners online and then meeting them for sex after minimal interaction/conversation, their widespread lack of condom use coupled with a tendency for many men to prefer having sex involving internal ejaculation, the multitude of risky sexual behaviors in which men were engaging, and widespread substance use/abuse in conjunction with sexual encounters—add up to a situation in which men who use the Internet to find partners for unprotected sex are placing themselves and their sex partners at great risk for contracting and/or transmitting HIV. The sheer variety of risky behaviors in which these men engage combine to form a very complicated web of behavioral risks. Each of these risk behaviors fulfills a specific need or set of needs physically, emotionally, and psychosexually, and as a result, each requires a unique approach to intervention and risk reduction. If HIV risk reduction efforts are to be successful among men who use the Internet to locate partners for unprotected sex, they will need to be comprehensive and creative, and capable of disentangling the multitude of risk factors and risk practices that commonly cooccur among men in this population. This will not be an easy task.

Acknowledgments

This research (officially entitled *Drug Use and HIV Risk Practices Sought by Men Who Have Sex with Other Men, and Who Use Internet Websites to Identify Potential Sexual Partners*) was supported by a Grant (5R24DA019805) from the National Institute on Drug Abuse. The author wishes to acknowledge, with gratitude, the contributions made by Thomas P. Lambing to this study's data collection and data entry/cleaning efforts. The author also thanks David Tilley for providing helpful comments on an earlier draft of this paper.

Endnotes

1. Due to differences from website to website in terms of the information made available to users about whether or not their emails were received and read, or whether they were removed by the web host's system prior to being read by the intended recipient, it is impossible to compute an accurate participation rate for *The Bareback Project*. Based on websites where enough information was available to users to allow for the participation rate to be calculated, the response rate was slightly greater than 10%. This could raise concern of selection bias and, therefore, the representativeness of the sample. Although it is difficult to be certain that the men who participated represent the men who did not, there is compelling evidence to suggest that differences between the two groups are minimal. Before *The Bareback Project* was started, the principal investigator conducted a large-scale content analysis with a random national sample of one of the main websites used by men to meet other men seeking unprotected sex partners (for additional information, see [19, 38, 72, 73]). The demographic composition of that sample and the one obtained in *The Bareback Project* closely match one another in terms of age representation, racial group composition, sexual orientation, and rural/suburban/urban location of residence. The two samples also resemble one another closely in terms of the types of sexual practices that men sought. The similarity of the two samples suggests that men who chose to participate in the present study represent those who did not, in terms of identifiable characteristics that are likely to be the best indicators of selection bias. Also, the demographic composition of men in *The Bareback Project* and the demographic composition of the male adult population-at-large are a fair approximation of one another in terms of their age breakdown [74] and rural/suburban/urban location of residence [75]. The present sample is better educated than men in the general population [74] and more likely to be HIV-positive (which is to be expected when one considers the population targeted in the present research).

2. It is interesting to note that the man reporting the largest number of sex partners over the course of his lifetime ($n = 20,000$) had actually maintained a written diary, which he has since computerized, detailing all of his lifetime sex partners. Ever since the time of his first sexual experience, he had kept detailed records of each different person with whom he had had any type of sexual contact. Therefore, rather than being an overestimation as one might be inclined to expect, the number of partners he reported was very close to

accurate. During the interview, he admitted to a slight rounding down of his lifetime number of partners, in the "off chance" that he may have double-counted a few persons accidentally. Also worth noting is the fact that this particular study participant was not the only person interviewed who had maintained sexual records. He was, as it turns out, one of several men who, during their interviews with the research team, casually mentioned keeping such records.

References

[1] G. Bolding, M. Davis, L. Sherr, G. Hart, and J. Elford, "Use of gay Internet sites and views about online health promotion among men who have sex with men," *AIDS Care*, vol. 16, no. 8, pp. 993–1001, 2004.

[2] S. S. Bull, M. McFarlane, L. Lloyd, and C. Rietmeijer, "The process of seeking sex partners online and implications for STD/HIV prevention," *AIDS Care*, vol. 16, no. 8, pp. 1012–1020, 2004.

[3] G. S. Ogilvie, D. L. Taylor, T. Trussler et al., "Seeking sexual partners on the internet: a marker for risky sexual behaviour in men who have sex with men," *Canadian Journal of Public Health*, vol. 99, no. 3, pp. 185–188, 2008.

[4] R. C. Berg, "Barebacking among MSM Internet users," *AIDS and Behavior*, vol. 12, pp. 822–833, 2008.

[5] E. G. Benotsch, A. M. Martin, F. M. Espil, C. D. Nettles, D. W. Seal, and S. D. Pinkerton, "Internet use, recreational travel, and HIV risk behaviors in men who have sex with men," *Journal of Community Health*, vol. 36, no. 3, pp. 398–405, 2011.

[6] T. W. Menza, R. P. Kerani, H. H. Handsfield, and M. R. Golden, "Stable sexual risk behavior in a rapidly changing risk environment: findings from population-based surveys of men who have sex with men in Seattle, Washington, 2003–2006," *AIDS and Behavior*, vol. 15, no. 2, pp. 319–329, 2011.

[7] P. N. Halkitis, J. T. Parsons, and L. Wilton, "Barebacking among gay and bisexual men in New York City: explanations for the emergence of intentional unsafe behavior," *Archives of Sexual Behavior*, vol. 32, no. 4, pp. 351–357, 2003.

[8] J. Kakietek, P. S. Sullivan, and J. D. Heffelfinger, "You've got male: internet use, rural residence, and risky sex in men who have sex with men recruited in 12 U.S. cities," *AIDS Education and Prevention*, vol. 23, no. 2, pp. 118–127, 2011.

[9] B. R. S. Rosser, J. M. Oakes, K. J. Horvath, J. A. Konstan, G. P. Danilenko, and J. L. Peterson, "HIV sexual risk behavior by men who use the internet to seek sex with men: results of the men's INTernet sex study-II (MINTS-II)," *AIDS and Behavior*, vol. 13, no. 3, pp. 488–498, 2009.

[10] M. A. Chiasson, S. Hirshfield, R. H. Remien, M. Humberstone, T. Wong, and R. J. Wolitski, "A comparison of on-line and off-line sexual risk in men who have sex with men: an event-based on-line survey," *Journal of Acquired Immune Deficiency Syndromes*, vol. 44, no. 2, pp. 235–243, 2007.

[11] E. Coleman, K. J. Horvath, M. Miner, M. W. Ross, M. Oakes, and B. R. S. Rosser, "Compulsive sexual behavior and risk for unsafe sex among internet using men who have sex with men," *Archives of Sexual Behavior*, vol. 39, no. 5, pp. 1045–1053, 2010.

[12] B. S. Mustanski, "Are sexual partners met online associated with HIV/STI risk behaviours? Retrospective and daily diary data in conflict," *AIDS Care*, vol. 19, no. 6, pp. 822–827, 2007.

[13] B. Mustanski and M. E. Newcomb, "Relationship characteristics and sexual risk-taking in young men who have sex with men," *Health Psychology*, vol. 30, pp. 597–605, 2011.

[14] C. Grov, J. A. DeBusk, D. S. Bimbi, S. A. Golub, J. E. Nanin, and J. T. Parsons, "Barebacking, the internet, and harm reduction: an intercept survey with gay and bisexual men in Los Angeles and New York City," *AIDS and Behavior*, vol. 11, no. 4, pp. 527–536, 2007.

[15] S. M. Jenness, A. Neaigus, H. Hagan, T. Wendel, C. Gelpi-Acosta, and C. S. Murrill, "Reconsidering the internet as an HIV/STD risk for men who have sex with men," *AIDS and Behavior*, vol. 14, no. 6, pp. 1353–1361, 2010.

[16] M. Berry, H. F. Raymond, T. Kellogg, and W. McFarland, "The Internet, HIV serosorting and transmission risk among men who have sex with men, San Francisco," *AIDS*, vol. 22, no. 6, pp. 787–789, 2008.

[17] G. Kok, H. J. Hospers, P. Harterink, and O. De Zwart, "Social-cognitive determinants of HIV risk-taking intentions among men who date men through the Internet," *AIDS Care*, vol. 19, no. 3, pp. 410–417, 2007.

[18] M. W. Ross, B. R. S. Rosser, and J. Stanton, "Beliefs about cybersex and Internet-mediated sex of Latino men who have Internet sex with men: relationships with sexual practices in cybersex and in real life," *AIDS Care*, vol. 16, no. 8, pp. 1002–1011, 2004.

[19] H. Klein, "HIV risk practices sought by men who have sex with other men, and who use internet websites to identify potential sexual partners," *Sexual Health*, vol. 5, no. 3, pp. 243–250, 2008.

[20] J. C. Forney and R. L. Miller, "Risk and protective factors related to HIV-risk behavior: a comparison between HIV-positive and HIV-negative young men who have sex with men," *AIDS Care*, vol. 24, pp. 544–552, 2012.

[21] C. Grov, S. A. Golub, and J. T. Parsons, "HIV status differences in venues where highly sexually active gay and bisexual men meet sex partners: results from a pilot study," *AIDS Education and Prevention*, vol. 22, no. 6, pp. 496–508, 2010.

[22] R. Needle, D. G. Fisher, N. Weatherby et al., "Reliability of self-reported HIV risk behaviors of drug users," *Psychology of Addictive Behaviors*, vol. 9, no. 4, pp. 242–250, 1995.

[23] American Psychiatric Association, *Diagnostic and Statistical Manual of Mental Disorders (DSM-IV-TR)*, American Psychiatric Association, Arlington, Va, USA, 2000.

[24] D. Binson, L. M. Pollack, J. Blair, and W. J. Woods, "HIV transmission risk at a gay bathhouse," *Journal of Sex Research*, vol. 47, no. 6, pp. 580–588, 2010.

[25] S. C. Kalichman and T. Grebler, "Reducing numbers of sex partners: do we really need special interventions for sexual concurrency?" *AIDS and Behavior*, vol. 14, no. 5, pp. 987–990, 2010.

[26] J. A. Kelly, Y. A. Amirkhanian, D. W. Seal et al., "Levels and predictors of sexual HIV risk in social networks of men who have sex with men in the Midwest," *AIDS Education and Prevention*, vol. 22, no. 6, pp. 483–495, 2010.

[27] M. A. Chesney, B. A. Koblin, P. J. Barresi et al., "An individually tailored intervention for HIV prevention: Baseline data from the EXPLORE study," *American Journal of Public Health*, vol. 93, no. 6, pp. 933–938, 2003.

[28] S. M. Noar, K. Carlyle, and C. Cole, "Why communication is crucial: meta-analysis of the relationship between safer sexual communication and condom use," *Journal of Health Communication*, vol. 11, no. 4, pp. 365–390, 2006.

[29] C. Courtenay-Quirk, K. J. Horvath, H. Ding et al., "Perceptions of HIV-related websites among persons recently diagnosed with HIV," *AIDS Patient Care and STDs*, vol. 24, no. 2, pp. 105–115, 2010.

[30] J. Kuriansky and S. Corsini-Munt, "Engaging multiple stakeholders for healthy teen sexuality: model partnerships for education and HIV/AIDS prevention," in *Sexuality Education: Past, Present, and Future*, E. Schroeder and J. Kuriansky, Eds., vol. 3 of *Principles and Practices*, pp. 311–334, Praeger Publishers, Westport, Conn, USA, 2009.

[31] M. Robinson and S. Robertson, "Young men's health promotion and new information communication technologies: illuminating the issues and research agendas," *Health Promotion International*, vol. 25, no. 3, pp. 363–370, 2010.

[32] D. Swendeman and M. J. Rotheram-Borus, "Innovation in sexually transmitted disease and HIV prevention: internet and mobile phone delivery vehicles for global diffusion," *Current Opinion in Psychiatry*, vol. 23, no. 2, pp. 139–144, 2010.

[33] D. Levine, J. McCright, L. Dobkin, A. J. Woodruff, and J. D. Klausner, "SEXINFO: a sexual health text messaging service for San Francisco youth," *American Journal of Public Health*, vol. 98, no. 3, pp. 393–395, 2008.

[34] F. Jin, J. Jansson, M. Law et al., "Per-contact probability of HIV transmission in homosexual men in Sydney in the era of HAART," *AIDS*, vol. 24, no. 6, pp. 907–913, 2010.

[35] L. A. J. Scott-Sheldon, K. L. Marsh, B. T. Johnson, and D. E. Glasford, "Condoms+pleasure=safer sex? A missing addend in the safer sex message," *AIDS Care*, vol. 18, no. 7, pp. 750–754, 2006.

[36] L. Palacios-Jimenez and M. Shernoff, *Facilitator's Guide to Eroticizing Safer Sex: A Psychoeducational Workshop Approach to Safer Sex Education*, Gay Men's Health Crisis, New York, NY, USA, 1986.

[37] W. O. Bockting, B. R. S. Rosser, and K. Scheltema, "Transgender HIV prevention: implementation and evaluation of a workshop," *Health Education Research*, vol. 14, no. 2, pp. 177–183, 1999.

[38] H. Klein, "Sexual orientation, drug use preference during sex, and HIV risk practices and preferences among men who specifically seek unprotected sex partners via the internet," *International Journal of Environmental Research and Public Health*, vol. 6, no. 5, pp. 1620–1635, 2009.

[39] C. A. Reisen, M. A. Iracheta, M. C. Zea, F. T. Bianchi, and P. J. Poppen, "Sex in public and private settings among Latino MSM," *AIDS Care*, vol. 22, no. 6, pp. 697–704, 2010.

[40] M. J. Mimiaga, S. L. Reisner, S. E. Bland et al., "Sex parties among urban MSM: an emerging culture and HIV risk environment," *AIDS and Behavior*, vol. 15, no. 2, pp. 305–318, 2011.

[41] G. P. Prestage, J. Hudson, I. Down et al., "Gay men who engage in group sex are at increased risk of HIV infection and onward transmission," *AIDS and Behavior*, vol. 13, no. 4, pp. 724–730, 2009.

[42] M. M. Taylor, G. Aynalem, L. V. Smith, J. Montoya, and P. Kerndt, "Methamphetamine use and sexual risk behaviours among men who have sex with men diagnosed with early syphilis in Los Angeles County," *International Journal of STD and AIDS*, vol. 18, no. 2, pp. 93–97, 2007.

[43] E. M. Gorman, K. R. Nelson, T. Applegate, and A. Scrol, "Club drug and poly-substance abuse and HIV among gay/bisexual men: lessons gleaned from a community study," *Journal of Gay and Lesbian Social Services*, vol. 16, pp. 1–17, 2004.

[44] R. J. Jacobs, M. I. Fernandez, R. L. Ownby, G. S. Bowen, P. C. Hardigan, and M. N. Kane, "Factors associated with risk for unprotected receptive and insertive anal intercourse in men

aged 40 and older who have sex with men," *AIDS Care*, vol. 22, no. 10, pp. 1204–1211, 2010.

[45] D. W. Purcell, G. E. Ibanez, and D. J. Schwartz, "Under the influence: alcohol and drug use and sexual behavior among HIV-positive gay and bisexual men," in *HIV+ Sex: The Psychological and Interpersonal Dynamics of HIV-Seropositive Gay and Bisexual Men's Relationships*, P. N. Halkitis, C. A. Gomez, and R. J. Wolitski, Eds., pp. 163–181, American Psychological Association, Washington, DC, USA, 2005.

[46] H. Klein, "Felching among men who engage in barebacking (unprotected anal sex)," *Archives of Sexual Behavior*, vol. 41, no. 2, pp. 377–384, 2012.

[47] M. I. Fernández, R. J. Jacobs, J. C. Warren, J. Sanchez, and G. S. Bowen, "Drug use and hispanic men who have sex with men in South Florida: implications for intervention development," *AIDS Education and Prevention*, vol. 21, no. 5, pp. 45–60, 2009.

[48] L. N. Schönnesson, J. Atkinson, M. L. Williams, A. Bowen, M. W. Ross, and S. C. Timpson, "A cluster analysis of drug use and sexual HIV risks and their correlates in a sample of African-American crack cocaine smokers with HIV infection," *Drug and Alcohol Dependence*, vol. 97, no. 1-2, pp. 44–53, 2008.

[49] C. Wei, S. H. Lim, T. E. Guadamuz, and S. Koe, "HIV disclosure and sexual transmission behaviors among an Internet sample of HIV-positive men who have sex with men in Asia: implications for prevention with positives," *AIDS and Behavior*, vol. 16, pp. 1970–1978, 2012.

[50] L. A. Hatfield, M. E. Ghiselli, S. M. Jacoby et al., "Methods for recruiting men of color who have sex with men in prevention-for-positives interventions," *Prevention Science*, vol. 11, no. 1, pp. 56–66, 2010.

[51] N. Crepaz, G. Marks, A. Liau et al., "Prevalence of unprotected anal intercourse among HIV-diagnosed MSM in the United States: a meta-analysis," *AIDS*, vol. 23, no. 13, pp. 1617–1629, 2009.

[52] S. E. Rutledge, "Formation of personal HIV disclosure policies among HIV-positive men who have sex with men," *AIDS Patient Care and STDs*, vol. 23, no. 7, pp. 531–543, 2009.

[53] R. Stall and F. Van Griensven, "New directions in research regarding prevention for positive individuals: questions raised by the Seropositive Urban Men's Intervention Trial," *AIDS*, vol. 19, supplement 1, pp. S123–S127, 2005.

[54] Substance Abuse and Mental Health Services Administration, "Results from the 2008 National Survey on Drug Use and Health: National findings (NSDUH series h-36, HHS publication number SMA-09-4434)," Office of Applied Studies, Rockville, Md, USA, 2009.

[55] J. W. Carey, R. Mejia, T. Bingham et al., "Drug use, high-risk sex behaviors, and increased risk for recent HIV infection among men who have sex with men in Chicago and Los Angeles," *AIDS and Behavior*, vol. 13, no. 6, pp. 1084–1096, 2009.

[56] P. N. Halkitis, P. P. Mukherjee, and J. J. Palamar, "Longitudinal modeling of methamphetamine use and sexual risk behaviors in gay and bisexual men," *AIDS and Behavior*, vol. 13, no. 4, pp. 783–791, 2009.

[57] S. J. Semple, S. A. Strathdee, J. Zians, and T. L. Patterson, "Sexual risk behavior associated with co-administration of methamphetamine and other drugs in a sample of HIV-positive men who have sex with men," *American Journal on Addictions*, vol. 18, no. 1, pp. 65–72, 2009.

[58] B. C. Kelly and J. T. Parsons, "Prevalence and predictors of nonmedical prescription drug use among men who have sex with men," *Addictive Behaviors*, vol. 35, no. 4, pp. 312–317, 2010.

[59] M. J. Mimiaga, S. L. Reisner, R. Vanderwarker et al., "Polysubstance use and HIV/STD risk behavior among Massachusetts men who have sex with men accessing Department of Public Health mobile van services: implications for intervention development," *AIDS Patient Care and STDs*, vol. 22, no. 9, pp. 745–751, 2008.

[60] J. J. Palamar, P. P. Mukherjee, and P. N. Halkitis, "A longitudinal investigation of powder cocaine use among club-drug using gay and bisexual men," *Journal of Studies on Alcohol and Drugs*, vol. 69, no. 6, pp. 806–813, 2008.

[61] R. E. Booth, B. K. Campbell, S. K. Mikulich-Gilbertson et al., "Reducing HIV-related risk behaviors among injection drug users in residential detoxification," *AIDS and Behavior*, vol. 15, no. 1, pp. 30–44, 2011.

[62] D. S. Metzger, G. E. Woody, and C. P. O'Brien, "Drug treatment as HIV prevention: a research update," *Journal of Acquired Immune Deficiency Syndromes*, vol. 55, supplement 1, pp. S32–S36, 2010.

[63] A. Jaffe, S. Shoptaw, J. A. Stein, C. J. Reback, and E. Rotheram-Fuller, "Depression ratings, reported sexual risk behaviors, and methamphetamine use: latent growth curve models of positive change among gay and bisexual men in an outpatient treatment program," *Experimental and Clinical Psychopharmacology*, vol. 15, no. 3, pp. 301–307, 2007.

[64] S. Shoptaw, C. J. Reback, S. Larkins et al., "Outcomes using two tailored behavioral treatments for substance abuse in urban gay and bisexual men," *Journal of Substance Abuse Treatment*, vol. 35, no. 3, pp. 285–293, 2008.

[65] E. W. Schrimshaw, M. Rosario, H. F. L. Meyer-Bahlburg, and A. A. Scharf-Matlick, "Test-retest reliability of self-reported sexual behavior, sexual orientation, and psychosexual milestones among gay, lesbian, and bisexual youths," *Archives of Sexual Behavior*, vol. 35, no. 2, pp. 225–234, 2006.

[66] L. M. Bogart, L. C. Walt, J. D. Pavlovic, A. J. Ober, N. Brown, and S. C. Kalichman, "Cognitive strategies affecting recall of sexual behavior among high-risk men and women," *Health Psychology*, vol. 26, no. 6, pp. 787–793, 2007.

[67] D. E. Morisky, A. Ang, and C. D. Sneed, "Validating the effects of social desirability on self-reported condom use behavior among commercial sex workers," *AIDS Education and Prevention*, vol. 14, no. 5, pp. 351–360, 2002.

[68] M. R. Kauth, J. S. S. Lawrence, and J. A. Kelly, "Reliability of retrospective assessments of sexual HIV risk behavior: a comparison of biweekly, three-month, and twelve-month self-reports," *AIDS Education and Prevention*, vol. 3, no. 3, pp. 207–214, 1991.

[69] L. E. Napper, D. G. Fisher, G. L. Reynolds, and M. E. Johnson, "HIV risk behavior self-report reliability at different recall periods," *AIDS and Behavior*, vol. 14, no. 1, pp. 152–161, 2010.

[70] K. A. Fenton, A. M. Johnson, S. McManus, and B. Erens, "Measuring sexual behaviour: methodological challenges in survey research," *Sexually Transmitted Infections*, vol. 77, no. 2, pp. 84–92, 2001.

[71] S. S. Weir, R. E. Roddy, L. Zekeng, and K. A. Ryan, "Association between condom use and HIV infection: a randomised study of self reported condom use measures," *Journal of Epidemiology and Community Health*, vol. 53, no. 7, pp. 417–422, 1999.

[72] H. Klein, "Differences in HIV risk practices sought by self-identified gay and bisexual men who use Internet websites to identify potential sexual partners," *Journal of Bisexuality*, vol. 9, no. 2, pp. 125–140, 2009.

[73] H. Klein, "Men who specifically seek unprotected sex partners via the internet: whose profiles are the most searched for by other site users?" *Journal of Gay and Lesbian Social Services*, vol. 22, no. 4, pp. 413–431, 2010.

[74] U.S. Census Bureau, *Profiles of General Demographic Characteristics 2000*, U.S. Government Printing Office, Washington, DC, USA, 2001.

[75] U.S. Census Bureau, *GCT-PH1. Population, Housing Units, Area, and Density: 2000*, U.S. Government Printing Office, Washington, DC, USA, 2001.

22

Evaluation of a Low-Threshold/High-Tolerance Methadone Maintenance Treatment Clinic in Saint John, New Brunswick, Canada: One Year Retention Rate and Illicit Drug Use

Timothy K. S. Christie,[1,2] Alli Murugesan,[1,3] Dana Manzer,[4] Michael V. O'Shaughnessey,[5] and Duncan Webster[6]

[1] Ethics Services, Horizon Health Network, Miramichi, NB, Canada E1V 1Y3
[2] Department of Bioethics, Dalhousie University, Halifax, NS, Canada B3K 6R8
[3] Dr. Reiman's Cancer Research Laboratory, University of New Brunswick, Saint John, NB, Canada E3B 5A3
[4] Uptown Clinic, St. Joseph's Hospital, Saint John, NB, Canada E2L 3L6
[5] British Columbia Centre for Excellence in HIV/AIDS, Vancouver, BC, Canada V6Z 1Y6
[6] Department of Medicine, Saint John Regional Hospital, Saint John, NB, Canada E2L 3L6

Correspondence should be addressed to Timothy K. S. Christie; timothy.christie@horizonnb.ca

Academic Editor: Ingmar Franken

Objective. To report the one-year retention rate and the prevalence of illicit opioid use and cocaine use in the Low-Threshold/High-Tolerance (LTHT) methadone maintenance treatment (MMT) clinic located in Saint John, New Brunswick, Canada. *Methods*. A description of the LTHT MMT clinic is provided. The one-year retention rate was determined by collecting data on patients who enrolled in the LTHT MMT clinic between August 04, 2009 and August 04, 2010. The prevalence of illicit drug use was determined using a randomly selected retrospective cohort of 84 participants. For each participant the results of six consecutive urine tests for the most recent three months were compared to the results of the first six consecutive urine tests after program entry. *Results*. The one-year retention rate was 95%, 67% of the cohort achieved abstinence from illicit opioids and an additional 13% abstained from cocaine use. *Conclusion*. The novel feature of the LTHT MMT clinic is that patients are not denied methadone because of lack of ancillary services. Traditional comprehensive MMT programs invest the majority of financial resources in ancillary services that support the biopsychosocial model, whereas the LTHT approach utilizes a medical model and directs resources at medical management.

1. Introduction

Most Canadian methadone maintenance treatment (MMT) programs have limited treatment capacity, hundreds of people on wait-lists and wait-times that exceed 6–12 months [1]. The result is that many people, who are motivated to seek treatment for their addiction, remain untreated. In Canada, the provision of MMT is regulated by Health Canada's guidelines, with each province and/or territory having the option of developing their own [2]. A review of the Federal Guidelines and those of seven provinces demonstrate that each adheres to the biopsychosocial model of MMT and

require, among other things, the provision of psychosocial counseling, random urine testing, and mechanisms for the involuntary discharge of patients [3–9].

This paper will report the evaluation results of the low-threshold/high-tolerance (LTHT) MMT clinic in Saint John, New Brunswick, Canada. The LTHT approach is novel because it utilizes a medical model rather than the traditional biopsychosocial model that predominates in Canada. This model incorporates recommendations of the Government of Canada "best practices" document with the foundational premise that the provision of MMT should not be contingent on the availability of resources for psychosocial treatment [10, 11].

The "low-threshold" aspect refers to the removal of barriers that limit or delay access to MMT. The referral process is open so clients can be referred from any source, including self-referral. Intake assessments are minimized; patients undergo a basic biopsychosocial evaluation and are admitted sequentially from the wait-list (although patients may be triaged in serious situations such as pregnancy). The "high-tolerance" aspect focuses on strategies designed to retain patients in treatment, for example, there is no mandated group or individual counseling, urine tests are scheduled not random, and the results are not used punitively as there is a "no involuntary discharge policy" relating to continued illicit drug use.

2. Objective

The objective is to report the one-year retention rate and the prevalence of illicit opioid use and cocaine use in the LTHT MMT clinic located in Saint John, New Brunswick, Canada.

3. Methods

3.1. One-Year Retention Rate. The one-year retention rate was determined by collecting data on each patient who received MMT from the LTHT clinic between August 04, 2009 and August 04, 2010. The total number of patients enrolled in the clinic during this time period was compared to the number of patients still in the program after 12 months. If a patient was no longer receiving methadone from the clinic, the reason(s) for his or her separation were determined. This was an intent-to-treat analysis, for example, regardless of whether the patient was on a stable dose of methadone or not, all patients who entered treatment during this time frame were included in the denominator, and only those still receiving MMT after 12 months were included in the numerator.

3.2. Illicit Opioid and Cocaine Use. The methods used to measure illicit opioid and cocaine use included (1) the development of inclusion and exclusion criteria, (2) the development of outcome measures, and (3) statistical analysis.

Inclusion and Exclusion Criteria. To measure the impact of the LTHT MMT clinic on illicit opioid and cocaine use, it was necessary to develop inclusion criteria that could control for variables that might impact on a participant's illicit drug use. For example, if a person was transferred to the LTHT MMT clinic from another MMT program, he or she might be abstinent from illicit drugs at program entry. Thus, the absence of illicit drug use could be explained independly of receiving treatment via the LTHT MMT clinic. Likewise, during the methadone induction phase (the period of time when a patient is being titrated to an adequate methadone dose), the patient will not yet receive the full benefit of the

methadone medication; continued illicit drug use is to be expected during this time period.

To control for this variability, the following inclusion and exclusion criteria were developed: (1) a participant could not be on a stable dose of methadone at program entry, and (2) participants must be on a stable dose of methadone after receiving treatment from the LTHT MMT clinic. A participant was considered to be on a stable dose of methadone at program entry (and ineligible for the study) if he or she had been transferred from another methadone program and had not received a single methadone dose adjustment greater than 10 mg within the first three months of entering the LTHT MMT clinic. Second, a patient was considered to be on a stable dose of methadone if he or she had been in treatment at the LTHT MMT clinic and had not received a methadone dose adjustment greater than 10 mg in the most recent three months.

Outcome Measurement. For each research participant, the results of six consecutive urine tests for the most recent three months were compared to the results of that participant's first six consecutive urine tests for the first three months after program entry; there was no overlap between these two time intervals. It was determined how many times each participant tested positive for illicit opioids or cocaine: one out of six times, two out of six times, three out of six times, four out of six times, five out of six times, or six out of six times. These results were compared to the same participants' first six urine test results at program entry.

Statistical Analysis. Paired *t*-tests were conducted to determine whether the mean number of positive tests was different between these two time intervals; an effect size was calculated using Cohen's D, and the alpha level was set at $P < 0.05$.

4. Results

4.1. One-Year Retention Rate. Between August 04, 2009 and August 04, 2010, 179 patients were enrolled in the LTHT MMT clinic. Uptake was immediate and dramatic: 122 patients entered treatment during the first three months of operation, and 153 were enrolled within five months. The average methadone dose was 70 mg; 66% were men, and the average age was 35 years. Of the 179 patients enrolled in the LTHT MMT clinic during the study period, 95% (n = 170) were still receiving methadone after one year. Of the nine people separated from the clinic at the time of analysis, three had voluntarily withdrawn their participation, three were incarcerated, two were transferred to primary care providers for continued MMT, and one person went into the witness protection program. Of the three people who voluntarily withdrew, two were females, their ages were 30, 45, and 47 years, and they were in treatment for 4, 7, and 10 months. The three patients incarcerated at the time of analysis were maintained on methadone while in jail and were to be readmitted to the LTHT MMT clinic upon their release, and the two patients who were transferred to other MMT providers continued to receive prescribed methadone.

TABLE 1

Population	Separated	Transfers from other programs	Induction phase	Eligible	Study sample
179 (100%)	9 (5%)	8 (4.5%)	28 (15.5%)	134 (75%)	84 (47%)

No information is available on the person who went into the witness protection program (for obvious reasons).

4.2. Randomly Selected Retrospective Cohort. Table 1 shows that out of the 179 patients in the LTHT MMT clinic, nine patients were separated from the clinic, eight were stable transfers from another MMT clinic, 28 were in the induction phase of treatment, 134 met the inclusion criteria (i.e., they were unstable at program entry and subsequently reached a stable dose of methadone), and 84 were randomly selected to be in the study. The random selection process started with a complete list of the 134 stable patients, the list was shuffled so that the order was random, then a random number generator produced a random list, and the corresponding patient was selected for inclusion until a sample of 84 people was generated.

All participants gave informed consent, and no one refused the invitation to participate. The average length of time in treatment was 16.2 months (range 9–18 months), the average methadone dose was 72.75 mg, 62% were men, and the average age was 35 years. These participants constitute 47% of all patients ever enrolled in the LTHT MMT clinic during the study period, and they are representative of the entire LTHT MMT clinic patient population in terms of age, gender, length of time in treatment, and methadone dose.

4.2.1. Opioid Positive Urine Tests. At program entry, the prevalence of illicit opioid use was 100%. Following entry into the program, initial urine screening showed that 23 participants tested positive for illicit opioids 1/6 times, 21 tested positive 2/6 times, 12 tested positive 3/6 times, 11 tested positive 4/6 times, five tested positive 5/6 times, and 12 tested positive 6/6 times. After stabilizing on methadone, the prevalence of illicit opioid use decreased to 33%: 56 research participants tested positive for illicit opioids 0/6 times, 15 tested positive 1/6 times, three tested positive 2/6 times, two tested positive 3/6 times, two tested positive 4/6 times, five tested positive 5/6 times, and one person tested positive 6/6 times. These participants were more likely to test positive for illicit opioids before stabilizing on methadone (mean = 2.88, SE = 0.19) than after stabilizing on methadone (mean = 0.79, SE = 0.15), $t(83) = -11.51$, $P < .001$, Cohen's D = −1.29. The decrease in positive tests was statistically significant ($P < .001$), and the effect size of −1.29 is considered large.

A comparison between the 56 research participants who consistently tested negative for illicit opioids with the 28 participants who tested positive at least once reveals no difference in methadone dose. The average methadone dose was 72.5 mg for those consistently testing negative and 73.21 mg for those testing positive at least once. A Mann-Whitney U Independent Samples Test determined that there is no statistically significant difference between these means ($P = .924$).

4.2.2. Cocaine Positive Urine Tests. At program entry, the prevalence of cocaine use was 55%. Following entry into the program, initial urine screening showed that 38 participants tested positive for cocaine 0/6 times, eight tested positive 1/6 times, six tested positive 2/6 times, four tested positive 3/6 times, six tested positive 4/6 times, nine tested positive 5/6 times, and 13 tested positive 6/6 times. After stabilizing on methadone the prevalence of positive cocaine tests decreased to 43%: 48 research participants tested positive for cocaine 0/6 times, eight tested positive 1/6 times, five tested positive 2/6 times, three tested positive 3/6 times, four tested positive 4/6 times, four tested positive 5/6 times, and 12 people tested positive 6/6 times. Although methadone has no biological effect on cocaine use, participants were more likely to test positive for cocaine before stabilizing on methadone (mean = 2.16, SE = 0.263) than after stabilizing on methadone (mean = 1.63, SE = 0.252), $t(83) = -2.56$, $P = .012$, Cohen's D = −0.23. The decrease in positive cocaine tests was statistically significant ($P = .012$), and the effect size of −0.23 is considered small.

5. Discussion

5.1. One-Year Retention Rate. Since there are no published data regarding the traditional biopsychosocial model in New Brunswick it is not possible to formally compare the two local models. However, a comparison may be made to the rates in British Columbia where they report a one-year retention rate between 40.5% and 52% [12–14, 16]. More recently the North American Opiate Medication Initiative (NAOMI) published an 87.8% one-year retention rate for the heroin prescription arm and a 54.1% one-year retention rate for the methadone arm [15]. The methadone arm in NAOMI had a "no involuntary discharge policy," which is a unique feature of the LTHT clinic making them somewhat comparable. However, an important qualification is that 92% of the illicit opioid use in Saint John, New Brunswick, involves the illegal use of prescription opioids for nonmedical purposes [16]. British Columbia has higher rates of heroin use, and NAOMI focussed exclusively on heroin users. Thus, there might be important differences among these patient populations that make direct comparisons inappropriate. Nevertheless, addiction to prescription opioids has been identified as an emerging epidemic in North America, and methadone is the appropriate medication for this condition [14, 17].

5.2. Illicit Drug Use. The 67% reduction in illicit opioid use is to be expected in a MMT program. In fact, the literature on this point is conclusive [18–21]. Interestingly, however, there is no difference in the average methadone dose between those patients who continued to use illicit opioids and those who abstained completely. Since there is no arbitrary limit to the methadone dose, continued opioid use among these patients is not likely to be attributed to inadequate dosing. Finally, there is evidence that retention in treatment and reduction in illicit opioid use are positively correlated with decreases in cocaine use, which is what has been observed in this cohort [22, 23].

In this study, the results of urine tests were used as a proxy measure for illicit opioid and cocaine use, with the tests being scheduled as opposed to random. Although there were no negative consequences associated with testing positive for illicit drugs, consistent with the "no involuntary discharge policy," it is possible that patients abstained from illicit drug use prior to submitting a urine specimen. For example, 95% of cocaine metabolite is excreted within 48 hours and 100% by 72 hours irrespective of the dose consumed. Thus, patients could have used cocaine prior to 72 hours before submitting to urine testing. Likewise, the opiate assay was designed to measure codeine, morphine, and hydromorphone at concentrations above 300 ng/mL, so lower concentrations may not have been detected by this test in some instances. Finally, since the current study did not have a control group, additional research is required in order to determine how the LTHT approach compares to other models of providing MMT. Ultimately, a well-designed controlled prospective clinical trial that formally compares the LTHT approach to differing MMT treatment modalities is required.

6. Conclusion

The one-year retention rate for the LTHT MMT clinic is 95%; 67% of participants achieved abstinence from illicit opioids, and an additional 13% abstained from cocaine use after stabilizing on methadone. The novel feature of the LTHT MMT clinic is that patients are not denied methadone because of lack of ancillary services. Traditional comprehensive MMT programs invest the majority of financial resources in ancillary services that support the biopsychosocial model, whereas the LTHT approach utilizes a medical model and directs resources at medical management. It is important to note, however, that patients at the LTHT clinic can receive ancillary services from other providers at the Uptown Clinic. For example, the clinic's nurse practitioner offers primary health care services, and the clinic is located in the Community Health Centre, which offers additional services. Access to an infectious diseases physician is also available at the Uptown Clinic, where there is a focus on communicable disease prevention and management as a component of the medical model.

Acknowledgments

The authors want to thank the editors and peer reviewers at the Journal of Addiction. Their critical comments and careful review have significantly improved this paper. The authors would also like to acknowledge the Health Promotion Research Fund for funding this project; the Uptown Clinic Steering Committee; the Saint John Police Force; the staff and patients at the Uptown Clinic; Dr. Jim Croll for his help with the statistical aspects of this study. Finally, the authors want to acknowledge the long standing support and contribution of Dr. Bob Newman from the International Centre for the Advancement of Addiction Treatment. Dr. Newman was instrumental in the design, development, and evaluation of the LTHT clinic.

References

[1] J. Luce and C. Strike, *A Cross-Canada Scan of Methadone Maintenance Developments*, 2011.

[2] Health and Welfare Canada, *The Use of Opioids in the Management of Opioid Dependence*, Minister of Supply and Services Canada, 1992.

[3] College of Physicians & Surgeons of Alberta, *Standards & Guidelines For Methadone Maintenance Treatment in Alberta*, College of Physicians an Surgeons of Alberta, 2005.

[4] College of Physicians and Surgeons of British Columbia, *Methadone Maintenance Handbook*, College of Physicians and Surgeons of British Columbia, 2009.

[5] College of Physicians & Surgeons of Nova Scotia, *Methadone Maintenance Treatment Handbook*, College of Physicians & Surgeons of Nova Scotia, 2012.

[6] College of Physicians & Surgeons of Ontario, *Methadone Maintenance Treatment Program Standards and Clinical Guidelines*, College of Physicians and Surgeons of Ontario, 4th edition, 2011.

[7] College of Physicians and Surgeons of Saskatchewan, *Saskatchewan Methadone Guidelines for the Treatment of Opiate Addiction*, College of Physicians and Surgeons and Saskatchewan Health, 2008.

[8] New Brunswick Addiction Services, *MMT Maintenance Treatment Polices and Procedures: New Beginnings*, 2009.

[9] Collège des Médecins du Québec, *The Use of Methadone in the Treatment of Opiate Addiction: Clinical Practice Guidelines*, College de Medecins du Quebec, 2000.

[10] Jamieson, Beals, Lalond and Associates, Inc, *Best Practices Methadone Maintenance Treatment*, Minister of Public Works and Government Services Canada, 2002.

[11] L. Amato, S. Minozzi, M. Davoli, S. Vecchi, M. M. Ferri, and S. Mayet, "Psychosocial combined with agonist maintenance treatments versus agonist maintenance treatments alone for treatment of opioid dependence," *Cochrane Database of Systematic Reviews*, no. 4, Article ID CD004147, 2008.

[12] J. F. Anderson and L. D. Warren, "Client retention in the British Columbia methadone program, 1996–1999," *Canadian Journal of Public Health*, vol. 95, no. 2, pp. 104–109, 2004.

[13] B. Nosyk, D. C. Marsh, H. Sun, M. T. Schechter, and A. H. Anis, "Trends in methadone maintenance treatment participation, retention, and compliance to dosing guidelines in British Columbia, Canada: 1996–2006," *Journal of Substance Abuse Treatment*, vol. 39, no. 1, pp. 22–31, 2010.

[14] B. Fischer, J. Rehm, S. Brissette et al., "Illicit opioid use in Canada: comparing social, health, and drug use characteristics of untreated users in five cities (OPICAN Study)," *Journal of Urban Health*, vol. 82, no. 2, pp. 250–266, 2005.

[15] E. Oviedo-Joekes, S. Brissette, D. C. Marsh et al., "Diacetylmorphine versus methadone for the treatment of opioid addiction," *New England Journal of Medicine*, vol. 361, no. 8, pp. 777–786, 2009.

[16] C. J. Strike, W. Gnam, K. Urbanoski, B. Fischer, D. C. Marsh, and M. Millson, "Factors predicting 2-year retention in methadone maintenance treatment for opioid dependence," *Addictive Behaviors*, vol. 30, no. 5, pp. 1025–1028, 2005.

[17] J. Mendelson, K. Flower, M. J. Pletcher, and G. P. Galloway, "Addiction to prescription opioids: characteristics of the emerging epidemic and treatment with buprenorphine," *Experimental and Clinical Psychopharmacology*, vol. 16, no. 5, pp. 435–441, 2008.

[18] V. P. Dole, M. E. Nyswander, and M. J. Kreek, "Narcotic blockade," *Archives of Internal Medicine*, vol. 118, no. 4, pp. 304–309, 1966.

[19] J. R. M. Caplehorn, M. S. Y. N. Dalton, M. C. Cluff, and A. M. Petrenas, "Retention in methadone maintenance and heroin addicts' risk of death," *Addiction*, vol. 89, no. 2, pp. 203–209, 1994.

[20] L. A. Marsch, "The efficacy of methadone maintenance interventions in reducing illicit opiate use, HIV risk behavior and criminality: a meta-analysis," *Addiction*, vol. 93, no. 4, pp. 515–532, 1998.

[21] S. M. Kelly, K. E. O'Grady, S. G. Mitchell, B. S. Brown, and R. P. Schwartz, "Predictors of methadone treatment retention from a multi-site study: a survival analysis," *Drug and Alcohol Dependence*, vol. 117, no. 2-3, pp. 170–175, 2011.

[22] I. Maremmani, P. P. Pani, A. Mellini et al., "Alcohol and cocaine use and abuse among opioid addicts engaged in a Methadone Maintenance Treatment Program," *Journal of Addictive Diseases*, vol. 26, no. 1, pp. 61–70, 2007.

[23] S. M. Stine, M. Freeman, B. Burns, D. S. Charney, and T. R. Kosten, "Effect of methadone dose on cocaine abuse in a methadone program," *American Journal on Addictions*, vol. 1, no. 4, pp. 294–298, 1992.

Parental Factors Associated with Mexican American Adolescent Alcohol Use

Cristina Mogro-Wilson

School of Social Work, University of Connecticut, 1798 Asylum Avenue, West Hartford, CT 06117-2698, USA

Correspondence should be addressed to Cristina Mogro-Wilson; cristina.wilson@uconn.edu

Academic Editor: Ingmar Franken

The purpose of this study is to further the understanding of how parenting and the relationship between the parent and the youth influence adolescent alcohol use in Mexican American families, with particular attention to acculturation. Results indicated that parental warmth is a strong factor in predicting adolescent alcohol use among Mexican adolescents. The parent-youth relationship played an important role in lowering alcohol use for Mexican American youth. Acculturation has an impact on the level of warmth, control, and the parent-youth relationship for Mexican American families. Findings indicate that there are unique family mechanisms for Mexican American families that should be considered when developing prevention and treatment options.

1. Introduction

Latinos constitute the largest and most rapidly growing ethnic group in the US [1]. Currently and over the past twenty years, non-Latino adolescent alcohol use has declined, yet alcohol use among Latino youth has remained high [2]. The Latino population continues to grow and is at a high risk because of the trends in demographics. Mexican Americans constitute 67% of the Latino population, or approximately 28 million individuals [3]. Latino youths have a higher high school dropout rate, a higher proportion of families living in poverty, and the highest fertility rate compared to other minority groups [1]. In addition, there are numerous alcohol-related problems reported by young drinkers, such as interpersonal problems, impaired school and work performance, risky sexual behaviors, and drunk driving [4–6]. For many reasons, such as limited access to the population and an increased diversity of the Latino population, research on Latino adolescent alcohol use is sparse and many studies group all Latino subgroups together, making it difficult to understand differences and similarities between groups [7, 8]. Study findings on a variety of health outcomes, including substance use, have shown differences by Latino subgroup [9, 10]. This study focuses on Mexican American youth because of the lack of specific knowledge on parenting in this subgroup of Latinos. In addition, various studies have shown that Mexican Americans, compared to other Latino subgroups such as Puerto Rican's, have unique family composition, cultural attitudes, and substance use [11, 12]. It has been demonstrated that family mechanisms, in particular parenting styles, may be of important influence on substance use tendencies among young individuals.

Baumrind's [13] theoretical framework of parenting delineated four dimensions to parenting styles: permissive, authoritarian, authoritative, and uninvolved. One of the critical ideas from Baumrind's four quadrants of parenting styles is that parenting revolves around issues of warmth and control. The categorization of these two characteristics, warmth and control, creates a typology of four parenting styles. *Permissive* parents are nondirective and are lenient and are warm and loving; *authoritarian* parenting is associated with low parental warmth and stricter rules; *authoritative* parenting is associated with high parental warmth and clear limits that are negotiated; *uninvolved* parent scan be rejecting and neglectful [14, 15].

Baumrind's [13] seminal studies showed that authoritative parenting, or warm and firm parenting, has higher levels of adolescent competence and psychosocial maturity than their peers who were raised by parents who were permissive, authoritarian, or uninvolved parents. Dozens of studies over the past fifteen years that all used different methods, samples, and measures reached the same conclusion that authoritative parenting is associated with advantages in adjustment, school performance, and psychosocial maturity [16, 17]. Research on parenting styles and alcohol use among non-Latinos indicates that authoritative parenting is associated with less alcohol use [18, 19]. The majority of research on parenting and adolescent outcomes has been conducted with European American families, and increasingly with families of color [20]. There has been surprisingly little empirical research on the role of parenting and the role it plays for alcohol use in Mexican American adolescents. In light of this, this paper will investigate the connection between parenting and alcohol use for Mexican American youth.

The literature characterizes Mexican American families as having strong loyalty and closeness to the extended family (*familismo*), interdependent relationships among different generations, and a hierarchical family structure with clear expectations for parent and child roles. This type of family structure is often characterized as authoritarian based on the strong emphasis on parental respect (*respeto*) and authority [14, 21, 22]. In addition to the hierarchical family structure where parents have authority [23, 24], the parent-youth relationships are also informed by cultural norms of *personalismo* and *simpatia*, which place an emphasis on warm personal relationships [23]. This dual cultural emphasis on warmth and control is consistent with an authoritative style. Some literature has also described Mexican American parents as relaxed and permissive toward their children, which has been interpreted as an acceptance of the adolescents' individuality [23, 25]. Parenting is embedded in the culture of a group, and in an effort to understand parenting, the cultural context must be considered.

Acculturation is the social and psychological influences that occur due to continuous contact between individuals from different cultures [26]. Parental acculturation has a strong influence on the adolescents' development [27]. Vega et al. [28] found that composite measures of adolescent and parent acculturation are better predictors of alcohol use than the gaps between adolescent and parent acculturation. Parenting styles may be more fluid than what the traditional cultural norms suggests and depend on parents' adherence to traditional values, acculturation level, and the larger context of their lives [22]. Within the cultural context, parenting practices among Mexican American families can range in a variety of ways, and it is not entirely clear how acculturation relates to parenting styles.

The parent-youth relationship is another important dynamic to consider when looking at family mechanisms, particularly in Latino families. The interactions, behaviors, and emotions exchanged between parents and their adolescents can be warm or hostile. The type of parenting style used is often a reflection of how the parents were raised. However, the parent-youth relationship is a unique set of interactions that has been linked to adolescent problem-solving behaviors and feelings of being able to control events that can affect him or her [29, 30]. The protective influences of Latino family centeredness and familismo include support, counseling, advice giving, and modeling of behaviors.

The support and advice giving in a Latino family builds a relationship between the youth and parent that is above and beyond the typical parenting style. The high quality of parent-youth relationships has been linked to the positive development of adolescents in multiple domains such as depressive symptoms, aggression, and substance use [31, 32]. Mexican American families are often considered to be highly child-centered, with parent-youth relationships often viewed as more important than the marital relationship [23]. The meaning and influence of parenting practices and the parent-youth relationship may differ across ethnic groups. Parental practices are often shaped by culture-specific norms and by ecological factors, such as the process of acculturation [33].

There have been few investigations on the relationship of parenting style to adolescent alcohol use among Mexican American youth specifically. A national sample on Latino adolescents utilizing the Add Health data indicated that high amounts of parental warmth, control, and parent-youth relationship decreased alcohol use [34]. However, acculturation of the parent (parent place of birth) did not influence parenting and the study did not investigate the findings for Mexican American youth [34]. A study of alcohol and other drug use among adolescents found that a positive relationship with the father was associated with less use of alcohol among the Latino subsample. Parental control or strictness was associated with lower substance use [35]. Another study of Latino preadolescents found lower rates of smoking initiation among youth who reported higher levels of parental monitoring and communication about problems with parents [36]. Research that included a subsample of Latino youth of approximately ages between 11 and 13 found that parental monitoring was associated with adolescents' lower use of drugs [37].

Thus, while parental control and warmth have been associated with less drug use, the research that was conducted thus far with Latino youth has several key limitations. First, research has been conducted with Latino samples that reflect substantial diversity with respect to culture, historical context, and history in the US This paper will address this gap by investigating Mexican American families. Second, the literature has not examined the relationship of acculturation level and the influence it may have on a parenting style and alcohol use for Mexican American families. Third, there has been little examination of the independent and combined influence of the role that the parent-youth relationship plays in relationship to parenting and its connection to alcohol use. The present study addresses these gaps in its investigation of the relationship between Mexican American parenting style, the parent-youth relationship, and adolescent alcohol use while taking into consideration the parents' acculturation level. Based on prior theoretical and empirical work, the study is guided by the following hypotheses.

H1: Mexican American parents who are high in control and those parents who are low in warmth (authoritarian parenting) will have adolescents who use alcohol less compared to those with high amounts of control and high warmth (authoritative parenting). The hypothesis is that Mexican American adolescents respond better to authoritarian parenting, as this is a traditional cultural norm.

H2: Those parents using high warmth will have a positive parent-youth relationship. Those parents who have a favorable view of their relationship with their adolescent will have adolescents who use alcohol less.

H3: Less acculturated parents use authoritarian parenting (more controlling). More acculturated parents use authoritative parenting (less controlling).

H4: Acculturated youth and families will have high levels of alcohol use, low levels of control, high levels of warmth, and a good parent-youth relationship.

2. Methodology

The data used for this paper is from the National Longitudinal Study of Adolescent Health (Add Health) based in the University of North Carolina at Chapel Hill. Add Health is a school based, longitudinal study of the health-related behaviors of adolescents and their outcomes in young adulthood. Add Health uses a clustered sampling design that is school-based so that the school is the initial point of contact between the researchers and the respondents. There are 132 schools in the core study. A self-administered questionnaire was taken in schools between September 1994 and April 1995 during a class period for grades 7–12. All of these students (83,105) were used as a sampling frame to identify a stratified (by grade and gender) random sample of 16,044 adolescents [38]. These 16,044 students comprise the core sample and were used for in-home interviews. All data used in this paper is taken from the in-home interview [39]. A parent, usually the mother, also completed a questionnaire. Ninety-five percent of the respondents for the in-home interview were female head of households, 88% of which were the biological mother; the remaining were grandmothers, step mothers, or aunts. One year later, the Wave 2 in-home sample was composed of adolescents who participated in the first wave of the in-home component and resulted in 10,547 participants [39]. The response rate for Wave 1 is 79%, and the response rate for Wave 2 is 88% [40]. For the purpose of this study only the adolescents who responded that they were Mexican American and had data on alcohol use behaviors for Waves 1 and 2 were used for this sample $n = 956$.

2.1. Measures

2.1.1. Alcohol Use. Adolescents were asked about how often they consume alcohol and how often they get drunk in the past 12 months, responses ranged from almost every day, three to five times a week, one or two days a week, two or three days a month, once a month or less or one or two days in the past year, or never. The drinking and getting drunk questions were asked in Wave 1 and Wave 2.

2.1.2. Parent Acculturation. Parents were asked if they were born in the United States.

2.1.3. Adolescent Acculturation. The adolescent was asked if they were born in the US.

2.1.4. Family Acculturation. The adolescent was asked what language they usually speak in their home.

2.1.5. Parental Control. Youth were asked if their parents allow them to make their own decisions about "(a) the time you must be home on weekend nights? (b) the people you hang around with? (c) what you wear? (d) how much television you watch? (e) which television programs you watch? (f) what time you got to bed on week nights? (g) what you eat?" A scale was created where the sum of the 7 questions was divided by 7, then multiplied by 100, giving a percentage. Those with a high percentage are highly controlled.

2.1.6. Parental Warmth. Youth were asked how warm and loving their mother/father was towards them options ranged 5 = strongly agree, 4 = agree, 3 = neither agree nor disagree, 2 = disagree, 1 = strongly disagree, where high numbers indicate high warmth. Mother and father warmth were averaged together with a Pearson correlation of .151, $P < .001$.

2.1.7. Parent-Youth Relationship. Parents were asked: "How often would it be true for you to make each of the following statements about your child" Indicator no. 1: you get along well with him/her; Indicator no. 2: you make decisions about his/her life together; Indicator no. 3: you feel you can really trust him/her. This was measured using a 5-point scale starting at always, often, sometimes, seldom, and never. Where higher numbers indicate a better relationship.

2.1.8. Peer Alcohol Use. Youth were asked how many of their three best friends drink alcohol at least once a month, and responses ranged from 0 to 3, peer alcohol use was used as covariate.

2.1.9. Income. Income was measured by a question in the parent questionnaire that asked about total income before taxes for everyone in the household, income was used as a covariate.

3. Results

The study sample consisted of 956 Mexican American adolescents ($n = 956$). Parental acculturation level that was measured by parent place of birth indicated that almost half of the parents were born inside the US (46%) with 54% born outside of the US Most of the Mexican American adolescents were born in the US (83%). About half of the adolescents spoke primarily English in the home (56%), indicating that 44% of the sample spoke primarily Spanish in the home. Gender was divided almost equally among adolescents with slightly more females with 52% and males with 48%. The adolescents in the sample ranged from 7th grade to 12th grade at Wave 1. Twelve percent of the sample were in the seventh grade, 12% in 8th grade, 13% in 9th grade, 24% in 10th grade, 19% in 11th grade, and 18% in 12th grade, and 3% of the sample refused to answer or was not in a school that had traditional grade levels. Income levels indicated that 64% of the families earned less than $34,000 annually (Table 1).

TABLE 1: Descriptive characteristics of Mexican American youth ($n = 956$).

Characteristic	Frequency	(%)
Place of birth: parent		
US	440	46%
Outside the US	516	54%
Place of birth: adolescent		
US	792	83%
Outside the U.S.	164	17%
Language Spoken at home		
English	538	56%
Spanish	418	44%
Sex		
Female	494	52%
Male	462	48%
Grade (at Wave 1)		
7th	112	12%
8th	114	12%
9th	121	13%
10th	230	24%
11th	180	19%
12th	167	18%
Not in school	1	0%
Refused	8	1%
School does not have grade levels of this kind	23	2%
Income		
$1,000–24,000	457	48%
$25,000–34,000	153	16%
$35,000–44,000	116	12%
$45,000–54,000	96	10%
$55,000–64,000	60	6%
$65,000–74,000	27	3%
$75,000–84,000	25	3%
Over $85,000	22	2%

TABLE 2: Parenting characteristics of Mexican American families ($n = 956$).

Parenting characteristic	Frequency	(%)
Parental warmth		
Very low warmth	28	3%
Low warmth	186	19%
Average warmth	142	15%
High warmth	296	31%
Very high warmth	304	32%
Parental control		
Not controlling	168	18%
Slightly controlling	595	62%
Very controlling	178	19%
Totally controlling	15	2%
Parent-youth relationship		
Get along well (PY1)		
Never	3	0.3%
Seldom	13	1%
Sometimes	101	11%
Often	314	33%
Always	525	55%
Make decisions together (PY2)		
Never	23	2%
Seldom	38	4%
Sometimes	230	24%
Often	316	33%
Always	349	37%
Trust them (PY3)		
Never	7	1%
Seldom	25	3%
Sometimes	117	12%
Often	218	23%
Always	589	62%

Parental warmth measured on a scale of 1 to 5 ranging from very low warmth to very high warmth had mostly parents indicating very high or high warmth (63%) and the rest (37%) indicting very low, low, or average warmth. Adolescents indicated that parental control on a scale of 0 to 100 that 18% were not controlling, 62% were slightly controlling, and 19% were very controlling with only 2% being totally controlling (Table 2).

The parent-youth relationship was measured by three different variables. The first, get along well together (py1), found most parents saying often or always (88%) with the remaining indicating never, seldom, or sometimes (12%). The second parent-youth relationship variable (py2), asking parents if they make decisions together with their adolescent, found that 70% often or always make decisions together and 30% never, seldom, or sometimes make decisions together. The third parent-youth relationship variable (py3) asked the parents if they trust their adolescent and found that 85% always or often trust them and 15% never, seldom, or sometimes trust them (Table 2).

3.1. Structural Equation Modeling Analysis.

Structural equation modeling (SEM) is used for an analysis of the effects between identified independent variables. The model for this analysis will be based in the existing research and theory. The data was analyzed using Mplus and the appropriate sample weights created by the AddHealth staff [38, 41, 42].

Multivariate normality was evaluated using Mardia's index. The P value for the multivariate index was statistically significant ($P < 0.05$). Examination of univariate indices of skewness and kurtosis revealed only two variables with absolute skewness values and kurtosis values above 2.0, the getting drunk variables from Wave 1 and Wave 2. Given the presence of nonnormality the Mplus analysis utilizing sample weights, a complex analysis was used using MLR, maximum likelihood estimation with robust standard errors, which is robust to nonnormality.

A variety of indices of model fit were evaluated resulting in good model fit. The Bollen-Stine bootstrapped chi-square test yielded a value of 88.665, with degrees of freedom of 36, and a P value of 0.001. The Root Mean Square Error of Approximation (RMSEA) was 0.039, which was less than 0.08 indicating good model fit. The P value for the test of close fit was 0.958, which was nonsignificant indicating good model fit [43]. The test of close fit provides a one-sided test of the null hypothesis that the RMSEA equals .05, and this is what is called a close-fitting model. The Comparative Fit Index was 0.986 which was higher than 0.95, indicating again good model fit [44]. The Tucker-Lewis Index (TLI) was 0.97, indicating a very good fit. The indices uniformly point towards good model fit. Inspection of the residuals and modification indices revealed no significant points of ill fit in the model. Figure 1 presents the parameter estimates incorporating sampling weights. The residuals are in standardized form and are reflective of unexplained variance in the endogenous variables.

Path coefficients for parent place of birth affecting parental control did result in statistical significant coefficients for Mexican American youth. On average, for parents born inside the US, parental control would decrease by .003 for Mexican American youth ($P < .001$) compared to those parents born outside the U.S. On average if English was spoken at home, parental control would decrease by .098 compared to those who spoke Spanish at home ($P < .001$). If English was spoken at home, the parent-youth relationship decreases by .043 compared to if Spanish was spoken in the home ($P < .001$). If the adolescent was born in the US, alcohol use at Wave 1 increased by .043 compared to those who were born outside the US ($P < .001$). If the adolescent was born in the US parental control decreased by .002 compared to if the adolescent was born outside the US ($P < .001$). If they were born in the US parental warmth increased by .027 compared to if the adolescent was born outside the US ($P < .001$).

For every one unit increase in parental warmth, the parent-youth relationship increases by 0.259 ($P < .001$). Parental control on the parent-youth relationship did not result in statistically significant coefficients. For every one unit increase in the parent-youth relationship, adolescent alcohol use is 0.189 units lower for Mexican American youth ($P < .001$). A one unit increase in parental warmth results in alcohol use at Wave 1 decreasing by 0.129 ($P < .001$). For Mexican American youth, parental control does not significantly influence the use of alcohol.

The covariate estimates for presentation purposes are not on the figure. For Mexican American youth, every additional friend who uses alcohol, parental control decreases by .007 ($P < .001$). For every additional friend who uses alcohol, alcohol use in Wave 1 increased by .678 ($P < .001$). Income did significantly influence parental warmth for Mexican American youth; for every one thousand dollar increase in income, parental warmth increased by 5.314 ($P < .001$). For every one thousand dollar increase in income, parental control decreased by .098 ($P < .001$).

4. Discussion

The results of this study contribute to the understanding of how family mechanisms, specifically parenting and the parent-youth relationship, influence the use of alcohol for

Mexican American adolescents and the impact of acculturation on these factors. Few studies are able to investigate within Latino subgroups. However, these subgroups are often very different in their cultural values and in their decision to use substances [7]. For these reasons, the model was tested for Mexican American youth. The dependent variable of alcohol use was measured once at Wave 1 and again one year later at Wave 2. None of the variables used in the model significantly predicted alcohol use at Wave 2. In this model, there is no prediction of change or no activity with intent to have an impact one year later. This may be due to the short-time period of one year from Wave 1 to Wave 2, and therefore sustained changes may have had difficulty becoming apparent. Therefore, all findings are relational and not causal.

One of the most interesting findings for Mexican American adolescents was the influence of acculturation on family mechanisms. Mexican American parents who are more acculturated, or born inside the US, and those who spoke English in the home had lower levels of parental control compared to less acculturated parents. This relationship was expected, given that if the parent is more acculturated their parenting style would become more similar to non-Latinos, and there would be less parental control. For Mexican American youth, if the adolescent was born in the US, there was more parental warmth and less control, compared to less acculturated youth. This finding confirms the idea that acculturation does have influence parenting for Mexican American families. Interestingly, a previous model testing a Latino sample showed that there was no relationship between parental acculturation and parental control [34]. The finding for Mexican American families indicates the increased influence of acculturation on parenting that does not exist in other studies looking at other subgroups of Latinos. This strengthens the rationale to continue to do research on subgroups of Latinos, as acculturation is creating differential effects on behaviors and outcomes. Various reasons for this difference in the level of acculturation on parenting necessitate further investigation, including the community characteristics and a more in-depth examination of the acculturation process for the parent, youth, and family.

Language spoken at home, a measure of family acculturation level, also had an influence on the parent-youth relationship. If English was spoken in the home, there was a decrease in the parent-youth relationship. This could possibly be contributed to a widening gap between the parent and youth as distance is created from the original culture. Traditional Latino families may have a stronger connection with their youth, and as the family moves toward being more acculturated and speaking more English in the home, the parent and the youth relationship suffers. Previous model testing did not show this relationship for a Latino sample [34]. The influence of language on the parent-youth relationship and the adolescent place of birth impact on parental warmth and control are unique to Mexican American families.

There have been very few research studies that show the impact of acculturation on parenting style. However, there is contradictory evidence. Some studies show that the gap between the child and parent acculturation levels lead to

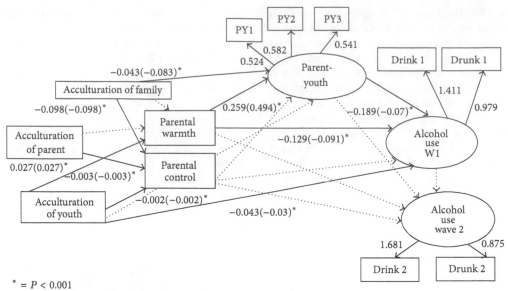

* = P < 0.001

Those arrows that are dotted had nonsignificant estimates.

Latent constructs are in circles, and all observed variables are in boxes.

Covariates used in this model are income and peer alcohol use.

Standardized estimates are presented on the arrows with unstandardized estimates in parenthesis.

All exogenous variables are considered to be correlated.

FIGURE 1: SEM model for explaining the relationship between parenting style, acculturation, and alcohol use in Mexican American adolescents.

more alcohol use, while others have found that the overall level of parent and child acculturation determines alcohol use [28, 45]. Martinez [46] found that family acculturation level is a better construct rather than differences in parent and adolescent acculturation when predicting substance use. This model does not support the finding of Martinez [46] where acculturation of the youth is the only direct predictor of alcohol use for adolescents.

Mexican American family mechanisms are influenced by acculturation factors. Similar to Delva et al. [7], who found that acculturation level was measured by preferred language spoken, Mexican adolescents were more likely to use alcohol or marijuana. Acculturation has an impact on level of warmth, control, and the parent-youth relationship for Mexican American families.

Although there is an effect of parent place of birth on parental control, parental control does not have a significant effect on alcohol use. However, it did have an effect for the entire Latino sample [34]. The large Latino sample ($n = 1887$) consisted of 51% Mexican American, 30% other subgroups such as Cubans and South Americans, and 19% Puerto Rican youth. The Mexican American subgroup could be pulling down the covariate estimate while the other subgroups in the Latino group are pulling the covariate up. This suggests differences among Latino subgroups around the understanding of parental control in relation to alcohol use. It is possible that there are cultural differences for the way parental control is practiced or the way that adolescents perceive parental control. The differences with the Mexican American youth compared to a Latino sample in Mogro-Wilson's [34] can be explained by the other subgroups not analyzed.

Parenting in a warm and loving manner, as interpreted by youth, was related to a decrease in alcohol use for Mexican-American youth. In addition the more warmth and love showed to the youth was also related to a better parent-youth relationship which decreases alcohol use. The importance of warmth found in this Mexican American sample is consistent with cultural norms that stress nurturing of the child in the context of a respect and a strong family [23, 34, 47]. The present study is unique in providing evidence for the role of the parent-youth relationship and the role of acculturation on warmth.

This research indicated that the stronger the parent-youth relationship Mexican American youth used less alcohol. The parent-youth relationship is an important construct in family mechanisms that can have an impact on alcohol use beyond typical parenting constructs of warmth and control. This finding highlights the importance of the parent-youth relationship in the use of alcohol and indicates the importance to target this construct in interventions and prevention. Parenting interventions should include aspects of building and strengthening parent-youth relationships, activities to foster the growth of the relationship, make decisions together, and build trust.

4.1. Limitations. Limitations of the study include the age of the data; the data for this study was collected in 1995; however, there has been little change in alcohol use over time for this population. Comparing the 1995 Add Health data to national alcohol use rates based on the Monitoring the Future Study, the rates used in the present study are similar to the national use rates [48]. The Monitoring the Future Study national use rates for Hispanic youth show in 2009 when asked if they have ever used alcohol, 19% of eighth graders responded that they had used alcohol, and 34% of tenth graders and 40% of twelfth graders indicated they had drank in the past year [10]. The Add Health sample of Mexican American adolescents used in this study indicates more alcohol usage with 35% of 8th graders reported using alcohol, 53% of tenth graders and 57% of twelfth graders. In addition to changes in alcohol use over time, there may also be changes in family dynamics that occur over time that are impossible to predict, and this adds to the limitations of the present study.

In addition to the date of data collection, there are measurement issues such as the construct of parental control. The measure used for parental control was unable to indicate negotiation, an important aspect of parenting, and this limits the findings. In addition, the parent-youth relationship would have benefited from a well-validated questionnaire such as the Alabama Parenting questionnaire or the Egna Minnen av Barndoms Uppfostran—My Memories of Upbringing (EMBU) [49, 50].

A limitation to the acculturation findings relates to how acculturation was measured. Measuring acculturation by language spoken at home and how long the individual has been in the country still holds validity. Many researchers continue to conceptualize and measure individual acculturation in a unilinear way [51, 52]. The variety of acculturation measures also shows that there is no consistent way to measure acculturation in the field. For these reasons and due to constraints of the secondary data set, acculturation was measured by place of birth and language spoken at home. However, this is a unidimensional way to measure acculturation, and the use of better measures of acculturation should be used in the future to see if the results are similar. Studies have demonstrated that proxy acculturation items, such as place of birth and language spoken at home, can be useful to assess acculturation in situations where use of a more comprehensive acculturation scale is impractical [52]. Language is considered the strongest single predictor of acculturation [53].

5. Conclusion

This study confirms the importance of the family as a protective factor for alcohol use in adolescence for Mexican Americans. Parenting and the relationship the parent has with their youth influences an adolescent's choice to use alcohol. The role of parents to reduce the risk taking behavior of alcohol use is a strong finding. The present study used combined scores of parental warmth and control of the mother and father; however, separating these differences to see what kind of contribution the mother versus the father in the role of parenting would be valuable. Extended research on other subgroups of Latinos would be useful in understanding the similarities and differences between Mexican American and other subgroups, such as Puerto Ricans. Further qualitative research would be useful in describing the parenting styles and practices in diverse groups of Mexican American families. It would be valuable to examine if parenting characterized by warmth is viewed as more consistent with Mexican American cultural norms. Further research that measures

acculturation bidimensionally and its influence on parenting and the parent-youth relationship would prove useful to the understanding of alcohol use.

Parental warmth can function as a protective factor for Mexican American families in preventing alcohol use. However, this is in the context of the parent-youth relationship, which is a necessary component to the model. Common beliefs about Latino families characterize parenting as strict, controlling, and abrasive. This model found no relationship between parental control and alcohol use for Mexican American families. Parental warmth plays a large role in adolescent alcohol use, as warmth increases the parent-youth relationship improves and alcohol use decreases. This paper supports the idea that Mexican American families have a protective quality of high warmth and a good parent-youth relationship, and as they acculturate the parent-youth relationship decreases and alcohol use increases.

Few interventions to prevent underage drinking have specifically targeted Latino youth or families [54, 55]. Further research is needed to design culturally appropriate interventions that are likely to be accepted among Latino families. Programs designed to improve parental warmth and caring behaviors toward the youth and programs to promote positive parent-youth relationships are likely to reduce adolescent alcohol use. Interventions that focus on relationship building, across the acculturation divide between the youth and parent, could help promote a positive parent-youth relationship. In addition focusing on trust building activities and making joint decisions between the parent and the youth could provide a protective factor from using alcohol in adolescence.

Acknowledgments

This research uses data from Add Health, a program project directed by Kathleen Mullan Harris and designed by J. Richard Udry, Peter S. Bearman, and Kathleen Mullan Harris at the University of North Carolina at Chapel Hill, and it was funded by Grant P01-HD31921 from the Eunice Kennedy Shriver National Institute of Child Health and Human Development, with cooperative funding from 23 other federal agencies and foundations. Special acknowledgment is due to Ronald R. Rindfuss and Barbara Entwisle for assistance in the original design. Information on how to obtain the Add Health data files is available at the Add Health website (http://www.cpc.unc.edu/addhealth). No direct support was received from grant P01-HD31921 for this analysis. This research was funded in part by the National Institute on Drug Abuse (NIDA) through the Child Welfare, Drug Abuse, and Intergenerational Risk (CWDAIR) Social Work Development Program at the School of Social Welfare, University at Albany (5R01-DA-015376-02).

References

[1] U.S. Census Bureau, 2010, U.S. Census Brief, http://www.census.gov/prod/cen2010/briefs/c2010br-02.pdf.

[2] L. D. Johnston, P. M. O'Malley, J. G. Bachman, and J. E. Schulenberg, *Monitoring the Future National Results on Adolescent Drug*

Use: Overview of Key Findings, 2009, National Institute on Drug Use, Bethesda, Md, USA, 2010.

[3] U.S. Census Bureau, 2011, American Community Survey B03001 1-Year Estimates Estimates Hispanic or Latino origin by specific Origin.

[4] S. A. Brown, M. McGue, J. Maggs et al., "A developmental perspective on alcohol and youths 16 to 20 years of age," *Pediatrics*, vol. 121, supplement 4, pp. S290–S310, 2008.

[5] National Institute on Alcohol Abuse and Alcoholism, *Underage Drinking*, U.S. Department of Health and Human Services, Rockville, Md, USA, 2006.

[6] Office of the Surgeon General, *The Surgeon General's Call to Action to Prevent and Reduce Underage Drinking*, Department of Health and Human Services, Washington, DC, USA, 2007.

[7] J. Delva, J. M. Wallace, P. M. O'Malley, J. G. Bachman, L. D. Johnston, and J. E. Schulenberg, "The epidemiology of alcohol, marijuana, and cocaine use among Mexican American, Puerto Rican, Cuban American, and other Latin American eighth-grade students in the United States: 1991–2002," *American Journal of Public Health*, vol. 95, no. 4, pp. 696–702, 2005.

[8] R. S. Zimmerman, W. A. Vega, A. G. Gil, G. J. Warheit, E. Apospori, and F. Biafora, "Who is Hispanic? Definitions and their consequences," *American Journal of Public Health*, vol. 84, no. 12, pp. 1985–1987, 1994.

[9] L. C. Gallo, F. J. Penedo, K. E. de Los Monteros, and W. Arguelles, "Resiliency in the face of disadvantage: do hispanic cultural characteristics protect health outcomes?" *Journal of Personality*, vol. 77, no. 6, pp. 1707–1746, 2009.

[10] L. D. Johnston, P. M. O'Malley, J. G. Bachman, and J. E. Schulenberg, "Monitoring the future national survey results on drug use, 1975–2005: volume 1, secondary school students," NIH Publication 06-5883, National Institute on Drug Abuse, Bethesda, Md, USA, 2006, http://www.monitoringthefuture.org.

[11] L. M. Estrada-Martínez, M. B. Padilla, C. H. Caldwell, and A. J. Schulz, "Examining the influence of family environments on youth violence: a comparison of Mexican, Puerto Rican, Cuban, non-Latino Black, and non-Latino White adolescents," *Journal of Youth and Adolescence*, vol. 40, no. 8, pp. 1039–1051, 2011.

[12] A. M. G. Wahl and T. M. Eitle, "Gender, acculturation and alcohol use among latina/o adolescents: a multi-ethnic comparison," *Journal of Immigrant and Minority Health*, vol. 12, no. 2, pp. 153–165, 2010.

[13] D. Baumrind, "Parental disciplinary patterns and social competence in children," *Youth and Society*, vol. 9, pp. 239–276, 1978.

[14] R. A. Bulcroft, D. C. Carmody, and K. A. Bulcroft, "Patterns of parental independence giving to adolescents: variations by race, age, and gender of child," *Journal of Marriage and Family*, vol. 58, no. 4, pp. 866–883, 1996.

[15] G. Gonzalez-Ramos, L. H. Zayas, and E. V. Cohen, "Child-rearing values of low-income, urban Puerto Rican mothers of preschool children," *Professional Psychology*, vol. 29, no. 4, pp. 377–382, 1998.

[16] L. Steinberg, "We know some things: parent-adolescent relationships in retrospect and prospect," *Journal of Research on Adolescence*, vol. 11, no. 1, pp. 1–19, 2001.

[17] L. Steinberg and A. S. Morris, "Adolescent development," *Annual Review of Psychology*, vol. 52, pp. 83–110, 2001.

[18] J. Lilja, S. Larsson, B. U. Wilhelmsen, and D. Hamilton, "Perspectives on preventing adolescent substance use and misuse," *Substance Use and Misuse*, vol. 38, no. 10, pp. 1491–1530, 2003.

[19] S. T. Ennett, K. E. Bauman, V. A. Foshee, M. Pemberton, and K. A. Hicks, "Parent-Child communication about adolescent tobacco and alcohol use: what do parents say and does it affect youth behavior?" *Journal of Marriage and the Family*, vol. 63, no. 1, pp. 48–62, 2001.

[20] V. C. McLoyd, A. M. Cauce, D. Takeuchi, and L. W. Wayne, "Marital processes and parental socialization in families of color: a decade review of research," *Journal of Marriage and Family*, vol. 62, no. 4, pp. 1070–1093, 2000.

[21] A. M. Cauce and M. D. Rodríguez, "Latino families: myths and realities," in *Latino Children and Families in the United States: Current Research and Future Directions*, J. Contreras, A. Neal-Barnett, and K. Kerns, Eds., pp. 3–25, Praeger, Westport, Conn, USA, 2002.

[22] L. H. Zayas and F. Solari, "Early childhood socialization in Hispanic families: context, culture, and practice implications," *Professional Psychology*, vol. 25, no. 3, pp. 200–206, 1994.

[23] C. J. Falicov, "Mexican families," in *Ethnicity and Family Therapy*, M. McGoldrick, J. Giordano, and N. Garcia-Preto, Eds., pp. 229–241, Guilford Press, New York, NY, USA, 3rd edition, 2005.

[24] K. M. Lindahl and N. M. Malik, "Marital conflict, family processes, and boys' externalizing behavior in Hispanic American and European American families," *Journal of Clinical Child and Adolescent Psychology*, vol. 28, no. 1, pp. 12–24, 1999.

[25] P. L. Escovar and P. J. Lazarus, "Cross-cultural child-rearing practices: implications for school psychology," *School Psychology International*, vol. 3, pp. 143–148, 1982.

[26] R. Redfield, R. Linton, and M. J. Herskovits, "Memorandum for the study of acculturation," *American Anthropologist*, vol. 38, pp. 149–152, 1936.

[27] J. M. Rodríguez and K. Kosloski, "The impact of acculturation on attitudinal familism in a community of Puerto Rican Americans," *Hispanic Journal of Behavioral Sciences*, vol. 20, no. 3, pp. 375–391, 1998.

[28] W. A. Vega, A. G. Gil, and E. Wagner, "Cultural adjustments and Hispanic adolescents," in *Drug Use and Ethnicity in Early Adolescents*, W. A. Vega and A. Gil, Eds., Plenum Press, New York, NY, USA, 1998.

[29] X. Ge, K. M. Best, R. D. Conger, and R. L. Simons, "Parenting behaviors and the occurrence and co-occurrence of adolescent depressive symptoms and conduct problems," *Developmental Psychology*, vol. 32, no. 4, pp. 717–731, 1996.

[30] G. Krampen, "Perceived childrearing practices and the development of locus of control in early adolescence," *International Journal of Behavioral Development*, vol. 12, no. 2, pp. 177–193, 1989.

[31] B. K. Barber, H. E. Stolz, and J. A. Olsen, *Parental Support, Psychological Control and Behavioral Control: Assessing Relevance Across Time, Culture and Method*, Blackwell Publishing, Boston, Mass, USA, 2005.

[32] K. E. Grant, B. E. Compas, A. F. Stuhlmacher, A. E. Thurm, S. D. McMahon, and J. A. Halpert, "Stressors and child and adolescent psychopathology: moving from markers to mechanisms of risk," *Psychological Bulletin*, vol. 129, no. 3, pp. 447–466, 2003.

[33] S. Voisine, M. Parsai, F. F. Marsiglia, S. Kulis, and T. Nieri, "Effects of parental monitoring, permissiveness, and injunctive norms on substance use among Mexican and Mexican American adolescents," *Families in Society*, vol. 89, no. 2, pp. 264–273, 2008.

[34] C. Mogro-Wilson, "The influence of parental warmth and control on Latino adolescent alcohol use," *Hispanic Journal of Behavioral Sciences*, vol. 30, no. 1, pp. 89–105, 2000.

[35] R. Coombs and J. Landsverk, "Parenting styles and substance use during childhood and adolescence," *Journal of Marriage and the Family*, vol. 50, pp. 473–482, 1988.

[36] S. Shakib, M. Mouttapa, C. A. Johnson et al., "Ethnic variation in parenting characteristics and adolescent smoking," *The Journal of Adolescent Health*, vol. 33, no. 2, pp. 88–97, 2003.

[37] D. J. Flannery, A. T. Vazsonyi, and D. C. Rowe, "Caucasian and hispanic early adolescent substance use: parenting, personality, and school adjustment," *Journal of Early Adolescence*, vol. 16, no. 1, pp. 71–89, 1996.

[38] K. Chantala and J. Tabor, *Strategies to Perform a Design-Based. Analysis Using the Add Health Data*, Carolina Population Center, University of North Carolina, Chapel Hill, NC, USA, 1999.

[39] R. Tourangeau and H. C. Shin, *National Longitudinal Study of Adolescent Health: Grand Sample Weight*, Carolina Population Center, University of North Carolina, Chapel Hill, NC, USA, 1999.

[40] K. M. Harris, F. Florey, J. Tabor, P. S. Bearman, J. Jones, and J. R. Udry, 2003, The National Longitudinal Study of Adolescent Health: Research Design, http://www.cpc.unc.edu/projects/addhealth/design.

[41] L. Muthen and B. Muthen, *Mplus User's Guide*, Muthen & Muthen, Los Angeles, Calif, USA, 1998–2001.

[42] K. Chantala, "Introduction to analyzing Add Health data," in *Proceedings of the Add Health Users Workshop National Institutes of Health*, Bethesda, Md, USA, July 2003.

[43] M. W. Browne and R. Cudeck, "Alternative ways of assessing model fit," in *Testing Structural Equation Models*, vol. 154, pp. 136–162, Sage Focus Editions, Beverly Hills, Calif, USA, 1993.

[44] K. A. Bollen and J. S. Long, Eds., *Testing Structural Equation Models*, Sage, Newbury Park, Calif, USA, 1993.

[45] J. Szapocznik and W. Kurtines, "Acculturation, biculturalism, and adjustment among Cuban Americans," in *Acculturation: Theory, Models and Some New Findings*, A. Padilla, Ed., pp. 134–160, Westview, Boulder, Colo, USA, 1980.

[46] C. R. Martinez, "Effects of differential family acculturation on Latino adolescent substance use," *Family Relations*, vol. 55, no. 3, pp. 306–317, 2006.

[47] C. Delgado-Gaitan, "Parenting in two generations of Mexican American families," *International Journal of Behavioral Development*, vol. 16, no. 3, pp. 409–427, 1993.

[48] L. D. Johnston, P. M. OMalley, J. G. Bachman, and J. E. Schulenberg, "Demographic subgroup trends for various licit and illicit drugs, 1975–2009," Monitoring the Future Occasional Paper No. 73, Institute for Social Research, Ann Arbor, Mich, USA, 2010, http://www.monitoringthefuture.org/.

[49] K. K. Shelton, P. J. Frick, and J. Wooton, "Assessment of parenting practices in families of elementary school-age children," *Journal of Clinical Child Psychology*, vol. 25, pp. 317–329, 1996.

[50] C. Perris, L. Jacobsson, and H. Lindstrom, "Development of a new inventory for assessing memories of parental rearing behaviour," *Acta Psychiatrica Scandinavica*, vol. 61, no. 4, pp. 265–274, 1980.

[51] M. Alegria, W. Sribney, M. Woo, M. Torres, and P. Guarnaccia, "Looking beyond nativity: the relation of age of immigration, length of residence, and birth cohorts to the risk of onset of psychiatric disorders for Latinos," *Research in Human Development*, vol. 4, no. 1-2, pp. 19–47, 2007.

[52] T. H. Cruz, S. W. Marshall, J. M. Bowling, and A. Villaveces, "The validity of a proxy acculturation scale among U.S. Hispanics," *Hispanic Journal of Behavioral Sciences*, vol. 30, no. 4, pp. 425–446, 2008.

[53] E. Arcia, M. Skinner, D. Bailey, and V. Correa, "Models of acculturation and health behaviors among Latino immigrants to the US," *Social Science and Medicine*, vol. 53, no. 1, pp. 41–53, 2001.

[54] L. O'Donnell, A. Myint-U, R. Duran, and A. Stueve, "Especially for daughters: parent education to address alcohol and sex-related risk taking among urban young adolescent girls," *Health Promotion Practice*, vol. 11, supplement 3, pp. 70S–78S, 2010.

[55] H. Pantin, G. Prado, B. Lopez et al., "A randomized controlled trial of familias unidas for hispanic adolescents with behavior problems," *Psychosomatic Medicine*, vol. 71, no. 9, pp. 987–995, 2009.

Permissions

List of Contributors

Jeffrey N. Weatherly
Department of Psychology, University of North Dakota, Grand Forks, ND 58202-8380, USA

Robert D. Keeley
Division of Community Health Services, Denver Health Medical Center, Denver, CO 80204, USA
Department of Family Medicine, University of Colorado at Denver Health Sciences Center, Aurora, CO 80045-0508, USA

Margaret Driscoll
Driscoll Consulting, 866 Paragon Dr., Boulder, CO 80303, USA

Benjamin Goddard, Leanne S. Son Hing and Francesco Leri
Department of Psychology, University of Guelph, 50 Stone Road East, Guelph, ON, CanadaN1G 2W1

Monideepa B. Becerra, Patti Herring and Helen Hopp Marshak
Department of Health Promotion and Education, School of Public Health, Loma Linda University, 24951 North Circle Drive, Loma Linda, CA 92350, USA

Jim E. Banta
Department of Health Policy and Management, School of Public Health, Loma Linda University, 24951 North Circle Drive, Loma Linda, CA 92350, USA

Steven C. Matson and Andrea E. Bonny
Department of Pediatrics, The Ohio State University College of Medicine, Columbus, OH, USA
Division of Adolescent Medicine, Nationwide Children's Hospital, 700 Children's Drive, G353 Timken Hall, Columbus, OH 43205-2664, USA

Cathleen Bentley and Vicki Hughes Dughman
Department of Clinical Services and Care Coordination, Nationwide Children's Hospital, Columbus, OH, USA

Hui G. Cheng
Shanghai Mental Health Center, Shanghai Jiao Tong University, 3210 Humin Road, Shanghai 201108, China

Orla McBride
Division of Population Health Sciences, Department of Psychology, Royal College of Surgeons in Ireland, 123 Street Stephen's Green, Dublin 2, Ireland

Hugh Klein
Kensington Research Institute, 401 Schuyler Road, Silver Spring, Maryland, MD 20910, USA
Rollins School of Public Health, Emory University, Atlanta, GA 30322, USA

Claire E. Sterk and KirkW. Elifson
Rollins School of Public Health, Emory University, Atlanta, GA 30322, USA

Jennifer Tropp Sneider
Neurodevelopmental Laboratory on Addictions and Mental Health, McLean Hospital, 115 Mill Street, Mail Stop 204, Belmont, MA 02478-1064, USA
McLean Imaging Center, McLean Hospital, Boston, MA, USA
Department of Psychiatry, Harvard Medical School, Belmont, MA, USA

Staci A. Gruber
McLean Imaging Center, McLean Hospital, Boston, MA, USA
Department of Psychiatry, Harvard Medical School, Belmont, MA, USA
Cognitive and Clinical Neuroimaging Core, McLean Hospital, Belmont, MA, USA

Jadwiga Rogowska
Department of Psychiatry, Harvard Medical School, Belmont, MA, USA

Marisa M. Silveri
Neurodevelopmental Laboratory on Addictions and Mental Health, McLean Hospital, 115 Mill Street, Mail Stop 204, Belmont, MA 02478-1064, USA
McLean Imaging Center, McLean Hospital, Boston, MA, USA
Department of Psychiatry, Harvard Medical School, Belmont, MA, USA

Deborah A. Yurgelun-Todd
Department of Psychiatry, Harvard Medical School, Belmont, MA, USA
The Brain Institute, University of Utah Medical School, Salt Lake City, UT, USA

Sasha A. Fleary and Robert W. Heffer
Department of Psychology, Texas A&M University, MS 4235, College Station, TX 77843, USA

E. Lisako J. McKyer
Department of Health and Kinesiology, Texas A&M University, Dulie Bell, College Station, TX 77843, USA

Kenny Karyadi, Ayca Coskunpinar, Allyson L. Dir and Melissa A. Cyders
Indiana University-Purdue University, Indianapolis, IN, USA

RayM.Merrill, Riley J. Hedin, Arielle A. Sloan and Carl L. Hanson
Department of Health Science, Brigham Young University, Provo, UT 84602, USA

Anna Fondario
Violence and Injury Prevention Program, Utah Department of Health, Salt Lake City, UT 84114, USA

Tytti Artkoski and Pekka Saarnio
School of Social Sciences and Humanities, 33014 University of Tampere, Finland

Lisa J. Merlo
Department of Psychiatry, University of Florida, P.O. Box 100183, Gainesville, FL 32610-0183, USA

Amanda M. Stone
University of Florida, Gainesville, FL 32610, USA
Department of Emergency Medicine, Orlando Regional Medical Center, Orlando, FL 32806, USA

Alex Bibbey
University of Florida, Gainesville, FL 32610, USA
Department of Radiology, Duke University, Durham, NC 27705, USA

Steven Persaud and Jane A. Buxton
Communicable Disease Prevention and Control, British Columbia Centre for Disease Control, 655West 12th Avenue, Vancouver, BC, Canada V5Z 4R4
School of Population and Public Health, University of British Columbia, 2206 East Mall, Vancouver, BC, Canada V6T 1Z3

Despina Tzemis and Margot Kuo
Communicable Disease Prevention and Control, British Columbia Centre for Disease Control, 655West 12th Avenue, Vancouver, BC, Canada V5Z 4R4

Vicky Bungay
School of Nursing, University of British Columbia, 302-6190 Agronomy Road, Vancouver, BC, Canada V6T 1Z3

Andrew L. Cherry
School of Social Work, University of Oklahoma, Tulsa Campus, Tulsa, OK 74135, USA

Mary E. Dillon
University of Central Florida, Orlando, FL 32816, USA

Thomas M. Heffernan and Terence S. O'Neill
Collaboration for Drug and Alcohol Research (CDAR), Division of Psychology, Department of Psychology, Northumbria University, Newcastle upon Tyne NE1 8ST, UK

Hasan Ziaaddini,
Research Center for Health Services Management, Institute of Futures Studies in Health, Kerman University of Medical Sciences, Kerman, Iran

Tayebeh Ziaaddini
Research Center for Social Determinants of Health, Institute of Futures Studies in Health, Kerman University of Medical Sciences, Kerman, Iran

Nouzar Nakhaee
Neuroscience Research Center, Institute of Neuropharmacology, Kerman University of Medical Sciences, P.O. Box 76175-113, Kerman, Iran

Daikwon Han and Dennis M. Gorman
Department of Epidemiology & Biostatistics, School of Rural Public Health, Texas A&M University, College Station, TX 77843, USA

Robyn L. Richmond
School of Public Health and Community Medicine, University of New SouthWales, Kensington, Sydney, Australia

Devon Indig
School of Public Health and Community Medicine, University of New SouthWales, Kensington, Sydney, Australia
Centre for Health Research in Criminal Justice, Justice Health, University of New SouthWales, Suite 302, Level 2, 152 Bunnerong Road, Pagewood, NSW2035, Australia

Tony G. Butler
National Centre in HIV Epidemiology and Clinical Research, University of New SouthWales, Kensington, Sydney, Australia

Kay A.Wilhelm
School of Psychiatry, Faculty of Medicine, University of New SouthWales, Faces in the Street, St. Vincent's Health Urban Mental Health Research, St Vincent's Hospital, Level 4, O'Brien Centre, St Vincent's Hospital, 390 Victoria Street, Sydney, NSW2010, Australia

Vicki A. Archer
Centre for Health Research in Criminal Justice, Justice Health, University of New SouthWales, Suite 302, Level 2, 152 Bunnerong Road, Pagewood, NSW2035, Australia

Alex D.Wodak
Alcohol and Drug Service, St. Vincent's Hospital, Darlinghurst, NSW2010, Australia

Raimondo Maria Pavarin
Epidemiological Monitoring Center on Addiction, DSM-DP, ASL Bologna, Via S. Isaia 94/A, 40100 Bologna, Italy

Dario Consonni
Unit of Epidemiology, Department of Preventive Medicine, Fondazione IRCCS Ca' Granda-Ospedale Maggiore Policlinico, Via San Barnaba, 8-20122 Milan, Italy

Hugh Klein
Kensington Research Institute, 401 Schuyler Road, Silver Spring, MD 20910, USA

Timothy K. S. Christie
Ethics Services, Horizon Health Network, Miramichi, NB, Canada E1V 1Y3
Department of Bioethics, Dalhousie University, Halifax, NS, Canada B3K 6R8

Alli Murugesan
Ethics Services, Horizon Health Network, Miramichi, NB, Canada E1V 1Y3
Dr. Reiman's Cancer Research Laboratory, University of New Brunswick, Saint John, NB, Canada E3B 5A3

Dana Manzer
Uptown Clinic, St. Joseph's Hospital, Saint John, NB, Canada E2L 3L6

Michael V. O'Shaughnessey
British Columbia Centre for Excellence in HIV/AIDS, Vancouver, BC, Canada V6Z 1Y6

Duncan Webster
Department of Medicine, Saint John Regional Hospital, Saint John, NB, Canada E2L 3L6

Cristina Mogro-Wilson
School of Social Work, University of Connecticut, 1798 Asylum Avenue, West Hartford, CT 06117-2698, USA

9 781632 396341